Recent A ...

Surge y
27

Recent Advances in Surgery 26
Edited by I. Taylor and C. D. Johnson

ISBN 1-85315-551-9
ISSN 0143-8395

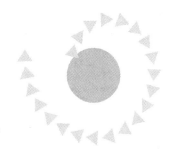

Recent Advances in

Surgery
27

Edited by

C. D. Johnson MChir FRCS
Reader and Consultant Surgeon
University Surgical Unit
Southampton General Hospital, Southampton, UK

I. Taylor MD ChM FRCS FMedSci FRCPS(Glas)Hon
Vice-Dean and Director of Clinical Studies
David Patey Professor of Surgery
Royal Free and University College
London Medical School
University College London, London, UK

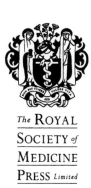

The ROYAL
SOCIETY *of*
MEDICINE
PRESS *Limited*

© 2004 Royal Society of Medicine Press Ltd

Published by the Royal Society of Medicine Press Ltd
1 Wimpole Street, London W1G 0AE, UK
Tel: +44 (0) 20 7290 2921
Fax: +44 (0) 20 7290 2929
Email: publishing@rsm.ac.uk
Website: www.rsmpress.co.uk

The authors are responsible for the scientific content and for the views expressed, which are not necessarily those of the Royal Society of Medicine, or of the Royal Society of Medicine Press Ltd. Medical knowledge is constantly changing. As new information becomes available, changes in treatment, procedures, equipment and the use of drugs become necessary. The editors and the publishers have, as far as possible, taken care to ensure that the information given in this text is accurate and up to date. However, readers are strongly advised to confirm that the information, especially with regard to drug usage, complies with current legislation and standards of practice.

British Library Cataloguing in Publication Data
A catalogue record for this book is available from the British Library
ISBN 1-85315-571-3
ISSN 0143-8395

Distribution in Europe and Rest of World:
Marston Book Services Ltd
PO Box 269
Abingdon
Oxon OX14 4YN, UK
Tel: +44 (0) 1235 465500
Fax: +44 (0) 1235 465555

Distribution in the USA and Canada:
Royal Society of Medicine Press Ltd
c/o Jamco Distribution Inc
1401 Lakeway Drive
Lewisville, TX 75057, USA
Tel: +1 800 538 1287
Fax: +1 972 353 1303
Email: jamco@majors.com

Distribution in Australia and New Zealand:
Elsevier Australia
30-52 Smidmore Street, Marrickville NSW 2204, Australia
Tel: +61 2 9517 8999
Fax: +61 2 9517 2249
Email: service@elsevier.com.au

Commissioning editor – Peter Richardson
Editorial assistant – Shirley Mukisa
Phototypeset by Phoenix Photosetting, Chatham, Kent, UK
Printed in Great Britain by Bell & Bain, Glasgow, UK

Contents

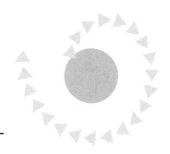

Contributors

Irfan Ahmed MD FRCS
Queens Medical Centre, University Hospital, Nottingham, UK

Åke Andrén-Sandberg MD PhD
Department of Gastrointestinal Surgery, Stavanger, Norway

Ian J. Beckingham FRCS(Gen)
Consultant Hepatobiliary and Laparoscopic Surgeon, Queens Medical Centre, University Hospital, Nottingham, UK

John A.C. Buckels CBE MD FRCS
Consultant Hepatobiliary and Liver Transplant Surgeon, Queen Elizabeth Medical Centre, Birmingham, UK

Richard A. Bulbulia MA FRCS
Specialist Registrar, Cheltenham General Hospital, Cheltenham, Gloucestershire, UK

Kevin Cassar MMEd MD FRCS(Ed)
Lecturer, University of Aberdeen, Specialist Registrar in General Surgery, Aberdeen Royal Infirmary, Foresterhill, Aberdeen, UK

Abhay Chopada FRCS
Royal Free and University College London Medical School, London, UK

Ian G. Finlay FRCS
Consultant Colorectal Surgeon, Lister Surgical Unit, Glasgow Royal Infirmary, Glasgow, UK

William R. Fleming MBBS FRACS
Consultant Surgeon, Austin Health, Victoria, Australia

Robert B. Galland MD FRCS
Consultant Surgeon, Royal Berkshire Hospital, Reading, UK

Christopher P. Gandy
Specialist Registrar in General Surgery, Yeovil District Hospital, Somerset, UK

Manj S. Gohel MRCS
Vascular Research Fellow, Cheltenham General Hospital, Cheltenham, Gloucestershire, UK

Nadey S. Hakim MD PhD FRCS FACS FICS
Consultant Surgeon and Surgical Director of the Transplant Unit, St Mary's Hospital, London, UK

Colin D. Johnson MChir FRCS
Reader in Surgery, University Surgical Unit, Southampton General Hospital, Southampton UK

Robin H. Kennedy FRCS
Consultant Surgeon, Yeovil District Hospital, Somerset, UK

Roger M. Kipling FRCA
Consultant Anaesthetist, Yeovil District Hospital, Somerset, UK

John Lynn MS FRCS
Consultant Endocrine Surgeon, Hammersmith Hospital, London, UK

Mark J. Midwinter MD FRCS
Surgeon Commander Royal Navy, Consultant Surgeon, Derriford Hospital, Plymouth, Devon, UK

Alexander Munro ChM FRCSEd
Formerly Professor of Clinical Surgery, University of Aberdeen, and Consultant Surgeon, Raigmore Hospital, Inverness, UK

Vijayaragaran Muralidharan MD FRCS
Senior Registrar, Liver Unit, Queen Elizabeth Hospital, Birmingham, UK

Vassilios E. Papalois MD PhD FRCS FICS
Consultant Transplant Surgeon, Transplant Unit, St Mary's Hospital, London, UK

Amjad Parvaiz FRCS
Specialist Registrar, Southampton General Hospital, Southampton, UK

Neil W. Pearce FRCS
Consultant in Hepatico-Biliary Surgery, Southampton General Hospital, Southampton, UK

Keith R. Poskitt MD FRCS
Consultant Surgeon, Cheltenham General Hospital, Cheltenham, Gloucestershire, UK

Robert A. Reichert MD FACS
Surgical Fellow, Academic Surgery, Breast Unit, Royal Marsden Hospital, London, UK

Nigel P.M. Sacks MS FRCS FRACS
Consultant Surgeon, Royal Marsden Hospital, London, UK

Grant Sanders FRCS
Specialist Registrar, Royal Devon and Exeter Hospital, Wonford, Exeter, Devon, UK

Bareen Shah FRCS
Consultant Surgeon, Ealing Hospital, London, UK

Fiona J. Slim
Senior Surgical Practitioner, Cheltenham General Hospital, Cheltenham, Gloucestershire, UK

Irving Taylor MD ChM FRCS FMedSci FRCPS (Glas) Hon
Vice-Dean and Director of Clinical Studies, Royal Free and University College London Medical School, London, UK

Sudeep K. Thomas MS FRCS
Clinical Research Fellow, Addenbrooke's Hospital, Cambridge, UK

John Thompson MS FRCS
Consultant Surgeon, Royal Devon and Exeter Hospital, Wonford, Exeter, Devon, UK

Mark R. Whyman MS FRCS
Consultant Surgeon, Cheltenham General Hospital, Cheltenham, Gloucestershire, UK

Gordon C. Wishart MD FRCS(Gen)
Consultant Breast and Endocrine Surgeon, Addenbrooke's Hospital, Cambridge, UK

John Thompson Grant Sanders

1

Blood transfusion and alternative approaches

Allogeneic transfusion confers a risk of immunomodulation, transmission of disease, allergic reaction, alloimmunisation and above all, clerical errors. It is likely that blood will become scarcer with increasing population age and the increased number of donor exclusions[1]. The risk of HIV and hepatitis B and C already excludes large numbers of potential blood donors. The introduction of a reliable test for new variant CJD and the appearance of pathogens such as SARS and West Nile virus will have a further impact on the blood supply.

REDUCING TRANSFUSION REQUIREMENTS

A number of methods have been utilised over the years in an attempt to decrease the use of allogeneic blood. These include meticulous surgical technique to reduce blood loss, agreed blood ordering schedules (ABOS), cross-matching on demand to reduce unnecessary wastage and a strict transfusion trigger, as well as autologous transfusion.

SURGICAL TECHNIQUE

Careful surgical technique minimises blood loss and recognises the importance of efforts to limit the use of blood to clinical necessity. Adjuncts such as cutting diathermy, harmonic scalpels and argon-beam coagulation are useful, but the best approach is to operate carefully with meticulous haemostasis.

TRANSFUSION TRIGGER

A 'transfusion protocol' decreases allogeneic transfusion by up to 43%[2]. Blood ordering schedules should be *agreed* between clinicians and the blood bank.

Mr John Thompson MS FRCS, Consultant Surgeon, Royal Devon and Exeter Hospital, Barrack Road, Wonford, Exeter, Devon EX2 5DW, UK

Mr Grant Sanders FRCS, Specialist Registrar, Royal Devon and Exeter Hospital, Barrack Road, Wonford, Exeter, Devon

Most operations can be performed with a group and antibody screen alone; as long as there are no abnormal antibodies, blood can be issued at 15–20 minutes notice using computerised or rapid spin crossmatch techniques. We have used this technique for elective aortic reconstruction for five years without problems.

The appropriate haemoglobin (Hb) level at which to transfuse patients is controversial. Clinical guidelines suggest that transfusion is rarely indicated if Hb > 10 g/dl and usually indicated if Hb < 6 g/dl in clinically stable patients not at risk of coronary artery disease.[3]

The TRICC (Transfusion Requirements in Critical Care) study[4] demonstrated that a restrictive transfusion strategy (Hb between 7 and 9 g/dl) is effective and possibly beneficial. Mortality at 30 days was no different in the 'restrictive' and 'liberal' groups (18.7% *versus* 23.3%; $P = 0.11$). However, in patients who were less acutely ill (APACHE 11 score ≤ 20), the mortality rate was 8.7% in the 'restrictive' arm and 16.1% in the 'liberal' arm ($P = 0.03$). Among those aged over 55 years, the mortality rate was 5.7% (restrictive) and 13.0% (liberal) ($P = 0.02$); this did not apply to those with clinically significant cardiac disease (many of whom were excluded from entry to the study). In addition, the hospital mortality rate was significantly lower in the 'restrictive' group (22.2% *versus* 28.1%; $P = 0.05$).

Jehovah's Witness[5] and haemodilution studies have also provided useful data. Healthy adults have no evidence of inadequate systemic oxygenation at Hb levels of 4.5–5.0 g/dl.[6] A retrospective cohort study[7] showed that those with a postoperative Hb of 7.1–8 g/dl had a mortality rate of 0% and a morbidity rate of 9.4%. These increased to 34.4% and 57.7% when the postoperative Hb was 4.1–5 g/dl. Odds of death increased 2.5 times with each gram decrease in Hb below 8 g/dl. There is no single Hb level below which all patients *require* a transfusion. The decision should consider age, comorbidity and vital signs.

Key point 1

- Blood transfusion should only be used where there is a clear *clinical* reason. Transfusion is usually indicated in fit patients when Hb < 6 g/dl.

Key point 2

- Arteriopaths and the elderly need a more liberal and individual approach to transfusion.

Key point 3

- Simple blood management techniques are the most effective means of reducing unnecessary transfusion.

AUTOLOGOUS TRANSFUSION

This describes any procedure whereby the patient's own previously donated (or shed) blood is retransfused. Recently the emphasis has shifted to an evaluation of the risks/benefits. A cardinal benefit is the 'peace of mind', knowing that patients are receiving blood free from contamination with HIV or other agents.[8]

PREOPERATIVE AUTOLOGOUS DONATION (PAD)

PAD is useful if the need for blood can be anticipated and a donation plan implemented.[9] The minimal predonation Hb level for autologous donation is 11 g/dl. Each unit of PAD (350–450 ml) decreases Hb by 1 g/dl and haematocrit (Hct) by 3 points.[10,11] If insufficient time is given to compensate for red cell loss, PAD offers little advantage. Candidates for total hip replacement (THR), in optimal clinical and haematological condition (Hb > 13.5 g/dl, Hct > 40%), donating 3 units over a 10-day period with intravenous iron, took 15–22 days to restore red cells lost with the first collection.[10]

Risks of donation

High-risk donors are those with coronary disease, cardiac failure, medication inhibiting cardiovascular compensation to hypovolaemia, aortic stenosis, transient ischaemic attacks and marked hypertension. Popovskyl et al.[12] found that 1 in 16 783 donations were associated with an adverse event requiring hospitalisation – 12 times as high a rate as with volunteer donors.

Risks of transfusion

In a retrospective review, adverse reactions after PAD composed 2.1% of all transfusion reactions and involved 0.16% of all PAD red cells,[13] although only 60% were thought to be directly related to PAD. Complications included haemolysis, endotoxic shock, febrile non-haemolytic transfusion reactions and transfusion of the wrong unit. Random misadministration carries a 36% probability of ABO incompatibility[14] and a 5% risk of a fatal acute haemolytic transfusion reaction.[14]

Key point 4

- Autologous blood is safer than bank blood, but the safest transfusion is the one you do not give!

Inclusion criteria

The Edinburgh Consensus Conference stated that PAD should be considered if the likelihood of transfusion exceeds 50%.[11] Blood losses are of course unpredictable,[15] despite attempts to stratify patients preoperatively.[16–18] One mathematical model, with a perioperative threshold Hct of 25%, in a 70 kg patient with a blood volume of 5000 ml and initial Hct of 45% donating 2–4 units, suggested that PAD could be harmful.[25] This assumes that compensatory erythropoiesis resulted in replacement of only two-thirds of the removed unit thereby dropping Hct by 1%. The same patient *not* predonating could lose 2500 ml without a transfusion, assuming a transfusion trigger of 7.5 g/dl.

In a meta-analysis of clinical studies[26] patients randomised to PAD were less likely to receive allogeneic blood, but more likely than control patients to receive *any* transfusion. In prostatectomy 3-unit PAD decreased allogeneic exposure compared with controls. However, the 10 controls were those who had been excluded from PAD, compared with 384 trial patients.[27] In total hip replacement[28] no patient needed allogeneic transfusion, but 69% in the PAD group were transfused autologous blood, illustrating the effect described in the mathematical model.

Key point 5

• PAD is usually impractical and may induce anaemia.

ACUTE NORMOVOLAEMIC HAEMODILUTION (ANH)

In ANH blood is collected in the anaesthetic room, whilst volume is maintained with clear fluids. As a result, the blood lost during surgery contains fewer red blood cells per millilitre. Blood is collected in standard blood bank bags containing acid citrate dextrose (ACD) and can be stored at room temperature for up to 6–8 hours, or at 4°C for up to 24 hours (blood for storage and reinfusion is spiked with an optimal additive solution known as SAG-M (saline adenine glucose–mannitol)).[29,30].

ANH has the advantage that it is simple; units are collected and stored in theatre, incurring no storage or testing costs, and minimising clerical error. In addition, the blood is fresh, containing functional platelets and clotting factors, and the lowered blood viscosity may improve oxygen delivery.[31]

Eligibility and safety
Fit patients with Hb > 11 g/dl expected to lose over 20% of their blood volume can be considered for ANH.[15,29] The drop in Hct is compensated for by an increase in cardiac output. Anaesthesia decreases oxygen consumption by 20%, but FiO_2 is increased to maintain oxygen delivery.

One in six surgical patients may be at risk for silent myocardial ischaemia – even those not thought to be at high risk on the basis of preoperative assessment.[32] However, the rheological effects of ANH may be beneficial.[31] Spahn *et al.*[33] demonstrated that ANH to an Hb of 8.8 ± 0.3 g/dl was well tolerated in 20 patients older than 65 years, as was an Hb of 9.9 ± 0.2 g/dl in patients with coronary artery disease receiving β-blockers.[34] However, Carvalho *et al.*[35] reported a case of life-threatening myocardial ischaemia in a patient undergoing ANH prior to abdominal aortic aneurysm repair.

ANH is contraindicated in patients with known myocardial disease[29] or who cannot raise cardiac output (previous infarction, calcium channel blockers or β-blockers). Furthermore, the effect of haemodilution on coagulation is still unknown, and any beneficial effect may be negated by increased bleeding.

Mathematical modelling has shown that the efficiency of ANH depends on (1) initial and target haematocrit, (2) ANH volume and (3) surgical blood loss.[36] Studies of the efficacy of ANH have not examined the effect on red cell mass.[37] Figure 1 illustrates the principle: ANH from an initial Hct of 0.45 would still allow up to 3500 ml of surgical blood loss, and the Hct could be maintained at ≥ 0.28.[40] Vamvakas and Pineda,[9] however, noted that an adult with an initial Hct > 0.45 could, without ANH, maintain a postoperative Hct > 0.25 and avoid transfusion, if there was an intraoperative blood loss of up to 3939 ml.

Efficacy of ANH

Consensus conferences   The Edinburgh Conferences in 1995[31],[41] and 1998[42,43] noted that there was still no evidence that ANH was effective, concluding that randomised controlled trials were required before ANH could be recommended.

Controlled trials   Sanders et al.[44] showed no reduction in the number of patients (29% and 30%) or units (total 92 and 93) transfused during major gastrointestinal surgery. The median ANH volume was 1350 ml. This conclusion was supported by preliminary data from a prospective randomised study in surgery for abdominal aortic aneurysm.[45]

A three-arm study[47] randomised patients undergoing cardiac surgery to cell salvage, ANH plus cell salvage or control. There were fewer transfusions in the cell salvage group compared with control, but there was no additional benefit with ANH.

Meta-analysis   Analysis of five randomised clinical trials looking at transfusion in ANH compared with PAD revealed no significant difference.[9,15] Bryson et al.[49] demonstrated that trials without a transfusion protocol showed

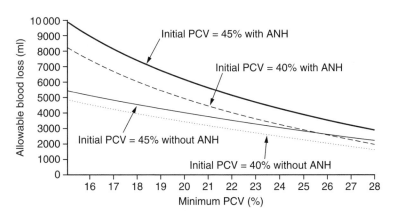

Fig. 1 Maximal allowable blood loss in a patient with a blood volume of 5000 ml and an initial packed cell volume value of 45% or 40%, with and without ANH.[40]

marked reductions in transfusions, but studies with a transfusion protocol did not.

Key point 6

- Emerging level I evidence does not support the efficacy of ANH.

INTRAOPERATIVE CELL SALVAGE (ICS)

ICS involves the collection and reinfusion of shed blood from the operative field or surgical drains. Shed blood is anticoagulated, filtered, washed, concentrated and returned. Unprocessed salvaged blood contains free haemoglobin and fibrin degradation products (FDP), red cell stroma and non-functional platelets, with negligible coagulation factors. Washing removes 95–98% of contaminants.

Although ICS is theoretically contraindicated in the presence of bacteria, malignant cells, amniotic or ascitic fluid,[9] recent work suggests that the risk of dissemination of malignant disease is minimal.[29,50]

ICS is safe; adverse reactions occurred at a rate of 0.027% (5/18 506) units during a 6-year period.[13] One death, due to air embolism during cell salvage, was reported between 1990 and 1995, in a total of 32 000 transfusions.[51]

Efficacy of cell salvage

Red blood cell conservation depends on the rate of haemorrhage and the willingness of the surgeon to use suction, not swabs.[10] ICS can be used in emergencies.[9] As surgical techniques improve, the blood available for ICS falls, but it is a valuable 'safety net' should unexpected heavy bleeding occur. The disposables for collecting blood are opened first. Only when sufficient blood for processing has been collected are the more expensive centrifuge components opened, which saves on cost – most systems become cost-effective at only 1 unit of blood.

Early work concluded that ICS could reduce the need for allogeneic blood,[52] a view upheld by the Edinburgh Consensus Conference in 1995.[41] By 1998,[42,53] evidence had accumulated that cell salvage was practical, safe, inexpensive, and potentially cost-saving. The International Study of Peri-operative Transfusion (ISPOT) group showed that ICS in cardiac and orthopaedic operations decreased allogeneic transfusion.[54]

ICS may be of greatest value, not because it hugely reduces the requirements for transfusion, but because help is immediately available in the event of rapid blood loss. However, cost-effectiveness has not been specifically addressed in any randomised trial.[53]

Key point 7

- ICS is effective in major blood loss cases and is a good safety net.

POSTOPERATIVE BLOOD RECOVERY (PBR)

PBR is used most commonly in cardiovascular and joint replacement surgery. Studies looking at efficacy have reached disparate conclusions,[15] but recent good-quality studies have shown reductions in blood transfusion and hospital stay following total knee replacement.[58]

Key point 8

- Postoperative reinfusion is safe and effective in orthopaedics.

'MEDICAL' TECHNIQUES

CONTROLLED HYPOTENSION

Induced hypotension reduces vascular resistance and hydrostatic pressure while maintaining cardiac output.[59] Haemodilution and hypervolaemia follow. One study[48] showed that hypotension with sodium nitroprusside reduced transfusion compared with ANH in prostatectomy.

ERYTHROPOIETIN (EPO)

EPO alone decreases allogeneic transfusion[60–62] especially in anaemic patients. EPO and iron are more effective.[63] EPO can increase Hct in patients undergoing ANH.[65] The role of EPO in PAD is limited. In 47 non-anaemic orthopaedic patients EPO did not reduce allogeneic transfusion,[66] and the Edinburgh Consensus concluded that the value and safety of EPO in PAD were unproven.[42] The use of EPO is confined to special cases such as Jehovah's Witnesses.

APROTININ

Aprotinin reduces transfusion and reoperation for bleeding in liver and cardiac surgery and may counteract aspirin-related bleeding.[68,69] However, it does not reduce blood exposure in elective[70] or ruptured[71] abdominal aortic aneurysm surgery.

OXYGEN CARRYING SOLUTIONS

Haemoglobin solutions and perfluorochemical emulsions (PFC)[72,73] include stroma-free human (10% diaspirin cross-linked) haemoglobin and xenobiotic products. All cause vasoconstriction that is related to the binding of nitric oxide.[72,73] PFC emulsion is licensed for the perfusion of coronary arteries after PTCA.[72,73] Problems, however, include short half-life, low oxygen-carrying capacity, poor shelf-life and temperature instability. Until further studies have been performed, these fluids remain experimental.

CONCLUSIONS

Meticulous surgical technique and the use of a transfusion protocol are good practice. PAD requires careful donor selection, venesection, storage and testing of blood, and correct retransfusion on a defined time scale, which is often impractical. Although there is little evidence to support it, EPO may improve this. There is no evidence that acute normovolaemic haemodilution decreases transfusion, unless it is extreme (2 litres); even then the amount conserved is modest. Most patients requiring transfusion will need more than is available by cell salvage. Its value therefore lies not in decreasing allogeneic exposure, but because it provides blood immediately available in the event of rapid blood loss. The efficacy of postoperative blood recovery remains uncertain. Controlled hypotension and the use of EPO have not been widely adopted. EPO may be used alongside other techniques, especially in the presence of anaemia. The efficacy of aprotinin has to be set against its high cost. Oxygen-carrying solutions remain largely experimental at present.

Key points for clinical practice

- Blood transfusion should only be used where there is a clear *clinical* reason. Transfusion is usually indicated in fit patients when Hb < 6 g/dl.

- Arteriopaths and the elderly need a more liberal and individual approach to transfusion.

- Simple blood management techniques are the most effective means of reducing unnecessary transfusion.

- Autologous blood is safer than bank blood, but the safest transfusion is the one you do not give!

- PAD is usually impractical and may induce anaemia.

- Emerging level I evidence does not support the efficacy of ANH.

- ICS is effective in major blood loss cases and is a good safety net.

- Postoperative reinfusion is safe and effective in orthopaedics.

References

1. Coursin DB, Monk TG. Extreme normovolemic hemodilution: How low can you go and other alternatives to transfusion? *Crit Care Med* 2001; **29**: 908–910.
2. Mallett SV, Peachey TD, Sanehi O, Hazlehurst G, Mehta A. Reducing red blood cell transfusion in elective surgical patients: the role of audit and practice guidelines. *Anaesthesia* 2000; **55**: 1013–1019.
3. Practice Guidelines for blood component therapy: A report by the American Society of Anesthesiologists Task Force on Blood Component Therapy. *Anesthesiology* 1996; **84**: 732–747.
4. Hebert PC *et al*. A multicenter, randomized, controlled clinical trial of transfusion requirements in critical care. Transfusion Requirements in Critical Care Investigators, Canadian Critical Care Trials Group. *N Engl J Med* 1999; **340**: 409–417.
5. Grebenik CR, Sinclair ME, Westaby S. High risk cardiac surgery in Jehovah's Witnesses. *J Cardiovasc Surg (Torino)* 1996; **37**: 511–515.

6. Lieberman JA *et al.* Critical oxygen delivery in conscious humans is less than 7.3 ml $O_2 \times kg^{-1} \times min^{-1}$. *Anesthesiology* 2000; **92**: 407–413.
7. Carson JL, Noveck H, Berlin JA, Gould SA. Mortality and morbidity in patients with very low postoperative Hb levels who decline blood transfusion. *Transfusion* 2002; **42**: 812–818.
8. Rutherford CJ, Kaplan HS. Autologous blood donation – Can we bank on it? *N Engl J Med* 1995; **332**: 740–742.
9. Vamvakas EC, Pineda AA. Autologous transfusion and other approaches to reduce allogeneic blood exposure. *Baillière's Best Pract Res Clin Haematol* 2000; **13**: 533–547.
10. Mercuriali F, Inghilleri G. Proposal of an algorithm to help the choice of the best transfusion strategy. *Curr Med Res Opin* 1996; **13**: 465–478.
11. Thomas MJ, Gillon J, Desmond MJ. Consensus conference on autologous transfusion. Preoperative autologous donation. *Transfusion* 1996; **36**: 633–639.
12. Popovsky MA, Whitaker B, Arnold NL. Severe outcomes of allogeneic and autologous blood donation: frequency and characterization. *Transfusion* 1995; **35**: 734–737.
13. Domen RE. Adverse reactions associated with autologous blood transfusion: evaluation and incidence at a large academic hospital. *Transfusion* 1998; **38**: 296–300.
14. Linden JV, Kruskall MS. Autologous blood: always safer? *Transfusion* 1997; **37**: 455–456.
15. Goodnough LT, Brecher ME, Kanter MH, AuBuchon JP. Transfusion medicine. Second of two parts – blood conservation. *N Engl J Med* 1999; **340**: 525–533.
16. Larocque B, Brien WF, Gilbert K. The utility and prediction of allogeneic blood transfusion use in orthopedic surgery. *Transfus Med Rev* 1999; **13**: 124–131.
17. Larocque BJ, Gilbert K, Brien WF. A point score system for predicting the likelihood of blood transfusion after hip or knee arthroplasty. *Transfusion* 1997; **37**: 463–467.
18. Larocque BJ, Gilbert K, Brien WF. Prospective validation of a point score system for predicting blood transfusion following hip or knee replacement. *Transfusion* 1998; **38**: 932–937.
19. Kanter MH *et al.* Preoperative autologous blood donations before elective hysterectomy. *JAMA* 1996; **276**: 798–801.
20. Yamada AH *et al.* Impact of autologous blood transfusions on patients undergoing radical prostatectomy using hypotensive anesthesia. *J Urol* 1993; **149**: 73–76.
21. Monk TG *et al.* Acute normovolemic hemodilution can replace preoperative autologous blood donation as a standard of care for autologous blood procurement in radical prostatectomy. *Anesth Analg* 1997; **85**: 953–958.
22. Kasper SM, Gerlich W, Buzello W. Preoperative red cell production in patients undergoing weekly autologous blood donation. *Transfusion* 1997; **37**: 1058–1062.
23. Goodnough LT, Price TH, Rudnick S, Soegiarso RW. Preoperative red cell production in patients undergoing aggressive autologous blood phlebotomy with and without erythropoietin therapy. *Transfusion* 1992; **32**: 441–445.
24. Mercuriali F *et al.* Use of erythropoietin to increase the volume of autologous blood donated by orthopedic patients. *Transfusion* 1993; **33**: 55–60.
25. Cohen JA, Brecher ME. Preoperative autologous blood donation: benefit or detriment? A mathematical analysis. *Transfusion* 1995; **35**: 640–644.
26. Forgie MA, Wells PS, Laupacis A, Fergusson D. Preoperative autologous donation decreases allogeneic transfusion but increases exposure to all red blood cell transfusion: results of a meta-analysis. International Study of Perioperative Transfusion (ISPOT) Investigators. *Arch Intern Med* 1998; **158**: 610–616.
27. Goodnough LM, Grishaber JE, Birkmeyer JD, Monk TG, Catalona WJ. Efficacy and cost-effectiveness of autologous blood predeposit in patients undergoing radical prostatectomy procedures. *Urology* 1994; **44**: 226–231.
28. Billote DB, Glisson SN, Green D, Wixson RL. A prospective, randomized study of preoperative autologous donation for hip replacement surgery. *J Bone Joint Surg Am* 2002; **84A**: 1299–1304.
29. Napier JA *et al.* Guidelines for autologous transfusion. II. Perioperative haemodilution and cell salvage. British Committee for Standards in Haematology Blood Transfusion Task Force. Autologous Transfusion Working Party. *Br J Anaesth* 1997; **78**: 768–771.
30. Goodnough LT, Monk TG, Brecher ME. Acute normovolemic hemodilution should replace the preoperative donation of autologous blood as a method of autologous-blood procurement. *Transfusion* 1998; **38**: 473–476.

31. Gillon J, Thomas MJ, Desmond MJ. Consensus conference on autologous transfusion. Acute normovolaemic haemodilution. *Transfusion* 1996; **36**: 640–643.
32. Muir AD *et al*. Preoperative silent myocardial ischaemia: incidence and predictors in a general surgical population. *Br J Anaesth* 1991; **67**: 373–377.
33. Spahn DR *et al*. Hemodilution tolerance in elderly patients without known cardiac disease. *Anesth Analg* 1996; **82**: 681–686.
34. Spahn DR, Schmid ER, Seifert B, Pasch T. Hemodilution tolerance in patients with coronary artery disease who are receiving chronic beta-adrenergic blocker therapy. *Anesth Analg* 1996; **82**: 687–694.
35. Carvalho B, Ridler BM, Thompson JF, Telford RJ. Myocardial ischaemia precipitated by acute normovolaemic haemodilution. *Transfus Med* 2003; **13**: 165–168.
36. Feldman JM, Roth JV, Bjoraker DG. Maximum blood savings by acute normovolemic hemodilution. *Anesth Analg* 1995; **80**: 108–113.
37. Kick O. The efficacy of acute normovolemic hemodilution. *Anesth Analg* 1998; **87**: 497–498.
38. Brecher ME, Rosenfeld M. Mathematical and computer modeling of acute normovolemic hemodilution. *Transfusion* 1994; **34**: 176–179.
39. Singbartl G, Singbartl K, Schleinzer W. Is acute normovolemic hemodilution cost-effective? *Transfusion* 1996; **36**: 849–850.
40. Goodnough LT, Brecher ME, Monk TG. Acute normovolemic hemodilution in surgery. *Hematology* 1997; **2**: 5–420.
41. Thomas MJ. Royal College of Physicians of Edinburgh Consensus Conference on autologous transfusion: final consensus statement. *Transfus Sci* 1996; **17**: 329–330.
42. Allain JP, Akehurst RL, Hunter JM. Royal College of Physicians of Edinburgh. Autologous transfusion, 3 years on: What is new? What has happened? *Transfusion* 1999; **39**: 910–911.
43. Gillon J, Desmond M, Thomas MJ. Acute normovolaemic haemodilution. *Transfus Med* 1999; **9**: 259–264.
44. Sanders G *et al*. A prospective randomised controlled trial of acute normovolaemic haemodilution (ANH) in major gastro-intestinal surgery and its effect on coagulation. *Blood* 2002; **100**: 209.
45. Ridler BMF, Thomas D, Teasdale A, Telford RJ, Thompson JF. Prospective randomised trial of ANH in elective aortic reconstruction. *Br J Surg* 2004; in press.
46. Matot I, Scheinin O, Jurim O, Eid A. Effectiveness of acute normovolemic hemodilution to minimize allogeneic blood transfusion in major liver resections. *Anesthesiology* 2002; **97**: 794–800.
47. McGill N, O'Shaughnessy D, Pickering R, Herbertson M, Gill R. Mechanical methods of reducing blood transfusion in cardiac surgery: randomised controlled trial. *BMJ* 2002; **324**: 1299.
48. Boldt J, Weber A, Mailer K, Papsdorf M, Schuster P. Acute normovolaemic haemodilution vs controlled hypotension for reducing the use of allogeneic blood in patients undergoing radical prostatectomy. *Br J Anaesth* 1999; **82**: 170–174.
49. Bryson GL, Laupacis A, Wells GA. Does acute normovolemic hemodilution reduce perioperative allogeneic transfusion? A meta-analysis. The International Study of Perioperative Transfusion. *Anesth Analg* 1998; **86**: 9–15.
50. Davis M, Sofer M, Gomez-Marin O, Bruck D, Soloway MS. The use of cell salvage during radical retropubic prostatectomy: does it influence cancer recurrence? *BJU Int* 2003; **91**: 474–476.
51. Linden JV, Tourault MA, Scribner CL. Decrease in frequency of transfusion fatalities. *Transfusion* 1997; **37**: 243–244.
52. Thompson JF, Webster JH, Chant AD. Prospective randomised evaluation of a new cell saving device in elective aortic reconstruction. *Eur J Vasc Surg* 1990; **4**: 507–512.
53. Desmond M, Gillon J, Thomas MJ. Perioperative red cell salvage: a case for implementing the 1995 consensus statement. *Transfus Med* 1999; **9**: 265–268.
54. Huet C *et al*. A meta-analysis of the effectiveness of cell salvage to minimize perioperative allogeneic blood transfusion in cardiac and orthopedic surgery. International Study of Perioperative Transfusion (ISPOT) Investigators. *Anesth Analg* 1999; **89**: 861–869.

55. Bell K, Stott K, Sinclair CJ, Walker WS, Gillon J. A controlled trial of intra-operative autologous transfusion in cardiothoracic surgery measuring effect on transfusion requirements and clinical outcome. *Transfus Med* 1992; **2**: 295–300.

56. Wong JC *et al*. Autologous versus allogeneic transfusion in aortic surgery: a multicenter randomized clinical trial. *Ann Surg* 2002; **235**: 145–151.

57. Clagett GP *et al*. A randomized trial of intraoperative autotransfusion during aortic surgery. *J Vasc Surg* 1999; **29**: 22–30.

58. Thomas D, Wareham K, Cohen D, Hutchings H. Autologous blood transfusion in total knee replacement surgery. *Br J Anaesth* 2001; **86**: 669–673.

59. Levack ID, Gillon J. Intraoperative conservation of red cell mass: controlled hypotension or haemodilution – not necessarily mutually exclusive? *Br J Anaesth* 1999; **82**: 161–163.

60. Effectiveness of perioperative recombinant human erythropoietin in elective hip replacement. Canadian Orthopedic Perioperative Erythropoietin Study Group. *Lancet* 1993; **341**: 1227–1232.

61. Faris PM, Ritter MA, Abels RI. The effects of recombinant human erythropoietin on perioperative transfusion requirements in patients having a major orthopaedic operation. The American Erythropoietin Study Group. *J Bone Joint Surg Am* 1996; **78**: 62–72.

62. Sowade O *et al*. Avoidance of allogeneic blood transfusions by treatment with epoetin beta (recombinant human erythropoietin) in patients undergoing open-heart surgery. *Blood* 1997; **89**: 411–418.

63. Corwin HL *et al*. Efficacy of recombinant human erythropoietin in the critically ill patient: a randomized, double-blind, placebo-controlled trial. *Crit Care Med* 1999; **27**: 2346–2350.

64. Goodnough LT, Monk TG, Andriole GL. Erythropoietin therapy. *N Engl J Med* 1997; **336**: 933–938.

65. Monk TG *et al*. A prospective randomized comparison of three blood conservation strategies for radical prostatectomy. *Anesthesiology* 1999; **91**: 24–33.

66. Goodnough LT *et al*. Increased preoperative collection of autologous blood with recombinant human erythropoietin therapy. *N Engl J Med* 1989; **321**: 1163–1168.

67. Bezwada HP, Nazarian DG, Henry DH, Booth RE, Jr. Preoperative use of recombinant human erythropoietin before total joint arthroplasty. *J Bone Joint Surg Am* 2003; **85A**: 1795–1800.

68. Levi M *et al*. Pharmacological strategies to decrease excessive blood loss in cardiac surgery: a meta-analysis of clinically relevant endpoints. *Lancet* 1999; **354**: 1940–1947.

69. Munoz JJ, Birkmeyer NJ, Birkmeyer JD, O'Connor GT, Dacey LJ. Is ε-aminocaproic acid as effective as aprotinin in reducing bleeding with cardiac surgery? A meta-analysis. *Circulation* 1999; **99**: 81–89.

70. Ranaboldo CJ *et al*. Prospective randomized placebo-controlled trial of aprotinin for elective aortic reconstruction. *Br J Surg* 1997; **84**: 1110–1113.

71. Robinson J, Nawaz S, Beard JD. Randomized, multicentre, double-blind, placebo-controlled trial of the use of aprotinin in the repair of ruptured abdominal aortic aneurysm. On behalf of the Joint Vascular Research Group. *Br J Surg* 2000; **87**: 754–757.

72. Dietz NM, Joyner MJ, Warner MA. Blood substitutes: fluids, drugs, or miracle solutions? *Anesth Analg* 1996; **82**: 390–405.

73. Scott MG, Kucik DF, Goodnough LT, Monk TG. Blood substitutes: evolution and future applications. *Clin Chem* 1997; **43**: 1724–1731.

Mark J. Midwinter

2

Abdominal compartment syndrome

Acute compartment syndromes as a result of increased pressure in the myofascial compartments of the extremities are well recognised. Once diagnosed, treatment by compartment decompression is necessary to avoid complications. In recent years a compartment syndrome associated with raised intra-abdominal pressure has been recognised and treated by decompression.

Historically, some effects of raised intra-abdominal pressure were reported as far back as the 19th century. In 1911 the literature was reviewed by Emerson.[1] It was noted that if the intra-abdominal pressure was raised above the range 19–33 mmHg (27–46 cmH$_2$O) in small animals (cats and guinea pigs) then death from respiratory failure ensued. The effects on renal function were later investigated in dogs.[2] In 1948 Gross[3] noted that closing the abdominal wall in neonates with large omphaloceles was frequently followed by respiratory and cardiovascular failure and subsequently death. It was postulated that this was due to 'abdominal crowding'. More recently, with the increasing number of laparoscopic procedures, the adverse effects of raised intra-abdominal pressure, particularly on the cardiovascular system, have been widely reported.[4,5]

It was not until recently that these observations were brought together and the profound effects of intra-abdominal hypertension in the critically ill patient recognised. The incidence of abdominal compartment syndrome (ACS) is unknown. Estimates vary from 1% to 33% in admissions to level 1 trauma units.[6,7]

MEASUREMENT OF INTRA-ABDOMINAL PRESSURE (IAP)

Both direct and indirect techniques for the measurement of IAP have been used. Direct methods include placing a catheter with an attached manometer

Mr Mark J. Midwinter MD FRCS, Surgeon Commander Royal Navy, Consultant Surgeon, Derriford Hospital, Plymouth, Devon PL6 8DH, UK

or pressure transducer in the peritoneal cavity. A commonly used example of this method is pressure measurement during laparoscopy. However, direct methods are rarely used to monitor IAP in other circumstances.

Indirect methods use pressure measurements elsewhere that reflect changes in the intra-abdominal pressure. Initially, this was performed by placing catheters percutaneously into the inferior vena cava.[8] This rather invasive method has been superseded by the use of urinary bladder pressure monitoring.[9] This has been validated against direct pressure measurements.[10] Bladder pressure monitoring may be intermittent or continuous; it is relatively simple and does not usually require any extra invasive procedure as most patients at risk of ACS will have a urinary catheter in situ.

An alternative indirect method is intragastric pressure measurement via a nasogastric tube, although this has not found widespread use.[11]

In the literature IAP measurements are quoted as either mmHg or cmH_2O. It should be noted that 1 mmHg is equal to 1.36 cmH_2O. All measurements here will be given in mmHg.

DEFINITIONS

Intra-abdominal hypertension (IAH) is defined as occurring when the IAP is raised above normal. Normal IAP is said to be atmospheric or subatmospheric.[1,12] However, normal IAP varies with position, body habitus and activity. A relationship between IAP and body mass index has been described.[13] Transient rises in IAP up to 80 mmHg have been observed in normal subjects. In postoperative patients IAP of between 3.0 and 10 mmHg are commonly observed without adverse consequences.

Abdominal compartment syndrome (ACS) is defined as the adverse physiological consequences that occur as a result of raised IAP and resolve following abdominal decompression. The IAP at which adverse cardiovascular consequences are observed has been reported as low as 15 mmHg.[14]

Key point 1

- IAP varies with position, activity and body mass index.

Key point 2

- IAPs of between 3.0 and 10 mmHg are commonly observed postoperatively without adverse effects.

PATHOPHYSIOLOGY

CARDIOVASCULAR

Using a canine model, it has been shown that venous return and cardiac output fall as IAP rises above 10 mmHg, despite normal arterial pressure.[8] Others have shown in a similar model that at an IAP of 40 mmHg, cardiac output and stroke volume were reduced by 36%.[15] A series of clinical reports have all shown improvement in haemodynamic parameters after abdominal decompression in patients with very elevated IAP (>30 mmHg).[16–18] The changes in cardiac output with IAP are more pronounced in hypovolaemia, and can be corrected to a degree with intravenous fluids.[19] Other cardiovascular parameters, such as pulse, blood pressure, central venous pressure and pulmonary capillary wedge pressure, although dependent on vascular volume, seem to be relatively unaffected by changes in IAP.[20]

RESPIRATORY

The respiratory effects of a raised IAP have been studied extensively.[8] With IAP >25 mmHg a significant increase in end-inspiratory pressure is required to maintain the same tidal volume. In anaesthetised dogs arterial pH and pO_2 decreased with an IAP of 40 mmHg.[15] Studies in humans have shown that patients with IAP >40 mmHg from both traumatic and non-traumatic causes had dramatic improvement in PaO_2 and a reduction in FiO_2 with abdominal decompression.[16] As a model of the change in pulmonary compliance with changes in IAP, Obeid *et al*.[21] investigated patients undergoing laparoscopic cholecystectomy. They found significant decreases in pulmonary compliance with IAP >16 mmHg.

RENAL

The effects of raised IAP on renal function have been documented by experimental and clinical observations. Animal models have shown that as IAP reaches 30 mmHg, anuria is induced.[16,22] This is reversible by abdominal decompression. The mechanisms of this effect include a decrease in renal plasma flow and glomerular filtration rate and are independent of the effect on cardiac output. Shunting of blood away from the cortex and into the medulla, direct compression of the renal veins, diminished renal arterial flow, increased renal vascular resistance, and increased levels of antidiuretic hormone, renin and aldosterone have all been demonstrated.

It has been observed in a prospective study that IAP increases to more than 20 mmHg postoperatively in one-third of patients.[11] This was associated with an increase in serum creatinine. A beneficial effect of abdominal decompression on renal function and urine output in patients with IAH has been reported.[17,18] An adverse effect of an IAP >25 mmHg on renal function following liver transplantation has been observed.[23] This was associated with a significantly higher mortality in the intensive care unit.

GASTROINTESTINAL

The effect of IAH on splanchnic blood flow has been investigated in anaesthetised pigs by Diebel *et al*.[24] While increasing the IAP but maintaining a constant arterial blood pressure, the mesenteric blood flow was measured using an ultrasound probe at the base of the mesentery and intramucosal pH by a tonometer in the ileum. Diebel *et al*. demonstrated that the mesenteric flow reduced to 61% and 28% of baseline at IAPs of 20 and 40 mmHg respectively. Intramucosal pH showed correspondingly severe acidosis. In a separate experimental series[25] the same group showed significant reduction in hepatic arterial and portal venous flow at an IAP of 20 mmHg. In a rat model using gas insufflation to induce IAH it has been shown that after 60 minutes with an IAP of 15 mmHg gut oxygen extraction, measured by portal vein and aortic oxygen content, was significantly increased.[26] Thirty minutes after deflation, free-radical production in the intestinal mucosa, liver, spleen and lungs was increased. Comparison with a control group demonstrated that rats exposed to IAH had significant *Escherichia coli* counts in the mesenteric lymph nodes, liver and spleen 3 hours after abdominal deflation, whereas rats not exposed to IAH had no bacteria detected.

A clinical study comparing patients undergoing laparoscopic and open cholecystectomy has shown significant decreases in hepatic circulation and gastric mucosal pH in the laparoscopic group.[27]

In the light of the experimental and clinical observations it has been postulated that splanchnic hypoperfusion, as a consequence of IAH, allows bacterial translocation to occur, and may predispose to sepsis and multiorgan dysfunction syndrome (MODS).

INTRACRANIAL PRESSURE

It has been noted that during laparoscopy significant elevation in intracranial pressure (ICP) can occur.[5] This has been confirmed in an animal model without head injury.[28] At an IAP of 25 mmHg a significant effect on cerebral perfusion pressure (CPP) independent of the systemic arterial pressure was observed. The same group reported similar findings in a patient with multiple trauma who developed ACS.[29] The CPP improved on abdominal decompression. The mechanism postulated for these effects is the rise in central venous pressure, which leads to a decrease in cerebral venous outflow and consequently an increase in intracranial vascular volume. However, others have found that central venous pressure is only marginally affected by IAH and abdominal decompression.[17,20]

ABDOMINAL WALL

It is well recognised that abdominal distension is associated with an increased risk of dehiscence and wound infections. It has been shown in a pig model that rectus sheath blood flow was reduced to 58% of baseline with an IAP of 10 mmHg and to 20% of baseline with an IAP of 40 mmHg, despite maintaining systemic mean arterial pressure.[30] The reduced perfusion of the abdominal wall may be a significant factor in the wound complications in these patients.

Key point 3

- The pathophysiology of IAH has been investigated widely in animal models with correlations observed in clinical studies.

> **Key point 4**
>
> - Intra-abdominal hypertension has significant physiological effects on the cardiovascular, respiratory, renal and gastrointestinal systems, as well as effects on intracranial pressure, cerebral perfusion and abdominal wall blood flow.

> **Key point 5**
>
> - The physiological effects are observed with IAP as low as 10 mmHg.

AETIOLOGY OF ABDOMINAL COMPARTMENT SYNDROME

Common causes of ACS are blunt and penetrating trauma to the abdomen, particularly involving hepatic, splenic or vascular injury.[31] The risk of ACS is especially high if there is both pelvic and abdominal trauma.[32] Packing as a method of controlling haemorrhage can also increase the risk of ACS. ACS may occur after elective abdominal surgery, particularly repair of abdominal aortic aneurysm or liver transplantation.[13,16,23,33] Any pathology that leads to oedema of the bowel, such as ischaemia followed by reperfusion or prolonged evisceration, will put the patient at risk of ACS if the abdomen is closed.

Non-operative and non-traumatic causes of ACS include bowel obstruction or ileus, pancreatitis and burns. The mechanism of ACS following a burn is not well understood, but appears to be related to the amount of intravenous fluid required for resuscitation.[19,34,35] Chronic ascites has been reported to be a cause of ACS, but the slow accumulation of ascities allows accommodation by stretching of the abdominal wall, and patients can tolerate large volumes of fluid without developing ACS. If the same fluid volume were to accumulate rapidly then ACS would result.[19,36]

> **Key point 6**
>
> - ACS can occur in patients following blunt or penetrating trauma, elective surgery and certain conditions without abdominal surgery.

DIAGNOSIS OF ABDOMINAL COMPARTMENT SYNDROME

Clinical abdominal examination is not a reliable method to assess the degree of IAH.[37] However, the presence of cardiorespiratory compromise, oliguria or anuria in a patient with adequate intravascular filling and a tense abdomen should raise the suspicion of ACS as a possible cause. A series of ACS patients reported from a level 1 trauma centre in Nashville, USA found that oliguria was never seen in the absence of ventilatory failure.[38] A raised IAP can be confirmed by measuring intravesical pressure as described above but, just as in acute compartment syndromes of the extremities, this should not delay abdominal decompression.

Key point 7

- A high index of clinical suspicion is important in order to consider the diagnosis of ACS, but clinical examination alone is poor at assessing the degree of IAH.

TREATMENT OF ABDOMINAL COMPARTMENT SYNDROME

Prevention of ACS by recognising patients at risk of IAH and avoiding forceful closure of the tense abdomen is clearly desirable. Prophylactically leaving the abdomen open should be considered in these patients.

In established ACS with multiorgan dysfunction syndrome, abdominal decompression is required. This should be a planned procedure, and requires some basic equipment, but can be performed in the intensive care unit or the operating theatre. Relief of IAH can have adverse consequences. The sudden decrease in systemic vascular resistance by opening up the splanchnic circulation with reperfusion of the gut and washing out metabolic products may lead to hypotension or cardiac arrest. The patient should have intravascular volume restored and monitored before decompression. Some authors describe giving hypertonic saline with mannitol and bicarbonate prior to decompression in an attempt to minimize the deleterious effects of reperfusion.[38] This is not practised in other units reporting their experiences.[6,39] Haemorrhage should be anticipated, and means to control this should be available, with packing if necessary. Temporary cover of the open abdomen may be achieved by a variety of means, one of the most popular being the use of an opened sterile 3 litre genitourinary irrigation bag, the so-called 'Bogata bag' (Fig. 1).[20] Vacuum dressings have recently gained popularity and allow better control of the fluid loss from the open abdomen.[40] If the patient's condition improves, consideration should be given to closing the abdomen. This can often be achieved between 4 and 10 days after decompression.[36,39] Later retraction of the abdominal wall musculature may make primary closure impossible, and plastic surgical procedures such as medial advancement of the rectus abdominus or non-absorbable mesh and split-thickness skin grafts may be necessary.

It has been recognised that a subset of patients with IAH treated by abdominal decompression failed to improve or had recurrence of the symptoms and signs of ACS.[40] These patients were characterised by a high intravenous fluid requirement. Continued IAP monitoring and changing the abdominal dressing configuration if IAP rises again is advised.

The treatment of IAH without established ACS is more controversial. Some authors have suggested that a threshold IAP of 25 mmHg should trigger abdominal decompression.[9,36] Despite the physiological effects at lower values

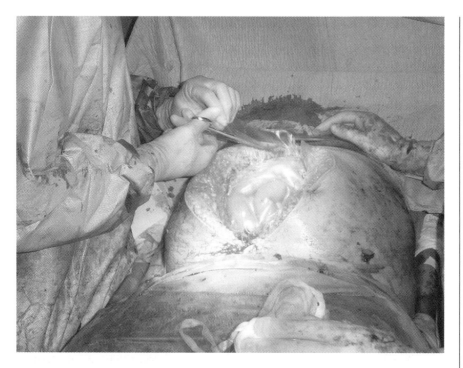

Fig. 1. Prophylactic placement of a 'Bogata' bag in a patient with penetrating abdominal trauma in order to avoid intra-abdominal hypertension.

of IAP, many patients will recover without adverse events from IAH. A grading of IAP has been suggested (Table 1).[39] These authors consider that patients with grade III or IV IAH require decompression. A recent prospective study of 706 patients with IAH, however, suggested that ACS did not occur until there was very marked IAH with pressures above 40 mmHg.[6] It is likely that the response of patients to IAH is complex and individual. Rather than being didactic about threshold levels of IAP for treatment, each patient at risk should be monitored,

Table 1. Grading of IAP as determined by intravesical pressure, and summary of clinical effects[39]

Grade	IAP (bladder pressure) in mmHg (in cmH₂O)	Clinical
I	7.3–11.0 (10–15)	None
II[a]	11.7–18.3 (16–25)	Oliguria, splanchnic hypoperfusion
III[b]	19.1–25.7 (26–35)	Anuria, increased ventilation pressures
IV[b]	> 25.7 (> 35)	As above and decreased pO₂

[a] Initial treatment aims to restore splanchnic and renal perfusion by hypervolaemic resuscitation.
[b] These patients will probably require urgent abdominal decompression.

and if adverse physiological consequences of IAH are observed then abdominal decompression should be considered. This should be performed before established MODS develops.

Key point 8

- ACS should be prevented by avoiding forceful closure of the abdomen.

Key point 9

- Hypovolaemia should be corrected prior to abdominal decompression.

Key point 10

- The IAP at which abdominal decompression should be performed remains controversial. Decompression should be considered in all patients with IAH who exhibit adverse physiological responses such as anuria or increasing ventilation pressure.

CONCLUSIONS

Abdominal compartment syndrome is associated with intra-abdominal hypertension and has profound physiological consequences. Patients developing ACS need to be recognised and treated. Monitoring IAP by means of intravesical pressure measurements is straightforward and can alert the clinician to rising IAP being associated with clinical deterioration. The key issue in IAH and ACS is prevention. This can be achieved in surgical patients by prophylactically leaving the abdomen open in patients at risk. It must be recognised, however, that ACS can develop in patients who have not undergone surgery.

Key points for clinical practice

- IAP varies with position, activity and body mass index.

- IAPs of between 3.0 and 10 mmHg are commonly observed postoperatively without adverse effects.

- The pathophysiology of IAH has been investigated widely in animal models with correlations observed in clinical studies.

Key points for clinical practice (continued)

- Intra-abdominal hypertension has significant physiological effects on the cardiovascular, respiratory, renal and gastrointestinal systems, as well as effects on intracranial pressure, cerebral perfusion and abdominal wall blood flow.

- The physiological effects are observed with IAP as low as 10 mmHg.

- ACS can occur in patients following blunt or penetrating trauma, elective surgery and certain conditions without abdominal surgery.

- A high index of clinical suspicion is important in order to consider the diagnosis of ACS, but clinical examination alone is poor at assessing the degree of IAH.

- ACS should be prevented by avoiding forceful closure of the abdomen.

- Hypovolaemia should be corrected prior to abdominal decompression.

- The IAP at which abdominal decompression should be performed remains controversial. Decompression should be considered in all patients with IAH who exhibit adverse physiological responses such as anuria or increasing ventilation pressure.

References

1. Emerson H. Intra-abdominal pressures. *Arch Intern Med* 1911; **7**: 754–784.
2. Thorington JM, Schmidt CF. A study of urinary output and blood-pressure changes resulting in experimental ascites. *Am J Med Sci* 1923; **165**: 880–886.
3. Gross R. A new method for surgical treatment of large omphaloceles. *Surgery* 1948; **24**: 277–292.
4. Ivankovich AD, Miletich DJ, Albrecht RF *et al*. Cardiovascular effects of intraperitoneal insufflation of carbon dioxide and nitrous oxide in the dog. *Anesthesiology* 1975; **42**: 281–287.
5. Josephs LG, Este-McDonald JR, Birkett DH, Hirsch EF. Diagnostic laparoscopy increases intracranial pressure. *J Trauma* 1994; **36**: 815–819.
6. Hong JJ, Cohn SM, Perez JM, Dolich MO, Brown M, McKenney MG. Prospective study of the incidence and outcome of intraabdominal hypertension and abdominal compartment syndrome. *Br J Surg* 2002; **89**: 591–596.
7. Ivatury RR, Porter JM, Simon RJ, Islam S, John R, Stahl WM. Intra-abdominal hypertension after life treatening penetrating abdominal trauma: prophylaxis, incidence, and clinical relevance to gastric mucosal pH and abdominal compartment syndrome. *J Trauma* 1998; **44**: 1016–1021.
8. Richardson JD, Trinkle JK. Hemodynamic and respiratory alterations with increased intra-abdominal pressure. *J Surg Res* 1976; **20**: 401.
9. Kron IL, Harman PK, Nolan SP. The measurement of intraabdominal pressure as a criterion for re-exploration. *Ann Surg* 1984; **199**: 28–30.
10. Iberti TJ, Kelly KM, Gentili DR *et al*. A simple technique to accurately determine intra-abdominal pressure. *Crit Care Med* 1987; **15**: 1140–1142.
11. Sugrue M, Buist MD, Hourihan F, Deane S, Bauman A, Hillman K. Prospective study of

intra-abdominal hypertension and renal function after laparotomy. *Br J Surg* 1995; **82**: 235–238.

12. Saggi BH, Sugerman HJ, Ivatury RR, Bloomfield GL. Abdominal compartment syndrome. *J Trauma* 1998; **45**: 597–609.

13. Sanchez NC, Tenofsky PL, Dort JM, Shen LY, Helmer SD, and Smith, RS. What is normal intra-abdominal pressure? *Am Surg* 2001; **67**: 243–248.

14. Schein M, Ivatury R. Intra-abdominal hypertension and the abdominal compartment syndrome. *Br J Surg* 1988; **85**: 1027–1028.

15. Barnes GE, Laine GA, Giam PY. *et al.* Cardiovascular responses to elevation of intra-abdominal hydrostatic pressure. *Am J Physiol* 1985; **248**: R208–213.

16. Cullen DJ, Coyle JP, Teplick R, Long MC. Cardiovascular, pulmonary, renal effects of massively increased intra-abdominal pressure in critically ill patients. *Crit Care Med* 1989; **17**: 118–121.

17. Fulda GJ, Stickles-Fulda E. Physiologic changes and outcome following surgical decompression for increased intra-abdominal pressure. *Crit Care Med* 1994; **22**: A68.

18. Widergren JT, Battisella FD. The open abdomen treatment for intra-abdominal compartment syndrome. *J Trauma* 1994; **37**: 158(abstract).

19. Mayberry JC, Welker KJ, Goldman, RK, Mullins, RJ. Mechanism of acute ascites formation after trauma resuscitation. *Arch Surg* 2003; **138**: 773–778.

20. Burch JM, Oritz VB, Richardson RJ, Martin RR, Mattox KL, Jordan GL. Abbreviated laparotomy and planned reoperation for critically injured patients. *Ann Surg* 1991; **215**: 476–484.

21. Obeid F, Saba A, Fath J. *et al.* Increases in intra-abdominal pressure affects pulmonary compliance. *Arch Surg* 1995; **130**: 544–548.

22. Richards WO, Scovill W, Shin B, Reed W. Acute renal failure associated with intra-abdominal pressure. *Ann Surg* 1983; **197**: 183–187.

23. Biancofiore G, Bindi ML, Romanelli AM, Bisa M, Boldrini A, Consani G, Filipponi F, Mosca F. Postoperative intra-abdominal pressure and renal function after liver transplantation. *Arch Surg* 2003; **138**: 703–706.

24. Diebel L, Dulchavsky S, Wilson RF. Effect of increased intra-abdominal pressure on mesenteric arterial and intestinal mucosal blood flow. *J Trauma* 1992; **33**: 45–49.

25. Diebel LN, Wilson RF, Dulchavsky SA, Saxe J. Effect of increased intra-abdominal pressure on hepatic arterial, portal venous and hepatic microcirculatory blood flow. *J Trauma* 1992; **33**: 279–283.

26. Eleftheriadis E, Kotzampassi K, Papanotas K, Heliadis N, Sarris K. Gut ischemia, oxidative stress and bacterial translocation in elevated abdominal pressure in rats. *World J Surg* 1996; **20**: 11–16.

27. Eleftheriadis E, Kotzampassi K, Botsios D. Splanchnic ischemia during laparoscopic cholecystectomy. *Surg Endosc* 1996; **10**: 324.

28. Bloomfield GL, Ridings PC, Blocher CR, Marmarou A, Sugerman HJ. Effects of increased intra-abdominal pressure upon intracranial and cerebral perfusion pressure before and after volume expansion. *J Trauma* 1996; **40**: 936–943.

29. Bloomfield GL, Dalton JM, Sugerman HJ, Ridings PL, DeMaria EJ, Bullock R. Treatment of increasing intracranial pressure secondary to the acute abdominal compartment syndrome in a patient with combined abdominal and head trauma. *J Trauma* 1995; **39**: 1168–1170.

30. Diebel L, Saxe J, Dulchavsky S. Effect of increased intra-abdominal pressure on abdominal wall blood flow. *Am Surg* 1992; **58**: 573.

31. Tiwari A, Haq AI, Myint F, Hamilton G. Acute compartment syndromes. *Br J Surg* 2002; **89**: 397–412.

32. Ertel W, Oberholzer A, Platz A, Stocker R, Trentz O. Incidence and clinical pattern of the abdominal compartment syndrome after 'damage-control' laparotomy in 311 patients with severe abdominal and/or pelvic trauma. *Crit Care Med* 2000; **28**: 1747–1753.

33. Harman PK, Kron IL, McLachlan HD., Freedlender AE, Nolan SP. Elevated intra-abdominal pressure and renal function. *Ann Surg* 1982; **196**: 594–597.

34. Greenhalgh DG, Warden GD. The importance of intra-abdominal pressure measurements in burned children. *J Trauma* 1994; **36**: 685–690.

35. Ivy ME., Possenti PP., Kepros J, Atweh NA, D'Aiuto M, Palmer J et al. Abdominal compartment syndrome in patients with burns. *J Burn Care Rehabil* 1999; **20**: 351–353.
36. Ivatury R, Diebel L, Porter JM, Simon RJ. Intra-abdominal hypertension and the abdominal compartment syndrome. *Surg Clin North Am* 1977; **77**: 783–800.
37. Kirkpatrick AW, Brenneman FD, McLean RF, Rapanos T, Boulanger BR. Is clinical examination an accurate indicator of raised intra-abdominal pressure in critically injured patients? *Can J Surg* 2000; **43**: 207–211.
38. Eddy V, Nunn C, Morris JA. Abdominal compartment syndrome. *Surg Clin North Am* 1997; **77**: 801–812.
39. Burch JM, Moore EE, Moore FA, Francoise R. The abdominal compartment syndrome. *Surg Clin North Am* 1996; **76**: 833–842.
40. Barker DE, Kaufman HJ, Smith LA, Ciraulo D, Richart CL, Burns RP. Vacuum pack technique of temporary abdominal closure: a 7 year experience with 112 patients. *J Trauma* 2000; **48**: 201–207.

I. Ahmed Ian J. Beckingham

3

Minimally invasive abdominal wall hernia repair

In the last 15 years the development and refinement of new techniques and assimilation of new and evolving medical technologies has turned laparoscopic inguinal hernia repair from an experimental to a widely performed procedure. Further improvements in prosthetic mesh technologies and new methods of mesh fixation are now expanding the role of laparoscopy to other types of hernia.

HISTORY

Hernia repair has evolved from hernia reduction[1] and primary closure of the hernial ring[2–4] through removal of the hernia sac combined with repair and reinforcements of the inguinal canal with non-absorbable darns.[5–7] A wide variety of techniques have been described, but overall recurrence rates in general remain around 10–20%.

Although it was never widely adopted by the surgeons at that time, the concept of reinforcing the inguinal canal with a prosthetic mesh was pioneered by Usher, who used a woven monofilament polypropylene mesh for inguinal hernia repair.[8,9] The concept of laparoscopic hernia repair has evolved from the work of René Stoppa, who suggested that *an extensive reinforcement of transversalis fascia without repair of the hernial defect was sufficient*.[10,11] The technique was modified by Lichtenstein, who popularised the concept of tension-free hernia repair.[12]

The first reported laparoscopic hernia repair was in 1982 by Ger.[13] Several other reports appeared in the literature advocating laparoscopic intra-

Irfan Ahmed MD FRCS, Queens Medical Centre, University Hospital, Nottingham

Mr Ian J. Beckingham Consultant Hepatobiliary and Laparoscopic Surgeon, Queens Medical Centre, University Hospital, Nottingham NG7 2UH, UK (for correspondence)

abdominal onlay techniques in the late 1980s. In the early 1990s Arregui and Doin described the transabdominal pre-peritoneal repair based on the Stoppa's principles.[14,15] Around the same time a new totally extraperitoneal approach was described, which offered the potential to avoid the risk of intrabdominal complications.[16,17] Laparoscopic transabdominal ventral hernia repair was also introduced in the 1990s, with improvement in recovery time, hospital stay and complications.[18]

The advantages and disadvantages of laparoscopic hernia repair are shown in Table 1.

Key point 1

- Laparoscopic hernia repair is associated with less postoperative pain, a faster recovery and quicker return to work than open hernia repair.

Key point 2

- Laparoscopic hernia repair is associated with less chronic groin pain and a lower recurrence rate.

TECHNICAL CONSIDERATIONS

Laparoscopic surgery remains dependent on the correct use of the available instrumentation and the use of prosthetic materials. The development of new dissecting tools and incorporation of various energy sources into laparoscopic surgery has given surgeons a greater choice and improved the ease of the

Table 1 Advantages and disadvantages of laparoscopic hernia repair

Advantages
- Less postoperative pain
- Fewer wound complications
- Reduced recovery time
- Improved cosmetic results
- Greater patient satisfaction
- Quicker operating time for bilateral hernias
- Easier operation in recurrent inguinal hernia
- Ability to treat bilateral hernia through one incision
- Lower incidence of chronic groin symptoms

Disadvantages
- Cannot be performed under local anaesthesia
- Steeper learning curve for surgeons
- Higher patient expectations
- Increased cost
- Higher incidence of visceral and vascular injuries
- Limited experience in obstructed/strangulated hernia surgery

procedure by enhancing the capability of tissue dissection and good haemostasis.

INSTRUMENTATION

Instrumentation used for grasping and dissection should be cost-effective and low-maintenance. Disposable, reusable and reposable instruments are available. Laparoscopic costs are strongly influenced by whether disposable or reusable instruments are used. It has been suggested that the ratio of the cost between reusable and disposable instrumentation is of the order of 2:1.[19] Recent concerns over prevention of transmission of prion material may increase the drive towards disposable instrumentation despite costs.

CANNULAS

Careful consideration of the cannula types and placement remains vital in laparoscopic hernia surgery. Misplacement of cannulae makes the procedure technically difficult. There remains a small but significant risk of cannula-related vascular or visceral injuries, which are cited as the major cause of mortality.[20] The principles of open establishment of pneumoperitoneum and placement of ports under direct visualisation will reduce injury to a minimum.

Various port designs incorporating balloons, sponges or cuffs around the port shaft to prevent leakage of pneumoperitoneum are helpful but not essential. Ports with a screw thread reduce the irritation of port slippage through the abdominal wall particularly in thin walled patients.

MESH

There is a wide range of synthetic and non-synthetic mesh available. Synthetic mesh can be single component, preformed or composite. Single-component mesh is made of either polypropylene, polyester or expanded polytetrafluoro-ethylene (ePTFE). Some newer mesh materials are available with impregnated silver and chlorhexidine to reduce the risk of infection. Polypropylene remains the most popular mesh in both open and laparoscopic surgery. ePTFE is the mesh of choice to be used intraperitoneally as it causes very little adhesion formation.

Preformed mesh is used to conform to the inguinal floor. *Composite* mesh is a two-layered mesh using ePTFE and Marlex. It is popular in ventral hernia repair, where it comes in direct contact with the bowel.

Non-synthetic mesh uses biological material from cadaver skin, porcine small intestine submucosa or porcine dermis. Experience with these newer materials is as yet very limited.

The selection of the mesh remains dependent on the site of mesh placement (extraperitoneal/onlay intra-abdominal), surgeon preference for mesh properties (e.g. stiffer, springy polypropylene mesh; floppy, conformable VYPRO mesh) and cost, since long-term follow-up data from laparoscopic series are insufficient to show differences in recurrence rates attributable to mesh type. The features that are desirable for mesh used in hernia repair are shown in Table 2.

Table 2 Features of the ideal prosthesis for hernia repair

- Permanent repair of the abdominal wall (no recurrence)
- Ingrowth characteristics resulting in a normal pattern of tissue healing and repair
- Easily assuming the conformity of the inguinal/abdominal wall
- Lack of predisposition to adhesion formation if placed intra-abdominally
- Resistance to infection
- Non-allergenic
- Low cost
- Easy handling
- Cuts easily without fraying
- See-through to allow accurate mesh placement over the defect

FIXATION OF MESH

Fixation devices have developed from the simple stapler used by Ger[13] in the first laparoscopic hernia repair in 1982 to more sophisticated stapling guns and tacking devices. Initially, the stapling guns required a second 10 mm port, but 5 mm tacking devices are now widely available.

Bioadhesives are the latest introduction; they include fibrin sealants and cyanoacrylate. Fibrin sealants and cyanoacrylate are not licensed for hernia fixation in the UK, although they are used for such purposes elsewhere in Europe.

VIDEO-ENDOSCOPIC SYSTEM

The quality of the image on the video-endoscopic system remains crucial for the operating surgeon. A high-quality image is essential when working in a confined extraperitoneal space. The use of the 30° laparoscope allows improved visualisation of the abdominal wall in ventral repairs and laterally in extraperitoneal repairs.

ERGONOMICS

Clinicians are learning the importance of surgical ergonomics with increasing experience. Attention to the minute details of postural mechanics can increase the ease of operation. During the learning curve for laparoscopic surgery there has been an increase in musculoskeletal complaints among laparoscopic workers.[21] Surgeon and assistant posture and attention to details in patient positioning and operating set-up can greatly enhance surgical efficiency.

TYPES OF HERNIAS FOR LAPAROSCOPIC REPAIR

Laparoscopic techniques have been described for all types of abdominal wall hernia.

INGUINAL HERNIAS

Inguinal hernia repair remains the most commonly performed operation in the elective general surgical practice.[22] Approximately 80 000 repairs are performed annually in the UK,[23] 100 000 in France[24] and 700 000 in the USA.[25]

Because inguinal hernia repair is performed so frequently, relatively modest improvements in clinical outcomes carry a significant impact on surgical practice.[26]

Successful repair of inguinal hernia can be accomplished in many ways. The concept of 'tension-free' open repair[12] has proved popular amongst surgeons. In this method a synthetic mesh is placed over the defect so that the hernia is repaired without the need to pull the tissues together under tension. Laparoscopic surgery has advanced the art of hernia repair by approaching the entire myopectineal orifice with its multiple openings and repairing it with minimal trauma.

Laparoscopic repair carries a certain advantage over conventional anterior herniorraphy. The recurrence rate and the incidence of chronic pain remains less in laparoscopic hernia repair[27] and rehabilitation is quicker.[28]

Approaches for inguinal hernia repair

The two most common types of laparoscopic inguinal hernia repair are transabdominal preperitoneal repair (TAPP) and totally extraperitoneal repair (TEP). The mode of operation in both these repairs follows the principle of placing the mesh in the preperitoneal space. As the result of this placement, the pressure that was contributing to hernia development now acts to keep the mesh in place and to prevent recurrence of the hernia.

The third form of repair is the original laparoscopic approach of onlay intraperitoneal inguinal hernia repair, which has now been superseded because of the unnecessary risk of mesh adherence.

TEP (totally extraperitoneal approach) In this repair, access to the preperitoneal cavity is achieved without incision of the peritoneal membrane. It requires an advanced knowledge of the posterior anatomy of the inguinal region (Fig. 1).

A 10 mm incision is made below the umbilicus. The anterior rectus sheath is identified and a 10 mm transverse incision is made, with care being taken to avoid damage to the underlying muscle. The rectus abdominus muscle is then retracted laterally and lifted anteriorly to expose the posterior rectus sheath. A 10 mm blunt trocar is then inserted beneath the rectus muscle, using the posterior rectus sheath to access the extraperitoneal space.

The extraperitoneal space is then dissected in one of two ways:

1. A balloon dissector can be inserted and inflated for a period of 2 minutes to open up the extraperitoneal space. The laparoscope can be inserted through the middle of the balloon to confirm correct placement. Following removal of the balloon, a 10 mm cannula with a smaller balloon incorporated within can be inserted to help maintain the extraperitoneal space. There can be occasional significant bleeds from the inferior epigastric vessels. Moreover, balloon devices are disposable and add a significant cost to the overall procedure.

2. The alternative technique uses the tip of the laparoscope to dissect sufficient space to insert two midline 5 mm trocars to then open up the extraperitoneal space under direct vision. This later technique is inexpensive and is likely to supersede the balloon dissection technique.

The two operating ports can be inserted both in the midline, one 1 cm superior to the symphysis pubis and one midway between the other two ports, or the second 5 mm port can be inserted laterally on the side of the hernia. The latter technique requires dissection of the hernia prior to insertion of the second port, whereas the two-midline-port technique permits two-handed dissection from the outset and allows dissection of both left and right sides in bilateral hernias without requirement for insertion of a fourth port (Fig. 1).

Once the ports have been inserted, dissection begins by exposure of Cooper's ligament on the pubic ramus by gently sweeping the tissues downwards. Any direct inguinal sac present will be reduced during this dissection and the femoral and obturator areas can be examined for hernias. If an indirect sac is present, it will be seen laterally. Dissection of the lateral compartment is started after identifying the epigastric vessels. The peritoneum is then dissected off the posterior surface of the abdominal wall and epigastric vessels. Dissection is carried out laterally up towards the anterior superior iliac spine to give a sizable extraperitoneal space.

Dissection of the hernial sac from the spermatic cord is achieved by identifying the sac on the superior–medial aspect of the cord and teasing it from the cord by blunt dissection. The hernial sac is reduced together with its contents. Long inguino-scrotal sacs can be transected and when necessary an

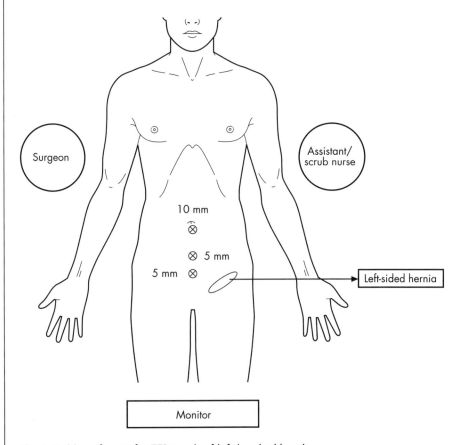

Fig. 1 Position of ports for TEP repair of left inguinal hernia.

endoloop can be applied to close the sac to prevent excessive pneumoperitoneum development. Once all hernial sacs have been reduced, the peritoneum is stripped back further from the posterior abdominal wall, testicular vessels and vas deferens to a few centimetres below the umbilicus.

For bilateral hernias, after one side has been dissected, the surgeon moves to the opposite side of the table but the laparoscope remains in the same position. The midline fat and peritoneal attachments (foveolar ligaments) are dissected to gain access to the opposite groin and the dissection proceeds in the same fashion. Dissection is facilitated by use of a 30° laparoscope at all stages of the operation but particularly in bilateral repairs.

When dissection is complete, the camera is removed and a 15×10 cm mesh is inserted after rolling it along its long axis. Once within the extraperitoneal space, the mesh is unfurled and pushed into place to cover across the midline, down beneath the pubic ramus and Cooper's ligament and across the posterior abdominal wall in the pocket where the peritoneum was stripped from the posterior wall. The mesh can be fixed by staples inserted into Cooper's ligament, along the medial and superior borders of the mesh (i.e. into the posterior surface of the rectus abdominus muscle), with care being taken to avoid the inferior epigastric vessels. Staples should *not* be inserted into the inferior border of the mesh (other than in Cooper's ligament) to avoid damage to the inguinal vessels medially, and to prevent inadvertent damage to cutaneous nerves laterally. A number of recent studies have shown that with correct placement of a large mesh, with care being taken to ensure that the mesh does not roll up as the gas is released, fixation is unnecessary in all but the larger direct hernias.[29]

Once the mesh has been placed, the gas is released under direct vision, holding the hernia sac superiorly and ensuring that the inferior border of the mesh does not roll up and cause an early recurrence. Any gas that has entered the peritoneal cavity is released by puncture of the posterior rectus sheath behind the rectus muscle. There is no need to close the anterior sheath defect (which is covered by the posterior sheath and the rectus muscle). Skin closure is with tissue glue or sutures.

TAPP (transabdominal preperitoneal approach) This technique requires entering the abdominal cavity to place the mesh in the preperitoneal space to cover the hernial orifices. The advantage of the transabdominal approach is familiarity of the intra-abdominal view and the larger space compared with the limited extraperitoneal space available in TEP approach.

After achieving the initial pneumoperitoneum using a Verres needle or the open technique via a supra-umbilical or umbilical port, two additional ports are placed lateral to the rectus sheath (Fig. 2).

The hernia is reduced into the peritoneal cavity. The dissection begins from the anterior superior iliac spine by lifting up a flap of peritoneum, well above the internal inguinal ring and above the rear wall of the inguinal canal as far as the median umbilical ligament. The small peritoneal vessels are coagulated during the dissection. Dissection continues in the avascular extraperitoneal plane by pushing the peritoneum with its surrounding preperitoneal fatty tissue away from the fascia transversalis and the rectus muscle. The dissection is continued to the middle of the symphysis to create a large enough space for

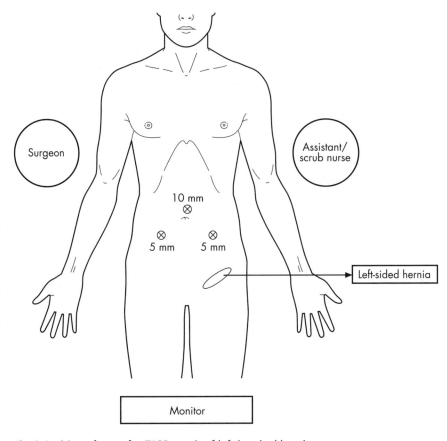

Fig. 2 Position of ports for TAPP repair of left inguinal hernia.

wrinkle-free placement of the mesh. In the inferior direction the medial compartment should be dissected as far as the iliac vessels to see the femoral hernial orifices.

After the dissection is complete, the epigastric vessels, internal inguinal ring, Hesselbach's triangle, Cooper's ligament, ileopubic tract, genital vessels and vas deferens should be clearly identified. A large 15 cm × 10 cm mesh is inserted. It should be placed sufficiently to overlap all the hernial orifices by at least 3 cm. Fixation is carried out with a staples in the area of Cooper's ligament, and superiorly and medially along the mesh border into the rectus muscle. After completion of the mesh fixation the peritoneal flap is carefully closed over the mesh, avoiding 'buttonholes' within the peritoneum that might allow mesh adherence or herniation of bowel. This can be achieved with staples or suture.

Key point 3
- Low recurrence rates are related to larger mesh size.

Postoperative management

Laparoscopic repair by either approach is comfortable so long as all efforts are made to remove free peritoneal gas. The wounds are small and there is no tissue ischaemia resulting from suturing of muscle tissue, nor is there tension from muscle repair. Bilateral hernias are as comfortable as unilateral repairs with this approach, and all patients can be discharged within a few hours of surgery subject to other medical and social issues. Patients are advised to resume normal activities as soon as comfortable. Driving is not permitted within 48 hours of a general anaesthetic, but after this time it is subject to any limitations imposed by the insurance company. In practical terms, patients can return to driving when they are completely pain-free from their operation (to permit an emergency stop). The majority will be back at work within a week of surgery.

Complications

Risks of anaesthesia   Laparoscopic repairs require a general anaesthetic, and patients are therefore exposed to the risks of this, which with modern anaesthesia is very low (1 in 185 000 – CEPOD 1987).[30]

Laparoscopic complications   Injury to the inguinal vessels can occur with either approach by inappropriate dissection, and in all cases it is preventable by avoiding dissection in the 'triangle of doom'. Bowel perforation and injury can occur in the TAPP approach with Verres needle injury, poor cannula placement technique or inadvertent diathermy contact. Bowel obstruction due to holes in the peritoneum allowing extraperitoneal bowel herniation or port site hernias also occur only after the TAPP approach.

Key point 4

- The key to the avoidance of complications is a thorough understanding of the anatomy of the posterior inguinal canal.

Bruising and haematoma formation   Postoperative bruising is common to all types of hernia repair. It may be around the port sites or in the inguinal canal. Haematomas can collect within the previous hernial sac and will therefore give the appearance of an early recurrence when reviewed. Differentiation can be achieved by seeking a history from the patient of postoperative bruising, the presence of a firm-to-hard irreducible mass in the inguinal canal and often an absence of the previous hernia discomfort. Further follow up at 2–3 months will show a reduction in size of the swelling as it resolves. Surgical intervention is not required except for an expanding haematoma in the immediate postoperative period.

Seroma formation   Most trials have suggested that the incidence of this complication is greater in laparoscopic surgery than in open surgery. Most seromas are self-limiting and resolve without any further intervention. This is probably dependent upon the type of mesh used, and may be less evident with softer, less irritant meshes.

Surgical emphysema   This is common particularly in the scrotum and abdominal wall. It may, however, extend through the subcutaneous planes into the chest, neck and facial tissues. Despite alarming appearances, it is harmless, and the carbon dioxide reabsorbs within 12–24 hours without any treatment.

Injury to nerves   Injury to cutaneous nerves in and around the inguinal canal may be responsible for chronic pain or numbness in the groin in all types of hernia surgery. The incidence is greatly reduced in laparoscopic repairs, as the ilioinguinal and hypogastric nerves are not encountered and there are no sutures with which to inadvertently ligate nerves.

Vascular injury   Bleeding from inferior epigastric vessels can be controlled laparoscopically by clips, and these vessels may be divided without significant postoperative problems. Bleeding from iliac vessels necessitates conversion to open surgery to investigate and repair. The importance of avoiding unnecessary dissection in this area cannot be overemphasised.

Infection   The rate of mesh infection remains very low with modern mesh production and sterilization techniques and does not represent a major problem in laparoscopic repairs. Antibiotic-impregnated mesh has recently become available.

Recurrence   This is not a major problem if the mesh is placed using the techniques described. The recurrence rate remains less than after open surgery.[31]

Testicular complications   Ischaemic orchitis and testicular atrophy can occur with any hernia surgery due to damage of the blood supply to the testis. The incidence appears to be lower with laparoscopic hernia repair than open repair. A few patients experience testicular pain as a result of trauma to the nerves travelling with the spermatic cord during dissection of a long indirect sac. This may last several months but eventually settles.

Bladder problems   The incidence of urinary retention is similar to that of open repair. Transient microscopic (or rarely macroscopic) haematuria can occur as a result of quite minor bladder manipulation and is of no significance. Bladder injury has been reported with both open and laparoscopic repairs.

Comparison of laparoscopic approach with open repair

A large EU meta-analysis recently compared the results of minimally invasive hernia repair with the traditional open mesh repair. This meta-analysis compared the results of 41 published trials. The conclusion was that the risks of haematoma formation and wound infection were less in the laparoscopic group. The duration of hospital stay was less and return to normal activity was quicker after laparoscopic surgery. The incidences of chronic pain, numbness and hernia recurrence were also less after laparoscopic repair. The incidence of haematoma formation was less after laparoscopic repair, but the risk of seroma formation was higher.[32]

The laparoscopic approach also often identifies additional hernias, some of which might well not have been seen at open surgery.[33] Thirty percent of patients have an indirect hernia in addition to a direct or femoral hernia, and 14% of recurrent hernias after open repair are a result of these missed hernias.[34] This is almost eliminated by the laparoscopic approach.[35]

Comparison of TEP and TAPP repair

The choice of either of the two approaches will depend largely on surgeon preference and expertise. The TAPP approach is less expensive than the TEP approach if balloon dissection and balloon ports are used. However, the TEP approach is cheaper if no balloon dissectors are employed and no staples are inserted. The TEP approach has a longer learning curve, but because the peritoneal cavity is not entered it has less potential for serious complications (vascular and bowel injury). The TAPP approach should be used for patients with incarcerated hernias as it allows adequate inspection of the sac contents to exclude ischaemic bowel.

Trials comparing these two approaches have reported a lower complication rate with TEP repair. Reports of iatrogenic bowel injury and adhesions are more common with TAPP repair. The incidence of postoperative pain is lower after TEP repair. There is no significant difference in recurrence rates.[36–38]

Key point 5

- TAPP and TEP repairs have similar outcomes with regard to recurrence rates, but TAPP is associated with a higher incidence of bowel and vascular complications than TEP.

NICE guidelines

The UK National Institute of Clinical Excellence (NICE) published the guidelines on laparoscopic hernia repair in January 2001. They are shown in Table 3. The report acknowledged that laparoscopic hernia repair was associated with less pain and a faster return to normal activity and work than the open technique. Its main argument for not recommending laparoscopic hernia repair for primary repairs was the increased cost of the laparoscopic approach. Modifications in technique (dispensing with the need for balloon

Table 3 NICE guidelines

- For repair of primary inguinal hernia, open (mesh) should be the preferred surgical procedure
- For the repair of recurrent and bilateral inguinal hernia, laparoscopic surgery should be considered
- When laparoscopic surgery is undertaken for inguinal hernia, the TEP procedure should be preferred
- Laparoscopic surgery for inguinal hernia should only be undertaken in those units with appropriately trained operating teams that regularly undertake these procedures

dissectors and staplers) will greatly reduce the cost of the procedure. New NICE guidelines are due for publication in August 2004.

FEMORAL AND PELVIC HERNIAS

These hernias are less common than inguinal hernias. They form about 2–4% of all groin hernias.[39] They remain amenable to laparoscopic repair through the same approach (TEP or TAPP) as inguinal hernia. Reduction of the hernia contents followed by mesh insertion, with or without fixation, is appropriate management.

Laparoscopy has a useful role to play in diagnosing and managing other rare pelvic hernias, including obturator, sciatic, supravesical, and prevascular hernias.

Key point 6

- Rare hernias are diagnosed increasingly frequently with the popularization of the laparoscopic technique.

VENTRAL HERNIA REPAIR

The term *ventral hernia* encompasses *incisional, epigastric, paraumbilical, umbilical, spigelian* and *traumatic hernias*. Incisional hernias form the largest group of ventral hernias and remain the most difficult to treat.

About 3–20% of all laparotomy patients will develop incisional hernias[12,40–42] and open primary repair has a high recurrence of 25–49%.[43–45] Introduction of open mesh repair has reduced the recurrence rate, but it remains between 1 and 23%.[46,47]

In 1991 LeBlanc reported the first successful series of laparoscopic ventral hernia repair.[18,46] Several large series have shown low recurrence rates (0–9%), faster postoperative recovery and shorter hospital stay, with low complication rates and higher patient satisfaction rates.[46–48]

An open cannulation technique is used to achieve a pneumoperitoneum through a 10 mm camera port placed laterally. Two 5 mm trocars are placed as far laterally from the hernial defect as possible (Fig. 3). A 30° laparoscope permits better visualisation of the anterior abdominal wall than a 0° laparoscope. Adhesions are divided under direct vision avoiding diathermy to reduce the risk of damage to bowel. The edges of the defect/defects are exposed. The hernial sac is left *in situ* intact.

The edges of the defect are accurately marked on the abdominal wall with a sterile marker pen and measured. The mesh is measured and cut to allow 3–5 cm greater than the defect. The prosthetic material is placed in the intra-abdominal position as an onlay. After insertion of the mesh into the peritoneal cavity it is fixed with staples and/or full-thickness sutures preplaced on the mesh and pulled through using a modified crochet hook device. These sutures anchor the mesh in the four corners with additional staples applied in two concentric rings to fix the mesh to the abdominal wall and reduce 'blowing

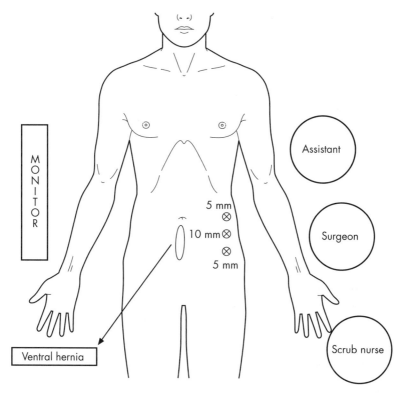

Fig. 3 Position of ports for ventral hernia repair.

through' of the mesh into the hernia defect itself ('double crown technique'). Fixation with staples alone may be associated with higher recurrence rates, particularly in larger hernias, since few of the staples penetrate more than 2–3 mm into the abdominal wall fascia.

Complications

Common complications are seroma formation, haemotoma and pain. Seromas are frequent probably because the peritoneum remains intact behind the mesh. Extraperitoneal mesh placement and destruction of the peritoneum with argon diathermy have been used to diminish the incidence of seroma formation. However, most seromas will reabsorb with time and aspiration should be avoided to reduce the risk of secondary infection. Wound problems, including port site hernia, may occasionally need re-operation.

Bowel injury is infrequent (0–5%) but remains a risk. Careful dissection without diathermy will reduce the risk.[49] Mesh infection may necessitate removal of the mesh.

The choice of mesh in ventral hernias has remained a point of discussion. The concerns with intra-abdominal onlay mesh remain the possibility of adhesion formation and subsequent fistula formation, particularly with traditional polypropylene meshes.[50] Adhesion formation to ePTFE mesh after intraperitoneal placement, however, is minimal,[51] and it has become the most widely used intraperitoneal mesh for onlay repairs despite its high cost, and has not been associated with bowel obstruction.

SERVICE PROVISION OF ABDOMINAL WALL HERNIA REPAIR

Economic issues remain an essential element in the decision making in the choice of hernia repair. Healthcare systems around the world in spite of resource constraint are facing steady increases in their expenditure due to advancement of technology and rising costs of disposable equipment and prosthetic implants. Patient awareness from media and the internet is driving a greater demand for newer techniques and technologies and this contributes to the rising popularity and increasing numbers of laparoscopic hernia repairs performed annually, despite the limitations of the NICE recommendations.

Key points for clinical practice

- Laparoscopic hernia repair is associated with less postoperative pain, a faster recovery and quicker return to work than open hernia repair.

- Laparoscopic hernia repair is associated with less chronic groin pain and a lower recurrence rate.

- Low recurrence rates are related to larger mesh size.

- The key to the avoidance of complications is a thorough understanding of the anatomy of the posterior inguinal canal.

- TAPP and TEP repairs have similar outcomes with regard to recurrence rates, but TAPP is associated with a higher incidence of bowel and vascular complications than TEP.

- Rare hernias are diagnosed increasingly frequently with the popularization of the laparoscopic technique.

REFERENCES

1. Ebbell B (transl.) The Ebers Papyrus. The Greatest Egyptian Medical Document. London: H. Milford and Oxford University Press, 1937: 17 and 123.
2. Marcy HO. A new use of carbolized catgut Ligatures. *Boston Med Surg J* 1871; **85**: 315.
3. Annandale T. A case in which a reduciable oblique and direct inguinal and femoral hernia existed on the same side and were successfully treated by the operation. *Edinburgh Med J* 1876; **21**: 1087–1091.
4. Cheatle GL. An operation for the radical cure of inguinal and femoral hernia. *Br Med J* 1920; **2**: 68–69.
5. Bassini E. Nuovo metodo per la cura ridicule dell'ernia inguinale. *Arch F Klin Chir* 1890; **40**: 429–476.
6. Halsted WS. *Bull Johns Hopkins Hosp* 1903; **149**: 211.
7. Shouldice EE. The treatment of hernia. *Ontario Med Rev* 1953: **20**: 670–684.
8. Usher FC, Gannon JP. Marlex mesh: a new plastic mesh for replacing tissue defects: I. Experimental studies. *Arch Surg* 1959; **78**: 131.
9. Usher FC. Hernia repair with knitted polypropylene mesh. *Surg Gynecol Obstet* 1963; **117**: 239.

10. Stoppa RE, Petit J. Henry X, Unsutured Dacron prosthesis in groin hernias. *Int Surg* 1975; **60**: 411–415.

11. Stoppa RE, Rives JL, Warlaumont CR et al. The use of Dacron in the repair of hernia of the groin. *Surg Clin N Am* 1993; **73**: 571–581.

12. Lichtenstein IL, Shulman AG, Amid PK, Montilier MM. The tension free hernioplasty. *Am J Surg* 1989; **157**: 188–193.

13. Ger R. The management of certain abdominal herniae by intraabdominal closure of the neck of the sac. *Ann R Coll Surg Engl* 1982; **64**: 342–344.

14. Arregui ME, Davis CD, Yucel O et al. Laparoscopic mesh repair of inguinal hernia using a preperitoneal approach. A preliminary report. *Surg Laparosc Endosc* 1992; **2**: 53–58.

15. Dion YM, Morin J, Laparoscopic inguinal herniorraphy. *Can J Surg* 1992; **35**: 209–212.

16. Phillips EH, Carroll BJ, Fallas MJ, Laparoscopic preperitoneal inguinal hernia repair with peritoneal incision. *Surg Endosc* 1993; **7**: 159–162.

17. McKernan BJ, Laws HL. Laparoscopic preperitoneal prosthetic repair of inguinal hernias. *Surg Rounds* 1992; **7**: 579–610.

18. LeBlanc KA, Booth WV, Laparoscopic repair of incisional hernias using expanded polytetrafluoroethylene: preliminary findings. *Surg Laparosc Endosc* 1993; **3**: 39–41.

19. Fengler TW, Panhlke H, Kraas E. Sterile and economic instrumentation in laparoscopic surgery. *Surg Endosc* 1998; **12**: 1275–1279.

20. Hashizume M, Sugimachi K. Needle and trocar injury during laparoscopic surgery in Japan. *Surg Endosc* 1997; **11**: 1198–1201.

21. Bergeur R, Smith WD, Davis S. Erogonomic problems associated with laparoscopic surgery. *Surg Endosc* 1999; **13**: 466–468.

22. Rutkow IM, Robbins AW. Demographic, classifactory, and socioeconomic aspects of hernia repair in the United States. *Surg Clin Nth Am* 1993; **73**(3): 413–426.

23. Kingsnorth AN, Gray MR, Nott DM. Prospective randomised trial comparing the Shouldice technique and plication darn for inguinal hernia. *Br J Surg* 1992; **79**.

24. Levard H, Boudet MJ, Hennet H, Hay JM. Inguinal hernia repair: a prospective multicentre trial on 1706 hernias. *Br J Surg* 1996; **83 suppl 2**: 72.

25. Schumpelick V, Treutner KH, Arlt G. Inguinal hernia repair in adults. *Lancet* 1994; **344**(8919): 375–379.

26. Simons MP, Kleijnen J, van Geldere D, Hoitsma HF, Obertop H. Role of the Shouldice technique in inguinal hernia repair: a systematic review of controlled trials and a meta-analysis. *Br J Surg* 1996; **83**(6): 734–738.

27. Liem MS, van Duyn EB, van der Graaf Y, van Vroonhoven TJ, Coala Trial Group: Recurrences after conventional anterior and laparoscopic inguinal hernia repair: a randomized comparison. *Annals of Surgery* 2003; **237**: 136–141.

28. Bringman S, Ramel S, Heikkinen TJ, Englund T, Westman B, Anderberg B; Tension-free inguinal hernia repair: TEP versus mesh-plug versus Lichtenstein: a prospective randomized controlled trial. *Annals of Surgery* 2003; **237**.

29. Hammond J, Mann G, Brooks A, Beckingham IJ. Laparoscopic totally extraperitoneal (TEP) hernia repair at a nice price. *Br J Surg* June 2003; Vol 90 (Suppl 1) 86.

30. Jenkins K, Baker AB. Consent and anaesthesia risk: Anaesthesia: Oct 2003; Vol 58: 10: 962.

31. EU Hernia Trialists Collaboration. Repair of groin hernia with synthetic mesh – meta-analysis of randomized controlled trails. *Ann Surg* 2002; **235**: 322–332.

32. McCormack K, Scott NW, Go PMNYH, Ross S, Grant AM on behalf of the EU Hernia Trialists Collaboration. Laparoscopic techniques versus open techniques for inguinal hernia repair (Cochrane Review). In: *The Cochrane Library*, Issue 3, 2003.

33. Crawford DL, Hiatt JR, Phillips EH. Laparoscopy identifies unexpected groin hernias. *Arch Surg* 1998; **64**: 976–978.

34. Flex E, Michas C, Gonzalez H. Laparoscopic hernioplasty: why it works. *Surg Endosc* 1997; **11**: 36–40.

35. Tetik C, Arregui M, Castro C. Complications and recurrences associated with laparoscopic repair of groin hernias: a multi-institutional retrospective analysis. In: Arregui M, Nagan RF, eds Inguinal hernias: Advances or Controversies? Oxford: Radcliffe Medical Press, 1994: 494–500.

36. Fitzgibbons RJ, Camps J, Cornet DA, Anniball R. Laparoscopic inguinal herniorrhaphy: Results of a multicenter trial. *Ann Surg* 1995; **221**: 3–13.

37. Phillips EH, Arregui M, Caroll BJ, et al Incidence of complications following laparoscopic hernioplasty. *Surg Endosc* 1995; **9**: 16–21.
38. Carbajo MA, Martin del Olm JC, Blanco JI, et al. Laparoscopic treatment vs. open surgery in the solution of major incisional and abdominal wall hernias with mesh. *Surg Endosc* 1999; **13**: 250–252.
39. Ruktow I. Epideomiologic, economic and sociologic aspect of hernia surgery in the United States in the 1990s. *Surg Clin N Am* 1998; **78**: 941–951.
40. Mudge M, Hughes LE. Incisional hernia: a 10 year prospective study of incidence and attitudes. *Br J Surg* 1985; **72**: 70–71.
41. Schoetz DJ, Coller JA, Veidenheimer MC. Closure of abdominal wounds with polydioxanone. A prospective study. *Arch Surg* 1988; **123**: 72–74.
42. Read RC, Yoder G. Recent trends in the management of incisional herniation. *Arch Surg* 1989; **124**: 485–488.
43. Hesselink VJ, Luijendijk RW, de Wilt JHW, Heide R, Jeekel J. An evaluation of risk factors in incisional hernia. *Surgery, Gynecology & Obstetrics* 1993; **176**: 228–234.
44. Van der Linden FT, van Vroonhoven TJ. Long term results after surgical correction of incisional hernia. *Neth J Surg* 1988; **40**(5): 127–129.
45. Stoppa RE. The treatment of complicated groin and incisional hernias. *World Journal of Surgery* 1989: **13**(5): 545–554.
46. LeBlanc KA, Booth WV, Whitaker JM, Bellanger DE. Laparoscopic incisional and ventral herniorrhaphy: our initial 100 patients. *Hernia* 2001; **5**: 41–45.
47. Moreno-Egea A, LironR, Girela E, Aguayo JL. Laparoscopic repair of ventral and incisional hernias using a new composite mesh (Parietex): initial experience. *Surg Laparosc Endosc Percutan Tech* 2001; **11**: 103–6.
48. Heniford BT, Park A, Ramshaw BJ, Voeller G. Laparoscopic repair of ventral hernias. Nine years experience with 850 consecutive hernias. *Ann Surg* 2003; **238**(3). 391–400.
49. Cassar K, Munro A. Surgical treatment of incisional hernia. *Br J Surg* 2002; **89**: 534–545.
50. Marchal F, Brunaud L, Sebbag H et al. Treatment of incisional hernias by placement of an intraperitoneal prosthesis: a series of 128 patients. *Hernia* 2000; **3**: 141.
51. Koehler RH, Begos D, Berger D, Carey S, leBlank K, Ramshaw B, Smoot R. Does ePTFE 'Dualmesh' limit intraabdominal adhesion formation in laparoscopic ventral hernia repair? A multiinstitutional reoperative experience. *JSLS* 2001; **5**: 348.

Alexander Munro Kevin Cassar

4

Repair of incisional hernia

Unfortunately, incisional hernia is a relatively common clinical problem after abdominal surgery. This complication has been reported in up to 11% of patients after open abdominal operations.[1] Most hernias occur in midline abdominal incisions since these are currently the most commonly used incisions for open abdominal procedures. An incisional hernia is defined as a bulge, both visible and palpable, through a previous abdominal incision. They may vary in size from a few millimetres to many centimetres and there may be single or multiple defects.

GENERAL FEATURES

AETIOLOGY

Incisional hernias that develop within a few months of an abdominal operation are likely to have occurred as a result of partial dehiscence of the deeper layers of the abdominal wound within the first few weeks after operation. Wound infection is an aetiological factor in at least some of these cases. Late incisional hernia may also develop in a wound that has been shown to be soundly healed several months or years after initial operation.

An important factor in the aetiology of incisional hernia is the type of suture used to close the wound. Perhaps the best material available is stainless steel wire, with wound failure rates of less than 1%,[2] but unfortunately most surgeons find the material difficult to handle. Monofilament non-absorbable sutures such as nylon and polypropylene are associated with low wound failure rates but do occasionally give rise to problems with wound pain and suture extrusion. Their use has to some extent been superseded by absorbable

Mr Alexander Munro ChM FRCSEd Professor of Clinical Surgery, University of Aberdeen, and Consultant Surgeon, Raigmore Hospital, Inverness IV2 3LX, UK (for correspondence)

Kevin Cassar MMEd MD FRCS(Ed) Lecturer, University of Aberdeen; Honorary Specialist Registrar, Aberdeen Royal Infirmary, Ward 36, Foresterhill, Aberdeen AB25 2ZN, UK

monofilament materials such as polydioxanone. Randomised controlled trial evidence suggests that this material is as good as non-absorbable suture material in terms of wound failure[3] but does not produce suture sinuses as frequently as non-absorbable materials. Catgut is associated with an unacceptably high rate of early wound failure and has largely been abandoned as a closure material.

Obesity is a factor in the causation of incisional hernia in some patients and the incidence of wound hernia increases with age. Insertion of a drain through a wound (a technique that is now rarely practised) appears to be associated with an increased incidence of incisional hernia.

Laparoscopic intervention is a further cause of incisional hernia; the resulting hernia is usually described as a 'port site hernia'. The incidence has been estimated as 1 in 550 cases: with increasing numbers of patients having laparoscopic surgery this problem is likely to be seen much more commonly in the future. They are mostly seen in the peri-umbilical area and are usually located in mid line incisions made for insertion of laparoscopic instruments 10 mm or more in diameter.

Finally 'button hole' incisional hernias, first described by Krukowski and Matheson[4] in 1987, are perhaps more common than was previously realised. They are often multiple and occur late, and may be due to the effect of continuous non-absorbable monofilament suture material 'sawing' through tissue. They are often elliptical defects whose long axis lies transversely across the abdomen with the medial corner close to the midline incision, and when explored surgically the suture material is seen at the inner corner of the defect.

SYMPTOMS AND SIGNS

Many patients with an incisional hernia do not have symptoms apart from a visible bulge centred on a previous incision, but for those who do the common symptoms include discomfort, particularly on bending, abdominal pain and episodes of intestinal obstruction, when the main symptoms include colicky abdominal pain and intermittent vomiting.

Examination of the patient who presents at the outpatient clinic with a lump related to a surgical wound in the abdomen should include both inspection and palpation of the abdomen in the supine and erect postures. If the patient presents acutely with colicky abdominal pain and there is a tender irreducible abdominal wall mass, strangulated incisional hernia should be considered as the most likely diagnosis and if plain abdominal radiographs confirm the presence of small bowel obstruction urgent operation will be necessary.

SURGICAL TREATMENT

PREOPERATIVE ASSESSMENT

In most patients the diagnosis will be obvious and investigations of the hernia are unnecessary. On the rare occasion when the diagnosis is in doubt, particularly if the patient is obese or the hernia is small, an ultrasound examination of the abdomen may be a useful investigation.

If the patient has a massive incisional hernia and there is evidence of respiratory insufficiency, the opinion of a consultant anaesthetist colleague should be sought before a decision is made about operation. In these circumstances the patient will require to have respiratory investigations including arterial blood gases and spirometry before operation. In addition some consideration of the likely effect of returning the hernial contents back inside the abdomen during repair of the hernia repair will be necessary as part of preoperative workup.

A major consideration is whether it is prudent to operate on the obese patient with an incisional hernia. There is very little evidence in the surgical literature on this point . Most surgeons advise weight reduction for the obese patient, but occasionally these patients present at a later date as an emergency with intestinal obstruction not having lost the required weight, making emergency operation technically difficult and hazardous for the patient.

WHICH OPERATION?

The procedure may be performed either laparoscopically or by open operation. Which route is chosen will largely depend on the operator's previous experience. The traditional technique of closure by approximating the margins of the defect on either side has been largely replaced by use of a prosthetic patch of either polypropylene mesh or expanded PTFE (polytetrafluoroethylene).

The laparoscopic approach is rapidly gaining ground and consists of dissecting the adhesions and reducing the sac contents into the abdomen. A patch is introduced into the abdomen through a port and placed in the defect with several centimetres' overlap at the margins to compensate for shrinkage. The prosthetic material is sutured to the margins of the defect.

OPEN OPERATION

Most surgeons will excise the previous scar together with a variable amount of redundant skin, enough to allow the skin edges to come together without tension. It is important to be aware that there may be very little subcutaneous fat present and occasionally the hernial sac containing bowel lies immediately deep to skin, making it vulnerable to damage with the scalpel. As soon as the hernial sac is identified, dissection proceeds along the surface of the sac until rectus sheath is clearly defined all the way around the perimeter of the base of the hernial sac.

At this stage it is useful to continue the dissection along the surface of rectus sheath around the abdominal wall defect using a unipolar or bipolar diathermy blade or scissors; at the same time the assistant applies traction on the wound edge using tissue forceps. We find it advantageous to dissect the plane between rectus sheath and the subcutaneous fat on both sides along the whole length of the previous incision for at least 4–5 cm lateral to the base of the hernial sac or the midline. This ensures that small additional 'button hole' incisional hernias have not been missed. If other defects in the abdominal wall are found, the bridge between the defect and the main hernia should be divided, thus creating one large defect.

Attention is now turned to the sac. In most circumstances it is probably best to open the sac and inspect the contents. Any adhesions between bowel and peritoneum require patient dissection for at least 5–6 cm lateral to the abdominal wall defect, avoiding damage to bowel, which in turn could increase the risk of wound infection. The sac is trimmed and the peritoneum closed using a continuous polypropylene or polydioxanone suture. If the bowel viability is in doubt as a result of small-intestinal strangulation, it is essential to divide all adhesions to the intestine and place the small intestine in a warm towel and wait for 10–20 minutes to see if normal intestinal colour returns. If bowel clearly needs resection, this should be done forthwith and in most cases a primary anastomosis will be possible. The abdomen is thoroughly lavaged with antibiotic solution (e.g. a cephalosporin) in normal saline.

The next step in the operation is to decide whether the defect is best repaired using the patient's own tissues or alternatively by inserting a synthetic patch. To some extent this will depend on the size of the defect and the resultant likely tension on any suture line.

Open suture repair

A variety of open suture techniques are available. The most basic of these includes simple fascial repair. The principle involves closure of the edges of rectus sheath on both sides of the wound using a continuous non-absorbable or slowly absorbable suture (e.g. polydioxanone), taking bites that include both anterior and posterior rectus sheath at least 2 cm in width with 1–2 cm spaces between sutures (Fig. 1). If the optimum strength of wound is to be achieved,

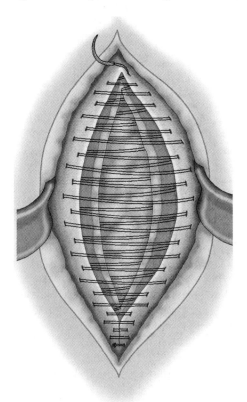

Fig. 1 Open suture technique for repair of incisional hernia using a continuous suturing method.

the suture length used should be at least four times the length of the wound. Tissues should be approximated but not strangulated by the suture. Other suture techniques include the Keel procedure (Fig. 2) and a Mayo repair with overlap of the rectus sheath edges. This technique may be supplemented with retention sutures.

The results reported using open suture techniques vary (Table 1) but it is of concern that the larger studies have all reported high recurrence rates. In the light of these results it is important that suture repair should only be performed when the fascial edges are suitable for suturing and come together without any tension. There should be no obvious risk factors for wound failure. Wound

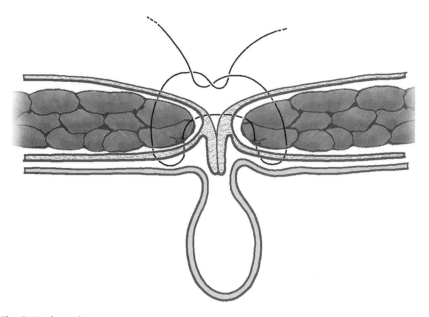

Fig. 2 Keel repair.

Table 1 Recurrence rates after open suture repair of incisional hernia

Reference	Year	Technique	No. of patients	Recurrence rate (%)	Follow-up (months)
Hope et al.[5]	1985	Da Silva method	27	0	30
Langer and Christiansen[6]	1985	Primary closure	154	31	48–120
George and Ellis[7]	1986	Keel or mass nylon	81	46	14
van der Linden and van Vroonhoven[8]	1988	Primary closure, two-layer fascial approximation, Mayo overlap repair	151	49	39
Naraynsingh and Ariyanayagam[9]	1993	Keel technique	85[a]	1	71
Gecim et al.[10]	1996	Primary closure	109[b]	45	7–92
Kuzbari et al.[11]	1998	Sliding door technique	10	0	26–66
Shukla et al.[12]	1998	Cardiff repair	50	0	52

[a] Only 23 had an incisional hernia; the remainder had para-umbilical, umbilical and epigastric hernias.
[b] Nine underwent mesh repair.

complications with primary suture techniques are common, ranging from 10% to 44%.

> **Key point 1**
>
> - Suture repair should only be performed when the fascial edges are suitable for suturing and come together without any tension. There should be no obvious risk factors for wound failure.

Open mesh repair

If good results are to be obtained, attention to detail is critical. It is important that the sac be widely dissected and opened, and that the bowel be dissected off the inner surface of peritoneum. Several prosthetic materials are available to cover the abdominal wall defect. There is general agreement that non-absorbable materials are better than absorbables. The most popular materials are polypropylene mesh and PTFE produced as a patch. Although these materials are both satisfactory, it is thought that if the wound has been contaminated during the operation, it is better to use polypropylene mesh rather than PTFE. The material may be placed intraperitoneally, subfascially or as an onlay patch. If the prosthesis is placed intraperitoneally and omentum is available, it should be placed between the mesh and bowel. This will prevent mesh from adhering to the small intestine, making it easier to dissect the bowel off the undersurface of the wound if the patient ever requires further laparotomy. Earlier concern that intraperitoneal placement might be associated with a substantial risk of septic complication has not been substantiated.

There is good evidence that mesh materials contract with time, so it is crucial that mesh is cut at least 3 cm larger than the abdominal wall defect so that there is a substantial overlap all the way around the defect. A popular method of repair is the 'sandwich' technique using two layers of mesh, one placed intraperitoneally and the other in front of the rectus sheath (Fig. 3). Interrupted sutures of polypropylene are passed through the anterior layer of prosthesis 3 cm medial to its lateral margin, through the abdominal wall 1–2 cm lateral to

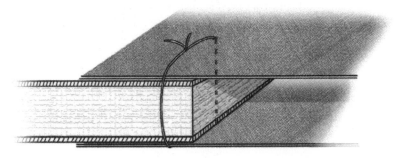

Fig. 3 'Sandwich' method for open mesh repair of incisional hernia. Two layers of mesh are used: (1) intraperitoneal and (2) onlay. The repair is done using interrupted sutures as shown.

the edge of the defect and then through the inner layer of mesh. The suture is passed back through the same layers in reverse order some 2 cm proximal or distal to the first passage so that the suture lies parallel to the wound edge.

A series of sutures is inserted in the same way on one side of the wound and then on the other and tied without tension. The mesh is trimmed appropriately before the second side of the wound is sutured.

An alternative method of applying the prosthetic material is to use it as an onlay prosthesis (Fig. 4). The peritoneum is closed and a piece of mesh is cut to a size at least 3 cm bigger than the abdominal wall defect. We generally use a continuous suture of polypropylene and stitch the mesh all the way around the defect using 1–2 cm bites. A further suture is then inserted approximating the perimeter of the prosthetic material and the rectus sheath. It is customary to insert a suction drain into the subcutaneous space before closing the skin incision.

There is little doubt that results obtained with prosthetic repair are associated with lower recurrence rates (0–10%) than when using open suture methods (Table 2). Further weight has been added to the evidence base in favour of prosthetic repair by a study recently reported by Luijendijk et al.[27] in which patients were randomised to either suture repair or prosthetic repair.

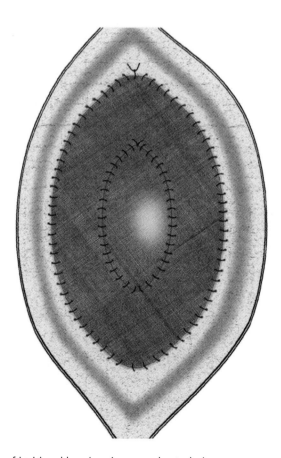

Fig. 4 Mesh repair of incisional hernia using an onlay technique.

Table 2 Recurrence rates after open mesh repair of incisional hernia

Reference	Year	Mesh used[a]	No. of patients	Recurrence rate (%)	Follow-up (months)
McCarthy and Twiest[13]	1981	Polypropylene	25	8	27
Matapurker et al.[14]	1991	Polypropylene	60	0	36–84
Temudom et al.[15]	1996	Polypropylene and PTFE	50	4	24
Gillion et al.[16]	1997	PTFE	158	4	37
McLanahan et al.[17]	1997	Polypropylene	106	4	24
Balen et al.[18]	1998	PTFE	45	2	39
Turkcapar et al.[19]	1998	Polypropylene	45	2	36
Whiteley et al.[20]	1998	Polypropylene	10	0	17
Arnaud et al.[21]	1999	Dacron	250	3	97
Bauer et al.[22]	1999	PTFE	98	10	72
Utrera Gonzalez et al.[23]	1999	PTFE	84	2	12–36
Chrysos et al.[24]	2000	PTFE	52	8	—
Ladurner et al.[25]	2001	Polypropylene	57	2	6–33
Martin-Duce et al.[26]	2001	Polypropylene	152	1	72

[a] PTFE, polytetrafluoroethylene.

Follow-up of at least 2 years was obtained. Recurrence was seen in 46% of patients who had suture repair compared with 23% of those who had prosthetic repair ($p = 0.005$). Wound complications with prosthetic repair also appear to be less common than with direct suture methods.

Key point 2

- Recurrence rates with mesh repair are much lower than with suture repair. Mesh repair is the technique of choice for most incisional hernias.

Laparoscopic incisional hernia repair

Although laparoscopic repair of incisional hernias has become widespread in North America, the technique has been slower to become established in the UK. The principle is to place a mesh or patch intraperitoneally, overlapping the defect in the abdominal wall. The mesh requires to be fixed to the under surface of the abdominal wall to prevent it becoming dislodged.

It is important to use laterally placed ports to ensure adequate distance from the site of the hernia. It is useful to have both a 0° and a 30° laparoscope available. With the abdomen well inflated, adhesive bands between intestine and the hernial sac are divided using diathermy scissors or an ultrasonic scalpel, taking great care not to damage bowel. The edge of the abdominal wall defect is identified clearly and the sac is left *in situ*. The size and shape of prosthetic material required may be outlined on the abdominal wall skin. It is important to use a patch big enough to overlap the defect by at least 3–4 cm.

The prosthetic material is introduced into the peritoneal cavity through a 10 mm port. Perhaps the most secure method of fixation is to use sutures inserted using a suture passer (Fig. 5). The principle is to pass a suture threaded into the eye of the suture passer, through a small incision in skin and the full thickness of abdominal wall and the mesh, into the peritoneal cavity. The suture remains in the peritoneal cavity while the suture passer is re-inserted into the peritoneal cavity to emerge in the abdominal cavity close to the point where the suture is. The suture is picked up in the suture passer and is brought back to the abdominal wall surface . The suture is tied, thus incorporating the mesh and the whole thickness of abdominal wall. This technique is particularly useful for fixing the corners of the patch. If this method is used for the whole procedure then the distance between sutures should be no more than 2 cm. Tacks or spiral staples can be used between sutures if desired.

Recurrence rates appear to be consistently low using laparoscopic mesh repair (Table 3) and wound complications are uncommon. Seroma rates (2–36%) vary widely from one study to another. They tend to settle with conservative management.

A number of studies have compared open mesh or patch repair with laparoscopic repair of incisional hernia. These studies have mostly included small numbers of patients, but the available evidence suggests that laparoscopic repair is as effective as open prosthetic repair and complications are less likely and hospital stay is shorter.[43]

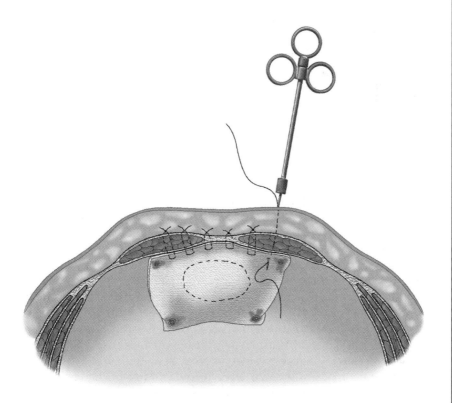

Fig. 5 Laparoscopic mesh repair of incisional hernia using a suture passer.

Table 3 Recurrence rates after laparoscopic incisional hernia repair

Reference	Year	Mesh used[a]	No. of patients	Recurrence rate (%)	Follow-up (months)
Park et al.[28]	1996	PTFE/ polypropylene	30	3	18
Costanza et al.[29]	1998	PTFE	16	5	18
Franklin et al.[30]	1998	Polypropylene	176	1	30
Toy et al.[31]	1998	PTFE	144	4	7
Koehler and Voeller.[32]	1999	PTFE	32	9	20
Kyzer et al.[33]	1999	PTFE	53	2	17
Sanders et al.[34]	1999	PTFE	11	9	12
Carbajo et al.[35]	2000	PTFE	100	2	30
Chowbey et al.[36]	2000	Polypropylene	202	1	35
Heniford and Ramshaw.[37]	2000	PTFE	100	3	22
Heniford et al.[38]	2000	PTFE	407	3	23
Szymanski et al.[39]	2000	Polypropylene	44	5	7
LeBlanc et al.[40]	2001	PTFE	96	9	51
Moreno-Egea et al.[41]	2001	Parietex[b]	20	0	10
Heniford BT et al.[42]	2003	PTFE	819	5	20

[a] PTFE, expanded polytetrafluoroethylene. [b] Sofradim, Villefranche sur Soane, France.

Key point 3

- Laparoscopic repair is as effective as open prosthetic repair and complications are less likely and hospital stay is shorter.

CONCLUSION

Incisional hernia is a common clinical problem for the surgeon who practises open abdominal surgery. The problem appears to be less common after laparoscopic surgery, although it is likely that it may become more frequent as more procedures are being tackled laparoscopically. Decision making regarding operation depends on the severity of symptoms and the fitness of the patient for operation. Combined assessment with a senior anaesthetist is useful in some marginal cases. If the defect is small and the edges come together without tension then suture repair using an absorbable suture such as polydioxanone or a non-absorbable monofilament suture such as polypropylene may be justified, but the trend in treatment has moved strongly towards prosthetic repair. This may be accomplished using an open operation to place the mesh. The material may be used as a 'sandwich' with one layer placed intraperitoneally and the other placed in front of the rectus sheath. Alternatively the mesh may be used as an 'onlay' prosthesis. Whatever technique is used, there must be 3 cm overlap between the edge of the defect and the edge of the prosthetic material. Good results obtained using open prosthetic repair may be matched or even bettered in terms of recurrence rates by laparoscopic placement of the prosthetic material, and hospital stay is shorter.

Key points for clinical practice

- Suture repair should only be performed when the fascial edges are suitable for suturing and come together without any tension. There should be no obvious risk factors for wound failure.

- Recurrence rates with mesh repair are much lower than with suture repair. Mesh repair is the technique of choice for most incisional hernias.

- Laparoscopic repair is as effective as open prosthetic repair and complications are less likely and hospital stay is shorter.

References

1. Mudge M, Hughes LE. Incisional hernia: A ten year prospective study of incidence and attitudes. *Br J Surg* 1985; **72**: 70.
2. Akman PC. A study of five hundred incisional hernias. *J Int Coll Surg* 1962; **37**: 125–142.
3. Krukowski ZH, Cusick EL, Engeset J, Matheson NA. Polydioxanone or polypropylene for closure of midline incisions: a prospective comparative trial. *Br J Surg* 1987; **74**: 828–830.
4. Krukowski ZH, Matheson NA. 'Button hole' incisional hernia: a late complication of abdominal wound closure with continuous non-absorbable sutures. *Br J Surg* 1987; **74**: 824–825.
5. Hope PG, Carter SS, Kilby JO. The da Silva method of incisional hernia repair. *Br J Surg* 1985; **72**: 569–570.
6. Langer S, Christiansen J. Long-term results after incisional hernia repair. *Acta Chir Scand* 1985; **151**: 217–219.
7. George CD, Ellis H. The results of incisional hernia repair: a twelve year review. *Ann R Coll Surg Engl* 1986; **68**: 185–187.
8. van der Linden FT, van Vroonhoven TJ. Long-term results after surgical correction of incisional hernia. *Neth J Surg* 1988; **40**: 127–129.
9. Naraynsingh V, Ariyanayagam D. Rectus repair for midline ventral abdominal wall hernia. *Br J Surg* 1993; **80**: 614–615.
10. Gecim IE, Kocak S, Ersoz S, Bumin C, Aribal D. Recurrence after incisional hernia repair: results and risk factors. *Surg Today* 1996; **26**: 607–609.
11. Kuzbari R, Worseg AP, Tairych G *et al*. Sliding door technique for the repair of midline incisional hernias. *Plast Reconstr Surg* 1998; **101**: 1235–1242.
12. Shukla VK, Gupta A, Singh H, Pandey M, Gautam A. Cardiff repair of incisional hernia: a university hospital experience. *Eur J Surg* 1998; **164**: 271–274.
13. McCarthy JD, Twiest MW. Intraperitoneal polypropylene mesh support of incisional herniorrhaphy. *Am J Surg* 1981; **142**: 707–711.
14. Matapurkar BG, Gupta AK, Agarwal AK. A new technique of 'Marlex-peritoneal sandwich' in the repair of large incisional hernias. *World J Surg* 1991; **15**: 768–770.
15. Temudom T, Siadati M, Sarr MG. Repair of complex giant or recurrent ventral hernias by using tension-free intraparietal prosthetic mesh (Stoppa technique): lessons learned from our initial experience (fifty patients). *Surgery* 1996; **120**: 738–743.

16. Gillon JF, Begin GF, Marecos C, Fourtanier G. Expanded polytetrafluoroethylene patches used in the intraperitoneal or extraperitoneal position for repair of incisional hernias of the anterolateral abdominal wall. *Am J Surg* 1997; **174**: 16–19.

17. McLanahan D, King LT, Weems C, Novotney M, Gibson K. Retrorectus prosthetic mesh repair of midline abdominal hernia. *Am J Surg* 1997; **173**: 445–449.

18. Balen EM, Diez-Caballero A, Hernandez-Lizoain JL *et al*. Repair of ventral hernias with expanded polytetrafluoroethylene patch. *Br J Surg* 1998; **85**: 1415–1418.

19. Turkcapar AG, Yerdel MA, Aydinuraz K, Bayar S, Kuterdem E. Repair of midline incisional hernias using polypropylene grafts. *Surg Today* 1998; **28**: 59–63.

20. Whiteley MS, Ray-Chaudhuri SB, Galland RB. Combined fascia and mesh closure of large incisional hernias. *J R Coll Surg Edinb* 1998; **43**: 29–30.

21. Arnaud JP, Tuech JJ, Pessaux P, Hadchity Y. Surgical treatment of postoperative incisional hernias by intraperitoneal insertion of Dacron mesh and an aponeurotic graft: a report on 250 cases. *Arch Surg* 1999; **134**: 1260–1262.

22. Bauer JJ, Harris MT, Kreel I, Gelernt IM. Twelve-year experience with expanded polytetrafluoroethylene in the repair of abdominal wall defects. *Mt Sinai J Med* 1999; **66**: 20–35.

23. Utrera Gonzalez A, de la Portilla de Juan F, Carranza Albarran G. Large incisional hernia repair using intraperitoneal placement of expanded polytetrafluoroethylene. *Am J Surg* 1999; **177**: 291–293.

24. Chrysos E, Athanasakis E, Saridaki Z *et al*. Surgical repair of incisional ventral hernias: tension-free technique using prosthetic materials (expanded polytetrafluoroethylene Gore-Tex Dual Mesh). *Am Surg* 2000; **66**: 679–682.

25. Ladurner R, Trupka A, Schmidbauer S, Hallfeldt K. The use of an underlay polypropylene mesh in complicated incisional hernias: successful French surgical technique. *Minerva Chir* 2001; **56**: 111–117.

26. Martin-Duce A, Noguerales F, Villeta R *et al*. Modifications to Rives technique for midline incisional hernia repair. *Hernia* 2001; **5**: 70–72.

27. Luidendijk RW, Hop WC, van den Tol MP *et al*. A comparison of suture repair with mesh repair for incisional hernia. *N Engl J Med* 2000; **343**: 392–398.

28. Park A, Gagner M, Pomp A. Laparoscopic repair of large incisional hernias. *Surg Laparosc Endosc* 1996; **6**: 123–128.

29. Constanza MJ, Heniford BY, Arca MJ, Mayes JT, Gagner M. Laparoscopic repair of recurrent ventral hernias. *Am Surg* 1998; **64**: 1121–1125.

30. Franklin ME, Dorman JP, Glass JL, Balli JE, Gonzalez JJ. Laparoscopic ventral and incisional hernia repair. *Surg Laparosc Endosc* 1998; **8**: 294–299.

31. Toy FK, Bailey RW, Carey S *et al*. Prospective, multicentre study of laparoscopic ventral hernioplasty. Preliminary results. *Surg Endosc* 1998; **12**: 955–959.

32. Koehler RH, Voeller G. Recurrences in laparoscopic incisional hernia repairs: a personal series and review of the literature. *JSLS* 1999; **3**: 293–304.

33. Kyzer S, Alis M, Aloni Y, Charuzi I. Laparoscopic repair of postoperation ventral hernia. Early postoperation results. *Surg Endosc* 1999; **13**: 928–931.

34. Sanders LM, Flint LM, Ferrara JJ. Initial experience with laparoscopic repair of incisional hernias. *Am J Surg* 1999; **177**: 227–231.

35. Carbajo MA, del Olmo JC, Blanco JI *et al*. Laparoscopic treatment of ventral abdominal wall hernias: preliminary results in 100 patients *JSLS* 2000; **4**: 141–145.

36. Chowbey PK, Sharma A, Khullar R, Mann V, Baijal M, Vashistha A. Laparoscopic ventral hernia repair. *J Laparoendosc Adv Surg Tech A* 2000; **10**: 79–84.

37. Heniford BT, Ramshaw BH. Laparoscopic ventral hernia repair: a report of 100 consecutive cases. *Surg Endosc* 2000; **14**: 419–423.

38. Heniford BT, Park A, Ramshaw BJ, Voeller G. Laparoscopic ventral and incisional hernia repair in 407 patients. *J Am Coll Surg* 2000; **190**: 645–650.

39. Szymanski J, Voitk A, Joffe J, Alvarez C, Rosenthal G. Technique and early results of outpatient laparoscopic mesh onlay repair of ventral hernias. *Surg Endosc* 2000; **14**: 582–584.

40. LeBlanc KA, Booth WV, Whitaker JM, Bellanger DE. Laparoscopic incisional and ventral herniorrhaphy: our initial 100 patients. *Hernia* 2001; **5**: 41–45.

41. Moreno-Egea A, Liron R, Girela E, Aguayo JL. Laparoscopic repair of ventral and

incisional hernias using a new composite mesh (Parietex): initial experience. *Surg Laparosc Endosc Percutan Tech* 2001; **11**: 103–106.

42. Heniford BT, Park A, Ramshaw BJ, Voeller G. Laparoscopic repair of ventral hernias: nine years' experience with 850 consecutive hernias. *Ann Surg* 2003; **238**: 391–400.

43. Goodney PP, Birkmeyer CM, Birkmeyer JD. Short-term outcomes of laparoscopic and open ventral hernia repair: a meta-analysis *Arch Surg* 2002; **137**: 1161–1165.

Richard A. Bulbulia Manj S. Gohel
Fiona J. Slim Mark R. Whyman Keith R. Poskitt

5

Surgical practitioners – Current roles and future prospects

The first surgical practitioner in the UK was appointed by the cardiac surgical team at The John Radcliffe Hospital in Oxford in 1989. Since then, they have become accepted and valued team members in a broad range of surgical specialities. In this chapter we will discuss the evolution of this new surgical team member, the roles surgical practitioners fulfil in surgical practice, and the benefits they provide to the patient, their surgical colleagues and the NHS. Finally, the potential future developments of this professional role will be explored.

HISTORICAL PERSPECTIVE

Surgical practitioners have been well established in the USA for a number of decades. They have a clearly defined role, training programme and career structure and are regulated by state licensing bodies. Cardiac surgeons at The John Radcliffe Hospital, Oxford developed this role in this country in 1989 with the approval of the Royal College of Surgeons of England and the Department of Health.[1] Cardiac surgery in general, and coronary artery bypass grafting (CABG) in particular, lends itself well to such a role. The cardiac surgeon's

Mr Richard A. Bulbulia MA FRCS, Specialist Registrar, Cheltenham General Hospital

Mr Manj S. Gohel MRCS, Vascular Research Fellow, Cheltenham General Hospital

Ms Fiona J. Slim Senior Surgical Practitioner, Cheltenham General Hospital

Mr Mark R. Whyman MS FRCS, Consultant Surgeon, Cheltenham General Hospital

Mr Keith R. Poskitt MD, FRCS, Consultant Surgeon, Cheltenham General Hospital, Sandford Road, Cheltenham, Gloucestershire GL53 7AW, UK (for correspondence)

assistant's role was primarily concerned with the harvesting and preparation of autologous venous conduits during CABG.

Despite initial scepticism and conservatism, this role proved to be a great success. By word of mouth, other cardiac surgeons learnt of this new development and centres across the UK appointed surgical practitioners to similar positions. By the mid 1990s surgical practitioners were appearing in other surgical specialities: general surgery, orthopaedics, urology, gynaecology, laparoscopic surgery and endoscopy.

The Royal College of Surgeons produced a discussion document in 1999 that was broadly supportive of this innovative role, but stressed the need for a formal and structured career pathway and the need for tight regulation of this new profession.[2] This discussion paper stimulated the creation of the National Association of Assistants in Surgical Practice (NAASP) in 2001. In collaboration with The Royal College of Surgeons, they have produced a core syllabus and a log book and, in conjunction with the Department of Health, are running a pilot scheme to train new surgical practitioners at a number of sites across the UK.

WHAT'S IN A NAME?

Surgical practitioners have had various titles over the years. These include surgeon's assistant, surgeon assistant, surgical assistant and first assistant (popular in America). Surgeon's assistant was the name favoured by the Royal College of Surgeons in their 1999 discussion document.[2] Recently, NAASP in consultation with the surgical community and the Department of Health have suggested that 'surgical practitioner' more accurately represents the potential scope of practice of this role and is their preferred title, which will be used throughout this chapter.

STIMULI FOR CHANGE

There are numerous reasons promoting the development and proliferation of surgical practitioners. The main driving force for change is the significant and ongoing changes in the labour market for healthcare professionals.

The New Deal[3] and European Working Time Directive[4] have resulted in an inexorable drive towards shift work and have reduced the presence of junior hospital doctors on surgical firms. By August 2004, junior hospital doctors will be restricted to working no more than 58 hours per week. Inevitably, these changes will impact negatively on both quality and continuity of care. This reduction in junior doctors' hours combined with the broadening scope of nurses' professional practice presents an opportunity to devolve tasks and responsibilities that were previously in the domain of medically qualified professionals to appropriately trained nurses.[5] The financial benefits of this approach are self-evident, shifting workload from a costly and dwindling group of junior doctors to nursing staff, who may be more cost-effective to employ and more abundant. Furthermore, an enhanced role for nurses is well received by patients and the public at large.

SURGICAL PRACTITIONERS' ROLES

The government's blueprint for reform of the National Health Service is the NHS Plan. This document stresses the value of team-based working:[6]

> 'Old-fashioned demarcations between staff mean some patients see a procession of health professionals ... Information is not shared and investigations are repeated ... Unnecessary boundaries exist between the professions which hold back staff from achieving their true potential.'

The 21st century surgical team includes medically qualified staff, specialist nurses, professions allied to medicine and, more recently, surgical practitioners. These team members are interdependent and, ideally, the team should enjoy a degree of autonomy within the hospital.

Key point 1

- Modern surgical care is best delivered by team-based working. Rigid demarcations between team members should be blurred and team members' roles should reflect their competence and ability, rather than title and tradition.

The surgical practitioner's multifaceted role must be viewed in the context of team-based working, and the account that follows is neither prescriptive nor exhaustive. One of the strengths of the surgical practitioner is the flexibility and responsive qualities they bring to their team and the institution in which they work.

Initially the surgical practitioner's domain was exclusively within the confines of the operating department. However, over time this role has evolved and expanded to incorporate pre- and postoperative care, and surgical practitioners have also taken on adjunctive roles in outpatient clinics and supportive roles in audit and research.

PREOPERATIVE CARE

Working in concert with consultant surgeons and surgical trainees, surgical practitioners are involved at the outset of the patient journey. Together, they see patients in the outpatient department at their initial assessment and participate in the consent process. They may meet again at the pre-assessment clinic, and, liaising with preregistration house surgeons, ensure that various preoperative tests have been performed and that it is appropriate to proceed with surgery. On the day of surgery the surgical practitioner reviews patients with the operating surgeon and any further patient concerns are addressed. The surgical practitioner ensures that a valid consent has been obtained and final preoperative tasks (such as marking the site of operation) are performed.

PERIOPERATIVE CARE

As a member of the surgical team, the surgical practitioner may have a variety of roles in theatre.[7] In addition to helping with patient positioning, preparation and draping, they may act as first assistant or carry out defined tasks under supervision. Examples of such tasks include vein harvesting and preparation for arterial bypass surgery, opening and closing wounds, varicose vein avulsions, and wound dressing. With increasing operative experience, competent surgical practitioners may progress to performing more complex tasks under close supervision.

Over time, the surgical practitioner may carry out complete procedures – initially with direct supervision and later with indirect supervision. Examples of such procedures include excision biopsies of skin lesions under local anaesthetic, temporal artery biopsy and skin grafting.

Surgical practitioners have also been involved in emergency surgical care. In an innovative development in one centre, the surgical practitioner, after a period of training and mentoring, ran an 'abscess list' where patients were seen by the on-call surgical team, listed for incision and drainage, and their admission arranged for the following morning.[8] This efficient and expedient approach has evident gains for both patient and institution.

POSTOPERATIVE CARE

The surgical practitioner may join the rest of the surgical team on postoperative ward rounds and, more frequently, see patients in whose care they have been involved in clinic. This provides patients with the opportunity to raise any concerns they may have with a familiar member of the surgical team and enables the surgical team to check the efficacy of their intervention. Complications of surgery, such as wound infections, can be accurately identified and meaningful local audit can be achieved. The information gained by such audit enables the surgical practitioner to produce and update valid patient information leaflets, further enhancing the consent process.

ADDITIONAL ROLES

Surgical practitioners can utilise their technical skills on the ward and in clinic. Examples of this include debridement of wounds, pinch skin grafting and botulinum toxin A injections for axillary hyperhidrosis. As an experienced member of the surgical team, they can also adapt to fulfil local needs: in our centre the surgical practitioner, working within the vascular outpatient clinic, runs a claudication clinic.

Key point 2

- Surgical practitioners can be responsive and flexible members of the surgical team, enabling the team and their institution to develop and reconfigure services to meet local demands.

LEGAL AND ETHICAL CONSIDERATIONS

The General Medical Council has provided clear guidelines for the delegation of tasks to other members of the surgical team. The delegation of tasks to non-medically qualified members of the surgical team is permissible provided it is in the best interest of the patients and that the competence of the person involved is assured. The consultant remains responsible for managing the patient's care.[9]

Surgical practitioners are covered by vicarious liability whilst performing duties for their NHS Trust. Furthermore, many have additional professional indemnity insurance through other trade unions.

BENEFITS OF SURGICAL PRACTITIONERS

PATIENTS' PERSPECTIVE

In our experience, the response of patients to this extended nursing role has been extremely positive. The continuity of care that they provide through the patient journey is invaluable and counteracts the hitherto high 'hand-off' rate, with patients seeing a consultant in clinic, a preregistration house surgeon in preadmissions clinic, a registrar on the day of surgery and another member of the surgical team for follow-up. The surgical practitioner provides a reassuring and constant presence throughout (Fig. 1).

Anecdotal evidence suggests that patients are generally unconcerned about the thought of staff members who are not surgeons performing their surgical procedures. It seems that it is medical 'insiders' and not the general public who are obsessed with titles and status, and patients are more interested in competence and communication skills.

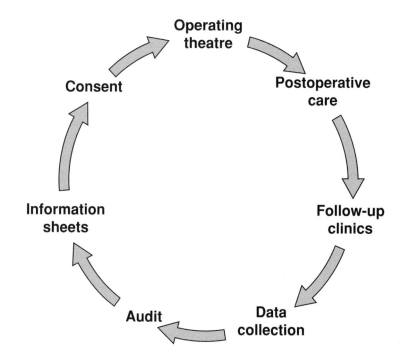

Fig. 1 The surgical practitioner role started predominantly in the operating theatre, but has expanded to encompass the full cycle of patient care.

SURGEON'S PERSPECTIVE

Once in post, the surgical practitioner rapidly becomes an invaluable member of the surgical team. With the rapid turnover of junior medical staff, they provide a stabilising influence, ensuring continuity and preservation of high standards of clinical care. Furthermore, they are sensitive to (and tolerant of) consultants' idiosyncrasies and ensure that new members of the surgical team are aware of individual consultant preferences. Consultants find the long-term presence of a trusted colleague most reassuring.

In response to the New Deal and European Working Time Directive, junior doctors' hours have been reduced significantly, and this trend will continue and become more pronounced over the next three years. This reduction in hours has a twofold impact on surgeons. Firstly, new recruits to the surgical team are needed simply to maintain current levels of productivity and standards, let alone to deliver the anticipated productivity gains. Secondly, the reduction in hours that surgical trainees actually spend on the 'shop floor' means that surgical training must be made more efficient, with training opportunities maximised. Surgical practitioners fulfil both these roles. They provide an extra, skilled pair of hands to the surgical team and may, if needed, substitute for surgical trainees. Working in parallel with trainees, they can, however, act as a potent facilitator for training.

TRAINEE'S PERSPECTIVE

Many of the activities of the surgical practitioner would appear to overlap with the traditional role of basic and higher surgical trainees. This has resulted in the erroneous perception that the surgical practitioner represents a threat to the junior surgeon, in direct competition for operative training opportunities. The early stages of the role inevitably require close consultant supervision. However, this period of intensive mentoring is limited and does not significantly detract from surgical training.

Our experience in Cheltenham has been that surgical practitioners can enhance training in three main ways.

Greater operating list efficiency creates more time for training
The addition of a trained surgical practitioner in theatre improves efficiency and facilitates one-to-one consultant training of junior surgeons (Fig. 2). In a local audit in Cheltenham we have found efficiency gains of 20 minutes per case in varicose vein surgery when the surgical practitioner is involved in theatre lists.

Staged withdrawal of supervision
One of the most exacting challenges facing both trainee and trainer is the progression from performing an operation with the supervising consultant scrubbed and acting as first assistant to operating with the trainer unscrubbed. Surgical practitioners can help 'bridge this gap'. The surgical practitioner acts as an informed first assistant to a competent senior trainee during major cases (Fig. 3). This allows the supervising surgeon to observe the trainee's progress in the operating department at times unscrubbed, if appropriate, and thus free from the temptation to 'help'. We have found that this approach greatly

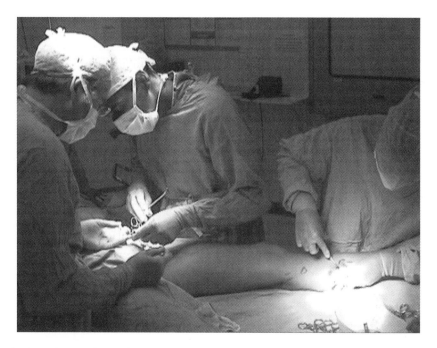

Fig. 2 During routine varicose vein surgery, the surgical practitioner is carrying out avulsions while the consultant is in direct supervision of the SHO performing the groin dissection.

facilitates specialist registrar training, allowing the trainee to gain operative confidence in major cases just prior to 'flying solo' as a newly appointed consultant surgeon.

The surgical practitioner as a trainer

The experienced surgical practitioner is an invaluable training resource, playing a key role in the training of junior surgeons in basic surgical techniques.

Key point 3

- The perception that surgical practitioners may detract from surgical training is wrong. They can help basic surgical trainees acquire operative skills and significantly facilitate training opportunities for higher surgical trainees.

Department of Health's perspective

The surgical practitioner's role chimes in harmony with the current agenda of health service reform in the UK.[6] Old demarcations between professions in the health service are being blurred or even dismantled. Tasks that were previously in the domain of doctors, an expensive and scarce resource, are being devolved to other members of the team. Examples of this devolution of care include breast and stoma-care nurses, ward nurse practitioners, phlebotomy services, nurse cannulation, nurse prescribing and death certification by senior nursing

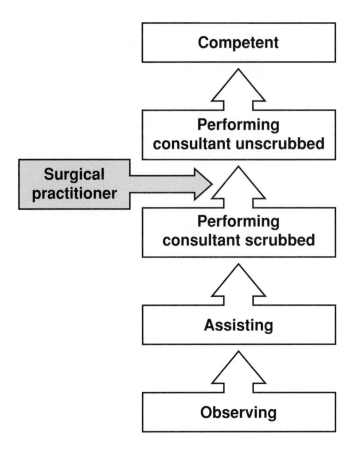

Fig. 3 The role of the surgical practitioner during the staged withdrawal of supervision of a trainee.

staff. A logical extension of this programme of devolution in the ward and in clinics is a similar programme within theatres.

Surgical practitioners enhance the delivery of care. Their involvement in clinic reduces potential 'bottlenecks' in the assessment of patients prior to surgery. In theatre the addition of an experienced and competent member to the pre-existing surgical team yields tangible productivity gains.

Key point 4

- Productivity gains in clinic and operating theatre are achieved without sacrificing quality. The surgical practitioner's presence throughout the patient journey ensures continuity of care, which is otherwise threatened by the drive towards shift work for junior surgeons.

FUTURE DEVELOPMENTS

Sir Terence English, in an editorial published in the *BMJ* in 1997,[10] broadly welcomed the development of surgical practitioners with a number of caveats.

The career structure and training needs of such practitioners needed clarification, and their precise status and authority in the surgical team needed definition.

Many of these concerns have been satisfactorily addressed in recent years, with one of the major developments being the creation of the National Association of Assistants in Surgical Practice (NAASP) in 2001. This national organisation, working in conjunction with The Royal College of Surgeons, has devised training and education programmes; a core syllabus and electronic logbook have been created. Team-based working is becoming increasingly accepted in the new NHS, and some of the concerns voiced by Sir Terence in 1997 about status and authority within the surgical team appear a little dated. As ever, the consultant surgeon remains in overall charge of all patients under his or her care. However, it is permissible to delegate tasks to competent and trusted medically and non-medically qualified members of the surgical team.

One of the great strengths of surgical practitioners is the responsiveness they afford the surgical team to react and respond to local needs of their healthcare environment. The surgical practitioner-led acute abscess service is one such example of local adaptation. In our unit we are currently exploring the potential productivity and quality gains of surgical practitioner-led 'one-stop' varicose vein assessment clinics. Other areas of development include the incorporation of surgical practitioners into a surgical on-call rota, whereby they could be called in to assist in emergency cases out of hours. This development could help trusts achieve working time compliance for some tiers of junior hospital doctors.

The UK government's agenda for the future development of this role is a little unclear. Their stated objective is to develop a consultant *delivered* programme of care for NHS patients. However, they have staked their electoral future on the enhanced delivery of healthcare. Some in Whitehall envisage the expansion of the surgical practitioner's role to involve increasing 'independent' operating. Specialities such as ophthalmology, with a high-volume – low-index case mix are particularly attractive for such an approach. Surgical practitioners performing lists of cataracts under remote supervision of ophthalmologists must seem a tantalising prospect with the potential to slash waiting lists for this procedure. It is, however, the authors' considered view that such a development, whilst superficially attractive and expedient, would ultimately be unwise. It would seem to run counter to the aspiration of consultant-delivered care and does not recognise the importance of teamwork in the delivery of quality care for surgical patients.

The Department of Health Modernisation Agency is currently running a New Ways of Working in Surgery Pilot based in Manchester and Imperial College, London. The aim of this scheme is to assess academic and non-academic training pathways for the surgical practitioner. These initiatives may help clarify an appropriate training programme for the role.

CONCLUSION

In conclusion, we enthusiastically endorse the continued development of surgical practitioners in the UK. They have the potential to create real productivity gains whilst protecting and enhancing quality patient care. They facilitate the training of junior surgeons rather than detract from it.

In the past few years we have witnessed the birth of a new profession. With the inception of the National Association of Assistants in Surgical Practice, surgical practitioners are regulating entry to the profession, defining and maintaining standards, and establishing formal training programmes. It is noteworthy that this has been achieved with close cooperation and overt support from the surgical community through The Royal College of Surgeons.

Key point 5

- Further developments of this role are envisaged. Close collaborative links exist between the National Association of Assistants in Surgical Practice, the Royal College of Surgeons and the Department of Health, and the evolution of the surgical practitioner can be considered an exemplar for the reform of traditional job structures within the NHS.

This surely presages the manner in which this valued new profession must interact within the NHS in the future. The working relationship between surgeons and surgical practitioners must be cooperative and complementary rather than competitive. Further development along these lines is eagerly anticipated as we strive to meet the challenges faced by the NHS in the 21st century.

Key points for clinical practice

- Modern surgical care is best delivered by team-based working. Rigid demarcations between team members should be blurred and team members' roles should reflect their competence and ability, rather than title and tradition.

- Surgical practitioners can be responsive and flexible members of the surgical team, enabling the team and their institution to develop and reconfigure services to meet local demands.

- The perception that surgical practitioners may detract from surgical training is wrong. They can help basic surgical trainees acquire operative skills and significantly facilitate training opportunities for higher surgical trainees.

- Productivity gains in clinic and operating theatre are achieved without sacrificing quality. The surgical practitioner's presence throughout the patient journey ensures continuity of care, which is otherwise threatened by the drive towards shift work for junior surgeons.

- Further developments of this role are envisaged. Close collaborative links exist between the National Association of Assistants in Surgical Practice, the Royal College of Surgeons and the Department of Health, and the evolution of the surgical practitioner can be considered an exemplar for the reform of traditional job structures within the NHS.

References

1. The Royal College of Surgeons of England and the Society of Cardiothoracic Surgeons of Great Britain and Ireland. *Cardiac Surgeons' Assistants; Guidelines for Heads of Departments.* London: RCSEng, 1994.
2. Royal College of Surgeons of England. *Assistants in Surgical Practice – A Discussion Document.* London: RCSEng, 1999.
3. NHS Management Executive. *Junior Doctors (1991) The New Deal.* London: Department of Health, 1991.
4. Council Directive 93/104/EC. Official Journal of the European Community 1993; L307: 18–24.
5. Department of Health. *A Health Service of all the Talents: Developing the NHS Workforce Consultation Document on the Review of Workforce Planning.* London: DoH, 2000.
6. Department of Health. *The NHS Plan. A Plan for Investment. A Plan for Reform.* London: DoH, 2000.
7. National Association of Theatre Nurses. *Future Ways of Working – Unleashing the Potential of Perioperative Practice.* August 2001.
8. Biggins J. The role of the RNSA in colorectal and general surgery. *Br J Periop Nurs.* 2002; **12**: 222–226.
9. General Medical Council. *Good Medical Practice,* 2nd edn. London: GMC, 1998.
10. English T. Medicine in the 1990s needs a team approach. *BMJ* 1997; **314**: 661–663.

Vijayaragaran Muralidharan   John A.C. Buckels

6

New perspectives in liver transplantation

Liver transplantation, once considered an experimental procedure undertaken as a desperate measure in the terminally ill patient, has become a widely accepted treatment for a variety of acute and chronic liver diseases. Greater understanding of the underlying disease process, development of surgical and anaesthetic techniques, reliable immunosuppression, and dependable postoperative care have contributed towards improved results with a 1-year survival rate of over 90% being achieved in the elective setting. This success has resulted in a disproportionate increase in demand, with estimates of between 15–80 per million population.[1] As such, there is an increasing need to improve the availability of organs and to minimise the need for re-transplantation. This chapter will focus on the current status of liver transplantation and stress the recent advances made, which include both surgical technique as well as changes in the management of specific disease states.

INDICATIONS FOR LIVER TRANSPLANTATION

Key point 1

- Broadly the indications for liver transplantation are classified as chronic liver failure, acute fulminant hepatic failure, primary hepatic malignancy and inborn errors of metabolism.

Vijayaragaran Muralidharan MD FRCS, Senior Registrar, Liver Unit, Queen Elizabeth Hospital, Birmingham

Mr John A.C. Buckels CBE MD FRCS, Consultant Hepatobiliary and Liver Transplant Surgeon, Queen Elizabeth Medical Centre, Edgbaston, Birmingham B15 2TH, UK (for correspondence)

CHRONIC LIVER FAILURE

The commonest indication for liver transplantation is end-stage chronic liver disease, which accounts for more than 80% of the procedure at most centres. The general criteria used to identify patients for transplant assessment are a combination of clinical and biochemical features. These vary depending on the aetiology of the underlying liver disease. Specific indications in cholestatic liver disease include intractable pruritus, intractable bone disease and recurrent cholangitis. By comparison, worsening synthetic function as evidenced by a serum albumin of less than 30.0 g/l or a prothrombin time longer than 4 s from normal are important indicators in hepatocellular disease states.[2] In addition to laboratory indicators, clinical events may precipitate the need for transplantation. These include hepatic encephalopathy, refractory ascites, and variceal bleeding.

Hepatic encephalopathy

This is usually diagnosed clinically by the presence of the typical flapping tremor or from its response to medical therapy. The diagnosis can be confirmed by an EEG. Early cases are easily missed, although minor alterations in speech and mood or mild confusion may raise suspicion. Often it is precipitated by specific events, including gastrointestinal haemorrhage, spontaneous bacterial peritonitis, excessive dietary protein consumption, constipation and sedative drugs. Recognition and removal of the causal agent, dietary protein restriction and medical therapy with lactulose and neomycin are often effective in treating acute episodes. Even mild encephalopathy has detrimental effects on quality of life and should lead to consideration for transplantation.

Ascites

Ascites in chronic liver disease can be effectively treated by a number of medical, surgical or radiological techniques. The new development of ascites should be investigated for the development of bacterial peritonitis, portal vein thrombosis or hepatic malignancy. Initial treatment involves dietary sodium restriction and diuretic therapy. Unresponsive patients may benefit from regular large-volume paracentesis with concurrent intravenous administration of 20% human albumin.[3] Although peritoneovenous shunting is effective in controlling ascites, potential risks include disseminated intravascular coagulation, sepsis and cardiac failure. It has few advantages over large-volume paracentesis and is not recommended for patients who are transplant candidates. A more recent and effective option is a transjugular intrahepatic portosystemic shunt (TIPS). The immediate risk of TIPS is worsening liver failure and hepatic encephalopathy, and advice from a skilled hepatologist should be sought before a TIPS is placed.[4] Unresponsive ascites is an indication for transplant assessment.

Spontaneous bacterial peritonitis (SBP)

This is a potentially lethal complication in cirrhotics with ascites. Many patients will present with evidence of sepsis, abdominal tenderness or decompensation, although these can be lacking. A high index of suspicion is required and patients should be treated with intravenous antibiotics. Not all will have a raised ascitic neutrophil count, and treatment is therefore pragmatic.[5] The occurrence of spontaneous bacterial peritonitis is a strong indication for transplant assessment, although surgery should be delayed until after a full course of treatment.

Variceal haemorrhage

This causes significant morbidity and mortality in patients with chronic liver disease. Between 35% and 80% of those with chronic liver disease develop varices, of whom 25–30% will experience haemorrhage. Two-thirds will subsequently rebleed, with a mortality rate approaching 35–50% for each episode.[6] Initial bleeds are treated with endoscopic banding, which is replacing sclerotherapy and is effective in 70–90% of cases. Non-selective beta-blockade reduces the risk of rebleeding, and also has an effect on bleeding from gastric varices.[6] TIPS should be considered for those in whom endoscopic control is unsuccessful, provided they have reasonable synthetic liver reserve. Recurrent variceal bleeding is a clear indication for transplant assessment and in appropriate cases a TIPS should be considered as bridging therapy.

Key point 2

- Clinical events may precipitate the need for transplantation. These include hepatic encephalopathy, refractory ascites, and variceal bleeding.

FULMINANT HEPATIC FAILURE

Acute fulminant hepatic failure (AFHF) can be defined as the onset of hepatic encephalopathy within 8 weeks of the onset of acute liver failure in the absence of pre-existing liver disease. When the encephalopathy commences between 8 weeks and 6 months it is termed late-onset or subacute. The commoner causes of AFHF are drugs (paracetamol overdose) and viral hepatitis, particularly non-A, non-B, non-C. AFHF patients who might benefit from liver transplantation are identified using published specific criteria, including the aetiological factor, age, acidosis, coagulopathy and the level of serum bilirubin.[7] Contraindications for liver transplantation include brain-stem dysfunction, uncontrolled sepsis and refractory hypotension.[8]

PRIMARY HEPATIC MALIGNANCY

Hepatocellular carcinoma (HCC) occurs in both cirrhotics and non-cirrhotics. The non-cirrhotic patient with a sporadic HCC usually presents with a large mass and late results of transplantation are poor (around 20%). This presentation is no longer an acceptable indication for transplantation. The majority of HCC occur on a background of cirrhosis (particularly hepatitis C, hepatitis B, haemochromatosis and alcoholic liver disease), and excellent results can be obtained from liver grafting if the tumour is diagnosed at an early stage (single tumours less than 5.0 cm or three tumours under 3.0 cm).[9]

Currently it is recommended that cirrhotics should undergo regular screening with ultrasound scans and α-fetoprotein (AFP) estimations. Although patients with Child's A cirrhosis might be potential resection candidates, the almost inevitable occurrence of later often multiple tumours suggest they should be also considered as transplant candidates. Patients with primary bile duct cancer (cholangiocarcinoma) are not transplant candidates due to the very high recurrence rates after grafting.

Key point 3

- Excellent results can be obtained from liver grafting if the tumour is diagnosed at an early stage (single tumours less than 5.0 cm or three tumours under 3.0 cm).

INBORN ERRORS OF METABOLISM

A number of inherited metabolic disorders may affect the liver in various ways. Enzyme defects in an otherwise normal liver may present with hepatic disorders (Wilson's disease) or may affect extrahepatic organs (familial hypercholesterolaemia) whereas extrahepatic defects may seriously affect the liver (protoporphyria). Conversely, generalised metabolic disorders that affect multiple organs may also manifest with liver disease (α_1-antitrypsin deficiency). The majority of these affect paediatric patients. Clinical presentations vary, and indications for liver transplantation in this selective group include liver failure, extrahepatic organ failure, development of HCC and severe symptoms affecting quality of life.[10]

SELECTION AND TIMING FOR TRANSPLANTATION

Selection of patients for transplantation remains difficult: both indications and contraindications are becoming more clearly defined and agreed. Consideration should be given if there is an expected length of life of less than 1 year (because of the liver disease) or a quality of life (because of the liver disease) that is unacceptable to the patient. The relative lack of donor livers means that not all those who might benefit from transplantation can be given a graft. Guidelines outlining selection have been developed;[11,12] however, these have not been updated and take little account of developments such as newer treatments for HCC and effective therapy to inhibit replication of hepatitis B or HIV.

The method of allocation of livers varies greatly between different systems: in the UK there are about 150 patients on the waiting list at any one time, with around 750 transplants performed annually. The waiting list mortality is about 10% per year and the median waiting time is 3–4 months. To ensure that listed patients have a reasonable expectation that they will receive a graft, and to ensure that designated transplant units work to a similar standard, a consensus group was set up.[13] This agreed that donor organs were a national resource and that patients should be listed only if they had a 50% probability or more of being alive 5 years after transplantation with a quality of life that is acceptable to the patient. In the USA, the situation is very different, with about 18 000 patients on the waiting list and around 4500 cadaveric transplants annually. Many patients are able to and do wait for periods of more than 2 years. To discourage listing patients too early, minimal criteria were introduced, but this did little to relieve the problem. To reduce the waiting list mortality and to ensure donor organs went to those who had greatest need, a new allocation system was introduced, based on the MELD (model for end-stage liver disease) or PELD (for children) system.[14] This score uses three laboratory values (creatinine, bilirubin and INR) and has been well validated to predict death within 90 days. Introduction of the MELD system has resulted in a reduction in the waiting list mortality, but as MELD does not well predict long-term outcome, additional measures will be needed.

Key point 4

- Patients should be listed for transplantation only if they have a 50% probability or more of being alive 5 years after transplantation with a quality of life that is acceptable to the patient.

SPECIFIC INDICATIONS

Recommendations on selection and timing are given for some of the more common indications.

Primary biliary cirrhosis (PBC)

Prognostic models have been developed for patients with this autoimmune disease that identify the ideal time for transplantation. The simplest of these utilises serum bilirubin, although others include age, bilirubin, albumin level and prothrombin time.[15] It is yet unknown whether medical therapy with ursodeoxycholic acid to improve liver biochemistry can delay or avert the need for transplantation.[16]

Primary sclerosing cholangitis (PSC)

This is a progressive cholestatic disorder associated with concurrent inflammatory bowel disease in around 70% of cases.[17] Patients may present with jaundice and cholangitis due to multiple biliary strictures or may be detected when asymptomatic with deranged liver biochemistry. Prognostic risk scores have been developed to aid with selection for transplantation.[18] Patients with PSC are at high risk of cholangiocarcinoma and if grafted after the development of malignancy they have a very poor outcome. Cases with clinical doubt should undergo guided biopsy of dominant strictures before acceptance onto the transplant waiting list.

Chronic viral hepatitis

Chronic hepatitis due to hepatitis C and hepatitis B viruses is an increasing problem in the West, although there have been major developments in antiviral therapy in the last decade that can control the diseases and avoid the need for transplantation. There is a major risk of HCC development in these patients, but if this is detected at an early stage, similar survival rates can be achieved after grafting as for those with benign disease.[19]

Treatment for hepatitis C currently uses combinations of interferon and ribavirin. Once there is hepatic decompensation, transplantation represents the only option, but there are significant risks of disease recurrence in the new liver, which often runs at an accelerated rate.[20] At present there are no effective post-transplant regimes of antiviral therapy but using younger donors to transplant hepatitis C patients may reduce the risks of recurrent disease.[21,22]

Hepatitis B can now also be treated with antiviral therapy using nucleoside analogues, which can prevent progressive liver damage. Patients who present with unresponsive or advanced disease can now be successfully transplanted due to the development of effective antiviral protocols utilising hepatitis B immunoglobulin and lamivudine.[23, 24]

Alcoholic liver disease

End-stage alcoholic liver disease is an increasingly accepted indication for transplantation but remains controversial because of possible recidivism and poor compliance. Nevertheless, the outcome after transplantation, in terms of both survival and quality of life, parallels that of patients transplanted for other chronic liver diseases.[25] Most programmes insist that patients have a period of abstinence of at least 6 months and that patients be assessed by a psychiatrist with expertise in alcoholism and undergo a formal alcohol rehabilitation programme prior to transplantation, as well as having a stable and supportive psychosocial environment. The relapse rate in the first few years after transplantation is about 40%, with up to 15% of patients returning to heavy drinking.[26]

Autoimmune hepatitis

This is now classified into three forms. Type 1 is the most common and is identified by the presence of anti-nuclear antibodies or anti-smooth muscle antibodies. Immunosuppressive therapy will prolong life, but there are dangers in long-term treatment with higher risks for those with the greatest cumulative doses. Forecasting the ideal time for liver grafting is difficult and advice from an expert hepatologist is mandatory. Liver transplantation improves survival,[27] but recurrence can occur and this group may require long-term steroids.

Key point 5

- Diseases that might recur in the transplanted liver are not a contraindication. For alcoholic liver disease patients should have a period of abstinence of at least 6 months, should be assessed by a psychiatrist with expertise in alcoholism and should undergo a formal alcohol rehabilitation programme prior to transplantation.

MANAGEMENT OF THE DONOR AND ORGAN RETRIEVAL

EVALUATION OF THE DONOR

This involves a detailed study of the past medical history and an assessment of the current clinical condition. While there is no upper age limit, the presence of or history of malignancy, intra-abdominal or systemic sepsis, or transmissible diseases would exclude organ donation. Non-metastatic brain and skin cancer are exceptions. Organ donors with bacterial meningitis have also been used for transplantation successfully, providing both donor and recipient receive adequate antimicrobial therapy.[28] Serological tests are performed to confirm negative results for HIV, HTLV-I, HBsAg, HBcAb and HCVAb. Exceptions to these criteria include the use of HbcAb- and HCVAb-positive donors for recipients with similar serology. Social background is also important and high-risk behaviour such as intravenous drug use may weigh against donation.

Important donor aspects include haemodynamic stability, episodes of cardiorespiratory arrest, inotrope requirements, electrolyte imbalances and liver function tests including prothrombin time. Once a donor has been accepted, management is conducted along specific protocols defined by the transplantation team. The final judgement of the donor liver is made at the retrieval operation, when its colour, texture and consistency can be adequately evaluated by an experienced surgeon. Assessing the approximate size of the donor organ, particularly when split or paediatric grafts are considered, excluding significant intra-abdominal pathology and determining the quality of perfusion of the explanted organ are additional important steps.

Marginal livers

This is a term that is used to describe organs that are stressed prior to storage by a combination of hypoxia, metabolic disturbances or ischaemia, and have an increased risk of early dysfunction. This may be secondary to hypotensive episodes in the donor, high vasopressor requirements or underlying liver pathology. This history in the donor together with subjective observation of the liver, particularly if the donor was elderly, aids in the suspicion of a marginal liver. However, with the increasing demand for organs, marginal livers from older patients can be used successfully but have a higher risk of ischaemia–reperfusion injury.[29] The selection of marginal livers requires a critical appraisal of the various donor factors, including liver function tests and the appearance of the graft itself. Although a number of tests have been studied, including the MEGX test, phophorus-31 magnetic resonance spectrometry and hyaluronic acid level in the graft caval effluent, they are yet to be proven superior to the subjective inspection of the donor organ by an experienced transplant surgeon. It should be stressed that marginal livers are not recommended for high-risk 'marginal recipients'.

Key point 6

- Overall the experience that marginal livers can be successfully used has meant a significant rise in the number of transplants performed.

The operative details of *donor hepatectomy* are given in specialist surgical texts. Almost all are beating-heart donors, although the organ shortage has recently led several teams to use non-heart-beating donors in the context of life support being withdrawn in theatre for appropriate cases followed by urgent hepatectomy. Evaluation of donor liver function is still under study and a significant proportion of potential grafts at present is not used.

ORGAN PRESERVATION

This underwent a revolution with the introduction of University of Wisconsin Solution (UWS). This allowed safe cold storage of donor livers for up to 24 hours, though 18 hours is a more practical upper time limit. This not only expanded the donor pool but also the time envelope in which the transplantation can be performed, allowing optimal preparation of the recipient with surgery performed on a semi-elective basis.

PERIOPERATIVE MANAGEMENT OF THE RECIPIENT

The management of patients undergoing liver transplantation has benefited from advances in anaesthesia and intensive care. As well as invasive monitoring to improve haemodynamic stability, anaesthetists are actively involved in near-patient testing of both biochemical and haematological parameters. Of the latter, thromboelastography (TEG) has had a significant impact by enabling the anaesthetist to monitor and treat post-reperfusion coagulopathy and to control the effects of excessive fibrinolysis by the use of kallikrein inhibitors, with a reduction in blood transfusion requirements.[30, 31]

SURGICAL TECHNIQUES

Since the first successful liver transplant was performed by Starzl in 1963, the technique for explantation of the recipient liver and implantation of the donor organ has been refined to reflect the changing clinical and technical requirements.

ADULT WHOLE-LIVER GRAFT

The operation is usually performed via generous bilateral subcostal incisions. Currently two different techniques are employed: removal of the liver with the intrahepatic vena cava or preservation of the recipient cava. In the former the need to perform full caval clamping can lead to haemodynamic instability, and this technique may require veno-venous bypass. With preservation of the recipient cava the donor cava can be anastomosed either to the stump of the hepatic veins or as a side-to-side cavo-cavostomy (piggyback technique).[32] During these anastomoses the recipient cava is only partially clamped, thus maintaining haemodynamic stability. Early in the hepatectomy a temporary end-to-side porto-caval shunt can be constructed to maintain stability and to prevent venous congestion of the bowel. [33]

For the biliary reconstruction, in most patients, an end-to-end anastomosis is fashioned using fine absorbable sutures between the obliquely cut donor and recipient ducts. Care is taken not to obstruct the lower end of the cystic duct, which can subsequently dilate and cause obstruction. T-tubes are no longer routinely used although one may be indicated in certain cases such as split grafts.[34] If the underlying disease is biliary atresia or PSC, a Roux-en-y choledocho-jejunostomy is required.

REDUCED-SIZE LIVER TRANSPLANTATION (RSLT)

RSLT was originally performed in 1984 as an innovative measure to increase the availability of grafts for paediatric recipients.[35] Mortality for children awaiting transplantation was high due to the scarcity of size-matched donor organs. This approach involves an *ex vivo* reduction in the donor liver, which is implanted in the orthotopic position after recipient hepatectomy. The commonest segments used are the left lateral segment (segments II and III), or the full left lobe based on size-matching of the donor and recipient organs. The original technique involved using a segment of donor inferior vena cava (IVC), but this was subsequently modified to exclude donor IVC by using the donor left hepatic vein to anastomose with the recipient IVC through an appropriately sized ostium. This approach has reduced mortality in the paediatric waiting list and most studies show patient survival to be equal or better than whole-graft paediatric recipients.[36]

SPLIT-LIVER TRANSPLANTATION (*EX VIVO* AND *IN SITU*)

This is the natural extension of RSLT, which enables the full use of the donor liver with a smaller left portion transplanted in a child and the larger right lobe in an adult. First performed in 1988, the acceptance and application as standard practice has increased the availability of cadaveric liver grafts by an estimated 25–28%.[37] Stringent criteria are needed to select donor livers for splitting due to the increased risk of preservation injury and complications related to the cut surface. Depending on the recipient size, there is a potential to vary the plane of separation. The right lobe graft (segments IV or V to VIII) is suitable for an adult, whereas a complete left lobe (segments II, III and IV) is suitable for a large child or small adult, while the left lateral segment is ideal for an infant. Splitting can be performed *ex vivo* or *in vivo*. For *ex vivo* splitting, standard organ procurement is performed, after which the graft is divided on the back table under slushed saline to prevent damage from warming. Back table cholangiography (and in some centres angiography) is used to delineate the biliary and vascular anatomy prior to splitting of the graft.[38] The *in situ* technique involves a left lateral segmentectomy or left hepatectomy in the heart-beating cadaveric donor, with the resected segment being perfused on the back table. This is followed by *in situ* cold perfusion of the right lobe. Both grafts are implanted using standard techniques described above. This technique has the advantage of reducing cold ischaemic time and the potential warming that may occur during *ex vivo* splitting but does significantly prolong surgery at the donor hospital.

Early results from split-liver transplantation were inferior, but rigorous selection criteria and limiting split grafts to elective recipients have improved the outcomes to comparable levels with whole-organ grafts.[37] Split-liver transplantation has achieved results comparable to RSLT in the paediatric recipient group and has the advantage of not diminishing the available donor pool for adult recipients.

The ultimate achievement for split-liver transplantation will be the capacity to use both hemigrafts for two adults. Initial experience is that left lobe recipients have a poorer outcome, although ongoing refinements may improve this.[39] Moreover, stringent recipient selection and accurate pairing for each potential donor may require regional matching and cooperation between experienced centres before this technique can be widely applied.[40]

Key point 7

- Split-liver transplantation has increased the availability of cadaveric liver grafts by an estimated 25–28%.

LIVING-DONOR LIVER TRANSPLANTATION (LDLT)

This was first performed successfully in 1989, with the first series being reported in 1991.[41] The donor operation, usually a left lateral segmental resection, is safe, with low morbidity and mortality rates. It has become a routine alternative to cadaveric transplantation in paediatric recipients and has resulted in a broadening of the recipient pool to include those in acute liver failure.[42]

More recently, LDLT has been adapted for adult recipients. Impediments to this include safety concerns for the donors and the adequacy of the hepatic mass. Two methods are used to calculate the adequacy of the graft volume: graft-to-recipient weight ratio; and the ratio of the graft volume as measured by CT or MRI volumetry with the recipient's estimated liver volume (ELV) obtained using a standard formula. The minimal safe graft volume based on this has been described as being between 30% and 50%. An insufficient graft volume results in the small-for-size syndrome, characterised by cholestasis, ascites and poor synthetic function and thought to be secondary to portal hyperperfusion.[43] Donor selection for LDLT needs to be rigorous in terms of informed consent and exclusion of medical conditions that may jeopardise the donor outcome.

Right lobe LDLT

The necessity for an adequate size led to the right lobe graft,[44] which is currently the fastest growing transplant technique. It is a complex procedure commencing with mobilisation of the liver from the retro-hepatic IVC. Hilar dissection identifies the right hepatic artery and portal vein while avoiding any exposure of the left hilar structures. Ultrasonography is performed to delineate the course of the middle and right hepatic veins and cholangiography to identify the biliary anatomy. Parenchymal dissection is performed using a CUSA (cavitron ultrasonic surgical aspirator) or a harmonic scalpel without inflow occlusion. Implantation in the recipient differs from RSLT in that the graft contains no IVC. Thus the donor right hepatic vein is anastomosed directly to the recipient right hepatic vein orifice. Biliary reconstruction is usually performed using a Roux-en-y hepaticojejunostomy.[45]

Adult LDLT using a right lobe graft is associated with a greater donor risk, with mortality rates between 0.3% and 0.5% and perhaps even as high as 1%,[46] compared with the 0.1–0.2% seen in left lobe LDLT for paediatric recipients. Transient hyperbilirubinaemia, 'transaminitis' and coagulopathy occur more frequently after donor right lobectomy. Biliary complications occur more frequently in recipients of right lobe LDLT compared with whole-graft cadaveric recipients. However, LDLT offers advantages over cadaveric donors, including short cold ischaemia times, healthy donors with normal liver function and the ability to perform transplantation prior to the recipient becoming critically ill.

In rare indications the recipient liver can be considered for grafting as a donor liver (domino procedure). This utilises livers from patients with hepatic metabolic disorders that cause systemic disease without affecting other liver functions. The main source is patients suffering from familial amyloid polyneuropathy, due to a single enzyme defect in their liver. As the recipient may take 20 or more years to develop amyloidosis, such grafts are suitable for implantation in the older recipient group, particularly in areas where the disease is prevalent.[47]

Key point 8

- Recently, live donor liver transplantation has been adapted for adult recipients. Impediments to this include safety concerns for the donors and the adequacy of the hepatic mass.

AUXILIARY LIVER TRANSPLANTATION

This has been proposed as an alternative technique in situations such as fulminant hepatic failure or for certain inborn errors of metabolism. For fulminant hepatic failure the concept is to transplant an adequate hepatic mass to allow recovery of the native liver without need for long-term immunosuppression. For inborn errors of metabolism the advantage is that acute graft failure would not be fatal. Initially, grafts were implanted in a heterotopic position, but more recently in the orthotopic site with a partial resection of the host liver to provide space. Small series have shown that immunosuppression can be withdrawn in many cases, but this approach has had limited application perhaps related to the technical issues of the surgery. Recently, living donors have been used for auxiliary partial orthotopic liver transplants, particularly for children with AFHF.[48]

REPEAT ORTHOTOPIC LIVER TRANSPLANTATION

This remains controversial, with issues relating to patient selection as well as the shortage of donor organs. The outcomes of repeat transplantation have improved in the past two decades, with patient and graft survival rates reaching 74% and 60% respectively at 1 year. The main indications are chronic rejection and hepatic artery thrombosis, but others include primary non-function, recurrent disease and biliary complications. Early re-transplantation has a relatively worse outcome when compared with late re-transplantation, in which graft survival rates are similar to first transplants. The outcomes reduce as the number of repeat transplants increase, and third or fourth grafts cannot usually be justified.[49]

IMMUNOSUPPRESSION

The range of immunosuppressive agents continues to grow and significant variations in regimes exist between differing centres. Most centres use a combination of drugs, which has the potential to limit toxicity and allow flexibility in tailoring treatments for individual patients and indications. Traditionally, triple therapy using prednisolone, azathioprine and cyclosporine gained general acceptance. Newer agents have supplanted cyclosporine with tacrolimus, which has been shown to provide better long-term outcomes. Most units still utilise prednisolone to treat rejection episodes as well as for early maintenance therapy, but it can usually be stopped within the first 3 months.[50] Azathioprine is still used by many centres, but is increasingly being replaced by mycophenolate mofetil (MMF). The main drawback of the calcineurin inhibitors (cyclosporine and tacrolimus) is nephrotoxicity, and lower-dose tacrolimus with MMF may preserve renal reserve. Recently, a macrolytic lactone, sirolimus, has been tested that is an effective substitute for the calcineurin inhibitors but does not produce nephrotoxicity. Unfortunately it has a negative impact on wound healing but may have a role to play in later long-term immunosuppression.

Early experience with polyclonal antibody preparations were disappointing, with high infectious complication rates. More specific CD25 antibodies hold greater promise as CD25 receptors are present only in activated cells. The murine–human chimeric preparation, basiliximab[51] and the humanised monoclonal antibody daclizumab[52] are both CD25 receptor-blocking antibodies and are currently undergoing clinical evaluation.

Key point 9

- Most immunosuppression regimes use a combination of drugs, which has the potential to limit toxicity and allow flexibility in tailoring treatments for individual patients and indications.

MANAGEMENT OF COMPLICATIONS

PRIMARY NON-FUNCTION

This may be due to unidentified pre-existing disease in the donor liver or to liver injury during retrieval and preservation, or it may be secondary to reperfusion injury. Although primary dysfunction is not uncommon, non-function is rare, occurring in only 2–3% of transplants. These patients can only be salvaged if an early regraft is possible. Early graft function has been shown to be a good predictor of long-term graft survival.[53]

POSTOPERATIVE HAEMORRHAGE

This has become less of a problem in liver transplantation. In addition to meticulous surgical technique, continuous monitoring of coagulation parameters during surgery, the use of antifibrinolytic agents, decompression of the splanchnic circulation by veno-venous bypass or temporary porto-caval shunt, and maintenance of the recipient's core temperature have all contributed to a significant reduction in transfusion requirements.[54]

ACUTE RENAL FAILURE

This is a common problem after liver transplantation. This is due to preexisting renal impairment, ischaemia–reperfusion injury, effects of postoperative sepsis or the side-effects of immunosuppressive therapy. Affected patients need renal support with either continuous veno-venous haemofiltration or haemodialysis during the 2–3 weeks before renal function recovers.

REJECTION

Acute cellular rejection

This characteristically occurs within the first 2 weeks after transplantation. Although 75–80% of patients will demonstrate histopathological evidence of acute cellular rejection, the incidence of biochemically apparent rejection is much lower, between 30–40%. It is diagnosed by percutaneous liver biopsy and is characterised by portal venous endophlebitis, portal infiltration, and bile duct inflammation and injury. Rejection is usually treated with a short course of high-dose steroid while optimising levels of calcineurin inhibitors. A single episode of acute cellular rejection has no impact on the incidence of chronic rejection and may have a favourable long-term outcome.[55] Response to therapy in most patients is prompt, but those with ongoing acute rejection may need repeated treatments and an increase in baseline immunosuppression.

Chronic rejection

This is more accurately defined as ductopenic rejection and may be seen a few weeks after the transplantation or may become evident months or years later. It is due to immunological injury to the bile ducts and has a variable response to treatment. Severe chronic rejection will usually require retransplantation but fortunately only occurs in around 10% of patients.

SEPSIS

This remains a major problem in immunosuppressed patients. Particular areas of concern, apart from the usual nosocomial infections, are cytomegalovirus (CMV) and fungal infections. Clinical CMV infection usually becomes apparent 4–8 weeks after transplantation. Fever associated with leucopenia is the common presentation, and rapid diagnosis is possible with PCR tests. The role of prophylactic ganciclovir for those receiving CMV-positive organs is still under study. Giving prophylaxis to those at risk can reduce invasive fungal infections.

BILIARY COMPLICATIONS

These include anastomotic and non-anastomotic strictures and bile leaks. Early investigation of biliary problems includes ultrasonography to identify biliary dilatation and to confirm hepatic arterial patency. Most biliary complications are usually managed by endoscopic retrograde cholangiopancreatography (ERCP) and stenting or less commonly by percutaneous drainage. Long-term problems usually present as recurrent cholangitis. Late biliary strictures are more likely to recur after radiological or endoscopic treatment and usually require surgical correction.

HEPATIC ARTERY THROMBOSIS

This is a devastating complication that occurs predominantly in the first month after transplantation, with leading centres reporting rates of around 2–3% in adults. It is often heralded by a massive rise in serum aminotransferases and can present acutely as acute fulminant hepatic or with biliary sepsis and strictures. Although a few cases have been rescued by thrombectomy, most require urgent re-transplantation. Delayed hepatic artery thrombosis is uncommon and may present with biliary sepsis or may remain asymptomatic. One-third of patients who suffer from silent delayed hepatic artery thrombosis remain well without requiring re-transplantation while 20% develop progressive graft failure.[56]

OUTCOMES AND THE FUTURE

In general, survival after transplantation is not greatly influenced by the underlying liver condition. The exceptions to this include fulminant hepatic failure, chronic viral hepatitis C and hepatobiliary malignancies. The overall survival rate at 1 year in most centres is around 90%, with almost 70% of patients surviving 10 years. The outcome for those transplanted for acute liver failure is lower at 60–70% at 1 year, although the survival curve for these patients is relatively flat with fewer later deaths than for other indications.[57]

Future progress with liver transplantation will require greater understanding of the natural history of liver disease together with the refinement of prognostic parameters to improve selection and timing. Hybrid bio-artificial devices and *ex vivo* perfusion techniques are being developed as bridging procedures for the critically ill patient with liver failure.

Development of selective immunosuppressive drugs and refinement of pre-emptive antimicrobial therapy require a clearer understanding of underlying mechanisms in allograft rejection and sepsis post transplantation. A number of promising new immunosuppressants as well as monoclonal antibodies targeted to adhesion molecules and other receptors are currently becoming available. Genetic engineering to achieve immune tolerance is another pathway forwards.

CONCLUSIONS

Orthotopic liver transplantation offers a well-established treatment for several irreversible acute and chronic liver diseases. The future is likely to see a further expansion of indications for transplantation that will overwhelm the limited donor supply. Significant effort and innovation will be required to increase the donor pool as well as to maximise the utilisation of each donor organ. There is considerable scope for a more selective approach to immunosuppression and control of sepsis. The financial cost of liver transplantation, as well as equitable allocation of scarce donor resources, are part of the ethical issues facing the transplant community.

Key points for clinical practice

- Broadly the indications for liver transplantation are classified as chronic liver failure, acute fulminant hepatic failure, primary hepatic malignancy and inborn errors of metabolism.

- Clinical events may precipitate the need for transplantation. These include hepatic encephalopathy, refractory ascites, and variceal bleeding.

- Excellent results can be obtained from liver grafting if the tumour is diagnosed at an early stage (single tumours less than 5.0 cm or three tumours under 3.0 cm).

- Patients should be listed for transplantation only if they have a 50% probability or more of being alive 5 years after transplantation with a quality of life that is acceptable to the patient.

- Diseases that might recur in the transplanted liver are not a contraindication. For alcoholic liver disease patients should have a period of abstinence of at least 6 months, should be assessed by a psychiatrist with expertise in alcoholism and should undergo a formal alcohol rehabilitation programme prior to transplantation.

- Overall the experience that marginal livers can be successfully used has meant a significant rise in the number of transplants performed.

- Split-liver transplantation has increased the availability of cadaveric liver grafts by an estimated 25–28%.

- Recently, live donor liver transplantation has been adapted for adult recipients. Impediments to this include safety concerns for the donors and the adequacy of the hepatic mass.

- Most immunosuppression regimes use a combination of drugs, which has the potential to limit toxicity and allow flexibility in tailoring treatments for individual patients and indications.

References

1. Modan B, Shpilberg O, Baruch Y *et al*. The need for liver transplantation: a nationwide estimate based on consensus review. *Lancet* 1995; **346**: 660–662.
2. Samuel D, Benhamou JP, Bismuth H. Criteria of selection for liver transplantation. *Transplant Proc* 1987; **19**: 2383–2386.
3. Gines P, Arroyo V, Vargas V *et al*. Paracentesis with intravenous infusion of albumin as compared with peritoneovenous shunting in cirrhosis with refractory ascites. *N Engl J Med* 1991; **325**: 829–835.
4. Lebrec D, Giuily N, Hadengue A *et al*. Transjugular intrahepatic portosystemic shunt (TIPS) vs paracentesis for refractory ascites: results of a randomized trial. *J Hepatol* 1996; **25**: 135–144.
5. Runyon BA. Monomicrobial nonneutrocytic bacterascites: a variant of spontaneous bacterial peritonitis. *J Hepatol* 1990; **12**: 710–715.
6. Stanley AJ, Hayes PC. Portal hypertension and variceal haemorrhage. *Lancet* 1997; **350**: 1235–1239.
7. O'Grady JG, Alexander GJM, Hayllar KN, Williams R. Early indicators of prognosis in fulminant hepatic failure. *Gastroenterology* 1989; **97**: 439–445.
8. Lidofsky SD. Liver transplantation for fulminant hepatic failure. *Gastroenterol Clin North Am* 1993; **22**: 257–269.
9. Wong LL. Current status of transplantation for hepatocellular cancer. *Am J Surg* 2002; **183**: 309–356.
10. Burdelski M, Rodeck B, Latta A *et al*. Treatment of inherited metabolic disorders by liver transplantation. *J Inherit Metab Dis* 1991; **14**: 604–618.
11. Lucey MR, Brown KA, Everson GT *et al*. Minimal criteria for placement of adults on liver transplant waiting list: a report of a national conference organized by the American Association for the Study of Liver Diseases. *Transplantation* 1998; **66**: 956–962.
12. Devlin J, O'Grady J. Indications for referral and assessment in liver transplantation: a clinical guideline. British Society of Gastroenterology. *Gut* 1999; **Suppl 6**: V11–V122.
13. Neuberger J, James O. Guidelines for selection of patients for liver transplantation in the era of donor-organ shortage. *Lancet* 1999; **354**: 1636–1639.
14. Wiesner RH, McDiarmid SV, Kamath PS *et al*. MELD and PELD: application of survival models to liver allocation. *Liver Transplant* 2001; **7**: 567–580.
15. Kim WR, Wiesner RH, Therneau TM *et al*. Optimal timing for liver transplantation in primary biliary cirrhosis. *Hepatology* 1998; **28**: 33–38.
16. Papatheodoridis GV, Hadziyannis ES, Deutsch M, Hadziyannis SJ. Ursodeoxycholic acid for primary biliary cirrhosis: final results of a 12-year, prospective, randomized, controlled trial. *Am J Gastroenterol* 2002; **97**: 2063–2070.
17. Chapman RW. The colon and PSC: new liver, new danger? *Gut* 1998; **43**: 595–598.
18. Dickson ER, Murtaugh P, Wiesner R. Primary sclerosing cholangitis. Refinement and application of survival models. *Gastroenterology* 1992; **102**: 1893–1902.
19. Mazzaferro V, Regalia E, Doci R. Liver transplantation for the treatment of small hepatocellular carcinomas in patients with cirrhosis. *N Engl J Med* 1996; **343**: 693–699.
20. Berenguer M, Prieto M, Rayon JM *et al*. Natural history of clinically compensated HCV-related graft cirrhosis following liver transplantation. *Hepatology* 2000; **32**: 852–858.
21. Singh N, Gayowski T, Wannstedt C *et al*. Interferon alpha for prophylaxis of recurrent viral hepatitis C in liver transplant recipients. *Transplantation* 1998; **65**: 82–86.
22. Wali MH, Heydtmann M, Harrison RF *et al*. Outcome of liver transplantation for patients infected by hepatitis C, including those infected by genotype 4. *Liver Transplant* 2003; **9**: 796–804.
23. Samuel D, Muller R, Alexander G *et al*. Liver transplantation in European patients with hepatitis B surface antigen. *N Engl J Med* 1993; **329**: 1842–1847.
24. Starkel P, Cicarelli O, Lerut J *et al*. Limited lamivudine and long term hepatitis B immunoglobulin immunoprophylaxis for prevention of hepatitis B recurrence after liver transplantation. *Transplantation* 2002; **74**: 408–410.
25. Krom RA. Liver transplantation and alcohol: who should get transplants? *Hepatology* 1994; **20**: 28S-32S.
26. Tang H, Boulton R, Gunson B *et al*. Patterns of alcohol consumption after liver transplantation. *Gut* 1998; **43**: 140–145.

27. Cattan P, Berney T, Conti F et al. Outcome of orthotopic liver transplantation in autoimmune hepatitis according to subtypes. *Transplant Int* 2002; **15**: 34–38.

28. Satoi S, Bramhall SR, Solomon M et al. The use of liver grafts from donors with bacterial meningitis. *Transplantation* 2001; **72**: 1108–1113.

29. Deschennes M, Forbes C, Tchervenkov J et al. Use of older donors is associated with more extensive ischaemic damage on intra-operative biopsies during liver transplantation. *Liver Transplant Surg* 1999; **5**: 357–361.

30. Ramsay MA. The use of antifibrinolytic agents results in a reduction in transfused blood products during liver transplantation. *Liver Transplant Surg* 1997; **3**: 665–669.

31. Kang Y. Transfusion based on clinical coagulation monitoring does reduce hemorrhage during liver transplantation. *Liver Transplant Surg* 1997; **3**: 655–659.

32. Tzakis A, Todo S, Starzl TE. Piggyback orthotopic liver transplantation with preservation of the inferior vena cava. *Ann Surg* 1989; **210**: 649–652.

33. Tzakis AG, Reyes J, Nour B et al. Temporary end to side portocaval shunt in orthotopic hepatic transplantation in humans. *Surg Gynecol Obstet* 1993; **176**: 181–183.

34. Randall HB, Wachs ME, Somberg KA et al. The use of T-tube after orthotopic liver transplantation. *Transplantation* 1996; **61**: 258–261.

35. Bismuth H, Houssin D. Reduced size orthotopic liver graft in hepatic transplantation in children. *Surgery* 1984; **95**: 367–370.

36. Broelsch CE, Stevens LH, Whittington PF et al. The use of reduced size liver transplants in children, including split livers and living related liver transplants. *Eur J Paediatr Surg* 1991; **1**: 166–171.

37. Azoulay D, Astarcioglu I, Bismuth H et al. Split liver transplantation. The Paul Brousse policy. *Ann Surg* 1996; **224**: 737–746.

38. Rela M, Vougas V, Muiesan P et al. Split liver transplantation: King's College Hospital experience. *Ann Surg* 1998; **227**: 282–288.

39. Azoulay D, Castaing D, Adam R et al. Split-liver transplantation for two adult recipients: feasibility and long-term outcomes. *Ann Surg* 2001; **233**: 565–574.

40. Mirza DF, Achilleos O, Pirenne J et al. Encouraging results of split-liver transplantation. *Br J Surg* 1998; **85**: 494–497.

41. Broelsch CE, Whitington PF, Emond JC et al. Liver transplantation in children from living related donors. Surgical techniques and results. *Ann Surg* 1992; **214**: 428–437.

42. Emre S, Schwartz ME, Shneider B et al. Living related liver transplantation for acute liver failure in children. *Liver Transplant Surg* 1999; **5**: 161–165.

43. Emond JC, Renz JF, Ferrell LD et al. Functional analysis of grafts from living donors. Implications for the treatment of older recipients. *Ann Surg* 1996; **224**: 544–552.

44. Fan ST, Lo CM, Liu CL et al. Safety of donors in live donor liver transplantation using right lobe grafts. *Arch Surg* 2000; **135**: 336–340.

45. Wachs ME, Bak TE, Karrer FM et al. Adult living donor liver transplantation using a right hepatic lobe. *Transplantation* 1998; **66**: 1313–1316.

46. Miller CM, Gondolesi GE, Florman S et al. One hundred and nine living donor liver transplants in adults and children: a single-center experience. *Ann Surg* 2001; **234**: 301–311.

47. Azoulay D, Samuel D, Castaing D et al. Domino liver transplants for metabolic disorders: experience with familial amyloidotic polyneuropathy. *J Am Coll Surg* 1999; **189**: 584–593.

48. Boudjema K, Bachellier P, Wolf P et al. Auxiliary liver transplantation and bioartificial bridging procedures in treatment of acute liver failure. *World J Surg* 2002; **26**: 264–274.

49. Yoong KF, Gunson BK, Buckels JA et al. Repeat orthotopic liver transplantation in the 1990s: Is it justified? *Transplant Int* 1998; **11(Supp 1)**: S221–223.

50. Padbury R, Gunson BK, Dousset B et al. Long-term immunosuppression after liver transplantation: are steroids necessary? *Transplant Int* 1992; **5**: S470–S472.

51. Calmus Y, Scheele JR, Gonzalez-Pinto I et al. Immunoprophylaxis with basiliximab, a chimeric anti-interleukin-2 receptor monoclonal antibody, in combination with azathioprine-containing triple therapy in liver transplant recipients. *Liver Transplant* 2002; **8**: 123–131.

52. Carswell CI, Plosker GL, Wagstaff AJ. Daclizumab: a review of its use in the management of organ transplantation. *Biodrugs* 2001; **15**: 745–773.

53. Porte RJ, Ploeg RJ, Hansen B *et al*. Long-term graft survival after liver transplantation in the UW era: late effects of cold ischemia and primary dysfunction. European Multicentre Study Group. *Transplant Int* 1998; **11(Suppl 1)**: S164–167.
54. Porte RJ, Molenaar IQ, Begliomini B *et al*. Aprotinin and transfusion requirements in orthotopic liver transplantation: a multicentre randomised double-blind study. EMSALT Study Group. *Lancet* 2000; **355**: 1303–1309.
55. Demetris AJ, Murase N, Delancey CP *et al*. The liver allograft, chronic (ductopaenic) rejection and microchimerism. What can they teach us? *Transplant Proc* 1995; **27**: 67–70.
56. Bhattacharjya S, Gunson BK, Mirza DF *et al*. Delayed hepatic artery thrombosis in adult orthotopic liver transplantation – a 12-year experience. *Transplantation* 2001; **71**: 1592–1596.
57. Schiod FV, Atillasoy E, Shakil AO *et al*. Etiology and outcome for 295 patients with acute liver failure in the United States. *Liver Transplant Surg* 1999; **5**: 29–34.

Amjad Parvaiz Neil W. Pearce

7

Cholangiocarcinoma

Cholangiocarcinoma is the term applied to primary malignant tumours of the biliary tract. They are categorised according to site into intrahepatic, gallbladder, hilar and distal bile duct cancers. The incidence of bile duct cancer in autopsy series ranges from 0.01% to 0.46%.[1] Despite its low occurrence, the diagnosis of cholangiocarcinoma should be considered in every case of obstructive jaundice. There is increasing evidence that suggests a steep, fourfold rise in the incidence of this condition over the last few decades; in particular intrahepatic cholangiocarcinoma now accounts for more deaths than hepatoma in the Western countries.[2] Cholangiocarcinoma has the potential to be diagnosed early, when it is small, localised, and amenable to an aggressive treatment approach. This chapter will concentrate on hilar bile duct cancers. Peripheral intrahepatic cholangiocarcinoma and gallbladder cancer will also be considered as closely related conditions that are diagnosed and managed in a similar way to hilar tumours. In contrast, carcinomas of the distal common bile duct present diagnostic and therapeutic problems more similar to carcinoma of the head of pancreas and are best considered with this condition.

Key point 1

- There is a fourfold rise in the incidence of cholangiocarcinoma over the last few decades. Intrahepatic cholangiocarcinoma now accounts for more deaths than hepatoma in the UK.

Mr Amjad Parvaiz FRCS, Specialist Registrar, Hepatobiliary Unit, Southampton General Hospital

Mr Neil W. Pearce FRCS, Consultant in Hepatico-Biliary Surgery, E Level, West Wing, MP 67, Southampton General Hospital, Southampton SO16 6YD, UK (for correspondence)

HISTORICAL BACKGROUND

The first bile duct resection for a malignant stricture was reported in 1954 by Brown and Myers,[3] and in the same year Edmondson and Steiner[4] first described primary liver cancers of biliary epithelial origin and reported a hilar variant. Klatskin's[5] classic description of hilar bile duct cancer followed in 1965 and focused attention on a rarely recognised disease, which has always since been associated with his name. At this time the condition was seldom diagnosed prior to laparotomy (or indeed autopsy) and the aim of surgery was palliative; operative intubation of the tumour was the accepted management. It was another decade before the first series of bile duct resections were reported, with a handful of long-term survivors.[6,7] The evolution of computed tomography (CT) changed preoperative evaluation and led to the increasing recognition of this disease prior to surgery, with subsequent early specialist referral and a consequent building of expertise in the hands of a few individuals. These pioneers were prepared to tackle this formidable challenge and move on from limited bile duct resection to radical lymphadenectomy, hepatic resection, vascular resection and reconstruction and ultimately liver transplantation[7–13] The last decade has seen the more widespread adoption of some of these techniques, and many series have reported high resection rates, good median survival data and an increasing proportion of long-term survivors.[11–20]

Key point 2

- Recently, with aggressive surgical approach, higher resection rates with good median survival have been reported.

GENERAL FEATURES OF CHOLANGIOCARCINOMA

AETIOLOGICAL FACTORS

The aetiology of most cholangiocarcinomas remains unknown; however, there are several well-known risk factors associated with this condition (Table 1).

Strong associations have been found between cholangiocarcinoma and gallstones, sclerosing cholangitis, ulcerative colitis, cystic abnormalities of the bile duct, liver flukes and the radiocontrast agent thorium dioxide (thorotrast).

Table 1. Factors associated with cholangiocarcinomas

Strong association	Possible association
Caroli's disease	Isoniazid
Choledochal cyst	Methyldopa
Liver fluke	Oral contraceptives
Ulcerative colitis	Asbestos
Primary sclerosing cholangitis	
Thorotrast	
Gallstones	

Possible mechanisms of carcinogenesis include chronic irritation, nitric oxide formation, intrinsic nitrosation and activation of drug-metabolising enzymes.

Although gallstones have been reported in one-third of patients with bile duct cancers,[21,22] a cause-and-effect relation has not been established. The incidence of cholangiocarcinomas in patients with ulcerative colitis ranges from 0.4% to 1.4% representing a severalfold increase in the risk of the general population. Crohn's disease is not associated with cholangiocarcinoma. Patients with ulcerative colitis and cholangiocarcinoma have cancers diagnosed at an age of 45–55 years, approximately two decades earlier than in patients without ulcerative colitis. The medical and surgical treatment of ulcerative colitis does not appear to influence the subsequent development of biliary tract cancer.

Reports have indicated a 0.25–28% incidence of cholangiocarcinoma in patients with congenital cystic abnormalities of the bile ducts.[23-25] In choledochal cysts, a causative role of pancreatic exocrine secretions, causing malignant transformation of the bile duct epithelium, has been postulated. In addition, bile stasis, stone formation and chronic inflammation within the cyst have also been implicated. The same factors play a role in the high incidence of cholangiocarcinoma in patients with Caroli's disease.[26]

In the Far East, infestation with the liver fluke *Opisthorchis viverrini* is a recognised cause of cholangiocarcinoma and *Clonorchis sinesis* has also been implicated. The parasites gain access to the host via the duodenum. The preferred site of infestation is in the intrahepatic bile ducts, where the adult trematodes can cause biliary obstruction and periductal fibrosis, hyperplasia and predispose to cholangiocarcinoma.

Key point 3

- The medical and surgical treatment of ulcerative colitis does not appear to influence the subsequent development of biliary tract cancer.

PATHOLOGY

More than 95% of bile duct cancers are adenocarcinomas, with a range from well-differentiated to poorly differentiated varieties. In addition to adenocarcinomas, several other histological types of bile duct cancers have been reported: squamous,[27] mucoepidermoid,[28] leiomyosarcoma,[29] cystadeno-carcinoma[30] and granular cell.[31] Autopsy results after death from cholangio-carcinoma have indicated the presence of metastatic disease in 75–80% of patients.[32] These usually involve regional lymph nodes, liver and peritoneum. Less commonly involved organs are lungs, bones, kidney and brain. At initial clinical presentation 15–30% of patients have metastatic disease.

CLINICAL FEATURES

The median age of patients at diagnosis of cholangiocarcinoma is from 60–70 years. Patients with cholangiocarcinoma secondary to ulcerative colitis or choledochal cyst present two decades earlier. Sex incidence is almost equal.[33] More than 90% of patients present with jaundice. Other common associated symptoms include upper abdominal pain, pruritus and weight loss. In patients with tumour located above the hepatic duct confluence, the right or left hepatic duct may be obstructed unilaterally. The classical presentation in this group of patients is with right upper quadrant pain and unilobar liver enlargement without jaundice. Biochemically, these patients have raised alanine aminotransferase (ALT) and alkaline phosphatase with little or no elevation in serum bilirubin levels.

Key point 4

- Biopsy of the suspected tumour is contraindicated in operable disease because of the high risk of needle track and peritoneal seeding

IMAGING AND ASSESSMENT OF CHOLANGIOCARCINOMA

The diagnosis of cholangiocarcinoma is challenging because it is often difficult to distinguish benign from malignant strictures. At the time of diagnosis most patients have advanced disease. There are four aims of preoperative assessment: confirmation of the diagnosis, assessment of local anatomy, exclusion of distant metastasis and assessment of physiological status.

IMAGING TECHNIQUES

For hilar cholangiocarcinoma diagnostic evaluation follows the standard approach for patients with obstructive jaundice. All patients have an initial ultrasound scan, to exclude simple gallstone disease. A dedicated contrast-enhanced multislice CT scan is performed in all patients to assess the region during the arterial, portal and hepatic phases of blood flow; scanning of the chest, abdomen and pelvis is mandatory to exclude lung or peritoneal metastases (Fig. 1).

Magnetic resonance (MR) imaging has gained popularity in recent years and it is our preferred investigation for the assessment of hepatic parenchymal and vascular involvement. Preoperative MR cholangiography has now superseded endoscopic retrograde cholangiopancreatography (ERCP) and percutaneous cholangiography as the first line of ductal imaging in our practice (Fig. 2), although in Japan selective cholangiography and percutaneous transhepatic cholangioscopy are advocated by some as imperative to the planning of the operative procedure.[11]

An isotope bone scan should be considered to further exclude disseminated disease. In cases of diagnostic uncertainty a positron emission tomography (PET) scan may also be helpful. PET uses [18F]fluoro-2-deoxyglucose (FDG) to assess metabolism in human tissue, thus highlighting areas of malignant disease. The combination of elevated CA19-9 value, digital image analysis and PET greatly assists in the differentiation of benign from malignant strictures.

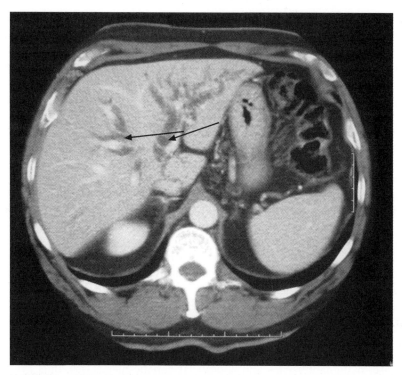

Fig. 1 CT image of hilar cholangiocarcinoma showing intra-hepatic duct dilatation (arrows).

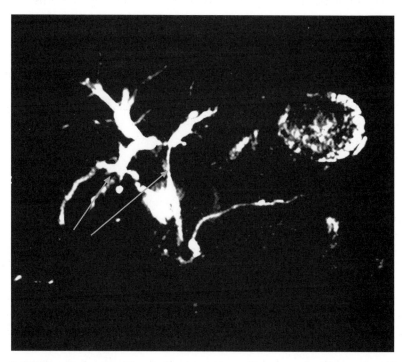

Fig. 2 MRC image showing hilar cholangiocarcinoma (long arrow) with intra-hepatic duct dilatation (short arrow).

In view of the difficulty in assessing these cases, all patients with non-metastatic disease should be referred to a specialist hepatobiliary surgical unit at the earliest opportunity. Biopsy of the suspected tumour is contraindicated in operable disease because of the high risk of needle tract and peritoneal seeding.

STAGING OF CHOLANGIOCARCINOMA

Hilar cholangiocarcinoma is most commonly described according to the Bismuth–Corlette classification (Fig 3)[8]. Although this describes the site of the stricture in the duct, it is of no value in staging in the modern era of radical resection, as it takes no account of the extent or pattern of vascular and parenchymal invasion, which are the main determinants of resectability and prognosis. Staging according to the UICC TNM classification[34] addresses some of these issues; however, several authors[13,16,18,35,36] have questioned the relevance of this to outcome after radical surgery and therefore its use in preoperative assessment. Currently there is no widely accepted staging system that has any consistent value in the preoperative assessment of resectability or prognosis in this disease.

STAGING LAPAROSCOPY

The primary role of staging laparoscopy is in identification of peritoneal disease, malignant ascites and superficial hepatic metastases, thus avoiding unnecessary laparotomy in patients with inoperable disease. One of the main

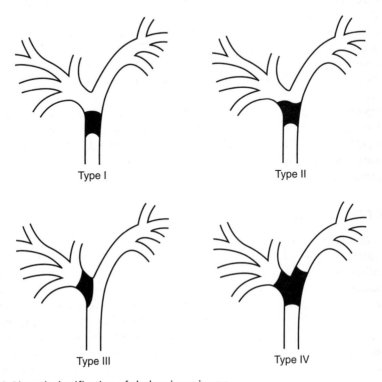

Type I

Type II

Type III

Type IV

Fig. 3 Bismuth classification of cholangiocarcinoma.

indications is after biopsy, which may have caused seeding; laparoscopy is helpful when there is radiological evidence suggesting locally advanced disease, making dissemination more likely. In our current practice we laparoscope the majority of cases.

The use of laparoscopic ultrasound may add further evidence of vascular and nodal involvement in experienced hands.[37,38] Its greatest benefit is in identifying choledocholithiasis and Mirizzi syndrome from bile duct or gallbladder cancer. With improved preoperative radiological imaging with multislice CT and MR, there are few cases where it yields additional information on staging, so it has not gained widespread popularity.

PREOPERATIVE MANAGEMENT

GENERAL ASSESSMENT

Routine blood tests should include full blood count, clotting profile, and renal and liver function tests, as well as hepatitis serology. It is our practice to check carcinoembryonic antigen (CEA) and CA19-9 as tumour markers. A serum CA19-9 value greater than 100 U/ml has a reported sensitivity and specificity for cholangiocarcinoma of approximately 75% and 80% respectively.[39] However, CA19-9 may rise rapidly in any form of biliary obstruction, whether malignant or benign, and in our experience false-positive results are common.

Serological evidence of viral hepatitis or a history of alcohol abuse combined with deranged liver function tests, raised prothrombin time or radiological evidence of cirrhosis should stimulate concern over functional hepatic reserve and the ability of the patient to withstand major hepatic resection. In these circumstances a biopsy of the planned liver remnant may be helpful. Further information on hepatic reserve may be obtained by measuring the indocyanine green retention rate at 15 minutes or calculating hepatic volume and proposed resection volume from three-dimensional reconstruction of CT or MR scan images.

Patients undergoing major hepatobiliary resection should be assessed for cardiovascular and respiratory function prior to surgery. Our standard practice is to perform routine echocardiography and reserve cardiac stress testing, coronary angiography and pulmonary function testing for those with relevant symptoms and signs.

PREOPERATIVE BILIARY DRAINAGE

The majority of patients with hilar cholangiocarcinoma are deeply jaundiced. Obstructive jaundice impairs hepatic function and therefore in our practice if the bilirubin is over 300 μmol/l, a period of preoperative biliary drainage is considered mandatory before embarking on major hepatic resection. Some authors[11] have questioned this practice in view of the reported increased incidence of infective complications and death after biliary tract intubation; this is an issue that has not yet been resolved. Our practice is to maintain patients on prophylactic antibiotics after drainage and keep the period of drainage as short as is practical to reduce the chance of cholangitis, although in many Japanese centres multiple transhepatic biliary drains are placed and left for a minimum of 6 weeks to allow hepatic functional recovery.[11] In practice many jaundiced patients have been stented endoscopically or percutaneously prior to referral to a specialist unit.

PORTAL VEIN EMBOLISATION

The majority of postoperative deaths following major liver resection relate to hepatic failure. The observation that right portal vein obstruction by tumour with resultant right lobe atrophy produced left lobar hypertrophy led to the development of selective portal vein embolisation to replicate this response preoperatively, thus increasing the volume of the liver remnant and reducing the risk of hepatic failure.[40,41]

CONTRAINDICATIONS TO RESECTION

Resectability rates reported from most Western centres have varied between 10% and 20%. In comparison, Japanese centres report much higher resection rates of 52–92%. This is achieved by their willingness to perform extensive resections, including vascular resection and reconstruction, radical lymphadenectomy and major hepatic resection. Adoption of these principles has changed the selection criteria for the surgery of cholangiocarcinoma (Table 2).

Table 2 Contraindications to resection of cholangiocarcinoma

- Lymph node metastases outside the planned field of resection, distant metastases or peritoneal deposits are absolute contraindications to resection
- Involvement of the main trunk of the hepatic artery or bilateral involvement of its branches should still be considered a contraindication for curative resection. Palliative resection and reconstruction may be offered in selected cases, but there is no realistic prospect of long-term survival
- Bilateral involvement of the biliary tree, beyond the second-order ducts, is not resectable. Nor is unilateral involvement at this level with contralateral portal vein occlusion or hepatic lobar atrophy
- Bilateral, second-order, portal vein branch involvement is not resectable
- Inadequate systemic physiological reserve to withstand surgery

SURGICAL TREATMENT OF HILAR CHOLANGIOCARCINOMA

Radical surgery remains the only means of possible cure in patients with cholangiocarcinoma. Many series[3,12,16,35,36,42] have identified the adverse impact of positive resection margins on survival rates after liver resection for hilar cholangiocarcinoma. In a multivariate analysis Neuhaus et al.[36] has identified radical surgical clearance as the single strongest predictor of 5-year survival after resection.

BILE DUCT RESECTION

Complete excision of the extrahepatic bile ducts must be performed, dividing the distal duct within the pancreatic head. The superior border of the head and neck of the pancreas defines the lower limit of the resection. All neural, lymphatic and connective tissue above this level, surrounding the hepatic artery and portal vein, is stripped from these vessels and resected *en bloc* with the bile duct. The proximal limit of the resection is determined by the level of suprahilar hepatic duct involvement and the extent of the hepatic resection. Duct resection margins should be sent for frozen section, prior to forming a Roux-en-Y hepatico-jejunostomy. The anastomosis is usually at the level of the hepatic sectional or segmental ducts.

HEPATIC RESECTION FOR HILAR CHOLANGIOCARCINOMA

Recent evidence strongly suggests that more extensive hepatic resections are associated with higher rates of R0 resection and a consequent better long-term survival.[17,43] The highest rates of histological clearance are obtained after right trisectionectomy with caudate lobectomy (segments 4–8 and 1).[36]

For technical reasons, in most cases of hilar cholangiocarcinoma the hepatic resection of choice is right trisectionectomy (segments 4–8) and caudate lobectomy. The greater length of the left hepatic duct and its position relative to the hepatic arteries allows wider surgical clearance with right-sided resections. Hence right trisectionectomy is often a less difficult and more radical operation than left hepatectomy, left trisectionectomy or central liver resection. Left-sided resections should be reserved for patients with predominant left liver involvement and in particular invasion of the segment 2 and 3 ducts or left portal vein or hepatic artery involvement.

CAUDATE LOBECTOMY

Caudate lobectomy is mandatory. A study of caudate anatomy by Nimura *et al.*[11] highlighted the frequency of caudate ductal involvement in hilar cholangiocarcinoma, with histological assessment revealing involvement in 44 of 45 consecutive curative resections. Many authors have appreciated the significance of these findings and presented large series advocating caudate lobectomy as standard practice for most hilar cancers, with resultant high rates of radical (R0) resection backing the technique.[11,13,14,36,44,45] In the series reported by Sugiura *et al.*[13] from the Keio group, the 5-year survival rate after resections including caudate lobectomy was 46% versus 12% in the no-caudate-lobectomy group.

Key point 5

- Radical surgery remains the only means of possible cure in patients with cholangiocarcinoma

---

RADICAL LYMPHADENECTOMY

Complete regional lymphadenectomy is essential for curative resection of hilar cholangiocarcinoma. *En bloc* removal of the regional nodes with the specimen removes the commonest site of metastasis from hilar cholangiocarcinoma. The extent of the lymphadenectomy should include clearance of the hilar, portal, common hepatic, posterior pancreatic and coeliac nodes. We also routinely perform para-aortic node clearance from the aorto-caval groove. Three recent series by Kosuge et al.,[16] Kitagawa et al.[15] and Neuhaus et al.[36] demonstrate that in patients undergoing radical lymphadenectomy, regional lymph node involvement does not significantly reduce 5-year survival. Kitagawa has also reported 5-year survivors with positive para-aortic nodes.

VASCULAR RESECTION AND RECONSTRUCTION

Portal vein involvement is not a contraindication to curative resection of hilar cholangiocarcinoma.[26] Indeed, recent work by Neuhaus et al.[36] suggests that portal vein resection is an independent predictor of 5-year survival after R0 hepatic resection (65% survival with vein resection *versus* 28% without). Invasion of the hepatic artery is a much poorer prognostic factor. Although hepatic artery resection and reconstruction is technically feasible, there are very few long-term survivors in this group.

PANCREATICODUODENECTOMY

En bloc pancreaticoduodenectomy in addition to major hepatectomy has been reported in cases with distal bile duct, duodenal or pancreatic invasion. It aids achievement of a radical clearance in patients with advanced disease, but with a substantial increase in morbidity. This radical surgery should be confined to exceptional cases in the hands of a few experts in specialist centres.

ORTHOTOPIC LIVER TRANSPLANTATION

Liver transplantation has been used in some centres with good results.[12,20,36] Although high rates of R0 resection are achievable with transplantation, any survival benefit is lost by the consequences of long-term immunosuppression. Liver transplantation therefore confers no real advantage over resection and is difficult to support at present in view of the small size of the donor pool.

Key point 6

- The role of radiotherapy and chemotherapy in the treatment of cholangiocarcinoma remains limited

---

ONCOLOGICAL TREATMENTS

The role of radiotherapy and chemotherapy in the treatment of cholangiocarcinoma is limited. Both modalities, either applied separately or in combination, have shown some promise, but have failed to show any survival benefit.

External-beam radiotherapy alone is of no value in cholangiocarcinoma. More recently, brachytherapy (an intracavity radiotherapy delivery system) has been used with some success. The delivery dose varies between 30 and 50 Gy, which can be supplemented with external-beam radiation of 30–45 Gy. Brachytherapy is delivered either by endoscopically placed nasobiliary tubes or by the transhepatic route.

Historically, cholangiocarcinoma has been regarded as chemoresistant. A local response rate up to 29% has been seen in patients treated with 5-fluorouracil (5-FU) and mitomycin C, alone or in combination with doxorubicin (Adriamycin) (FAM).[46] Recent interest has centred on the use of 5-FU and gemicitabine in combination with external- or internal-beam therapy, which has resulted in a reported response rate of 20%.[47] However, these are highly selected case series and no randomised controlled evidence exists, nor has any significant improvement in survival yet been reported.

CARCINOMA OF THE GALLBLADDER

As with cholangiocarcinoma, the incidence of carcinoma of the gallbladder is increasing. It is most commonly seen in elderly women, with a female-to-male ratio of 3 : 1.[48] The mean age of patients with carcinoma of gallbladder is around 65 years, with most cases presenting during the seventh and eighth decades of life.[48] Despite improvement in diagnostic tools, the outlook for patients with gallbladder cancer remains very poor.[49,50,51] The reported 5-year survival rate is between 3% and 5% in most European series.

AETIOLOGICAL FACTORS

The risk factors for the development of carcinoma of the gallbladder are better understood than those for cholangiocarcinoma. A long-standing history of gallstone disease is present in almost all cases of gallbladder cancer. There is a slightly higher incidence of carcinoma of gallbladder in people working in the rubber industry; however, the carcinogen has not been identified.[52] Porcelain gallbladder is a premalignant condition, with 10% of patients having foci of malignancy at the time of diagnosis. There is a strong familial element to the high incidence of gallbladder carcinoma seen in Asian populations, particularly in Pakistan and North West India.

PATHOLOGY AND STAGING OF GALLBLADDER CANCER

Adenocarcinoma of the gallbladder produces diffuse thickening of the wall of the gallbladder and is often very difficult to differentiate from severe cholecystitis. Rarely, squamous cell carcinomas and adenoacanthomas are also reported.

Gallbladder cancer is extremely aggressive. The mode of spread may be via lymphatic, vascular or perineural infiltration, direct extension into adjacent structures or intraperitoneal seeding. The lymphatic drainage from the gallbladder is almost identical to that of hilar cholangiocarcinoma. The cystic node is frequently involved early in the disease, with subsequent spread to the nodes in the hepatoduodenal ligament, superior and inferior pancreaticoduodenal nodes, and then via the coeliac and superior mesenteric nodes into the para-aortic chain. Precise knowledge of the anatomy of these lymphatics is crucial when radical lymphadenectomy is undertaken for resectable cases.

The liver is often involved via direct spread of the tumour into segments IV and V; subsequent intrahepatic seeding via the portal system is a very poor prognostic feature. Tumours may also directly invade the duodenum, pancreas and the hepatic flexure of the colon. Cancers sited in Hartmann's pouch can cause hepatic duct compression and are difficult to differentiate from hilar cholangiocarcinoma in appearance and behaviour. Peritoneal spread is common. In some cases this may be iatrogenic due to inadvertent perforation of the gallbladder during cholecystectomy for presumed gallstone disease.

The staging system proposed by Nevin et al.[53] is simple to remember and widely used (Table 3). The UICC TNM classification is more detailed, but, as with hilar cholangiocarcinoma, neither system is of great help when assessing resectability.

Table 3 Nevin's staging of gallbladder cancer[53]

Stage 1	Tumour confined to mucosa
Stage 2	Tumour breaches the muscularis mucosa
Stage 3	Tumour extends through the muscularis propria
Stage 4	Tumour involves the cystic duct node
Stage 5	Tumour involves the liver or other organ

DIAGNOSIS AND CLINICAL FEATURES

The clinical presentation of patients with carcinoma of gallbladder is very variable, ranging from the incidental finding of early carcinoma after cholecystectomy for the symptoms of gallstone disease, to obstructive jaundice or more general symptoms associated with advanced disease such as anorexia, weight loss and lethargy. The diagnosis is usually suggested by ultrasound and supported by CT. Gallbladder carcinoma should be suspected in patients with gallbladder symptoms if ultrasound suggests a thick-walled gallbladder, particularly if associated with an intraluminal mass or evidence of liver involvement. Under these circumstances routine cholecystectomy should not be undertaken. These patients should be imaged with CT and if suspicion persists referred to a specialist centre with facilities for liver resection (Figure 4). The subsequent work-up is almost identical to that for hilar cholangiocarcinoma. The greatest difficulty lies in differentiating between severe cholecystitis and carcinoma, which may have almost identical radiological features (Figure 5).

Although direct liver involvement usually does not pose any problems, peritoneal disease or extensive distant lymph node metastases are a contraindication to radical surgery. The incidence of lymph node metastasis at the initial presentation ranges from 25% to 75%.

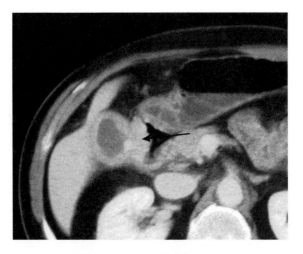

Fig. 4 Gallbladder carcinoma with stone in the Hartman's Pouch (arrow).

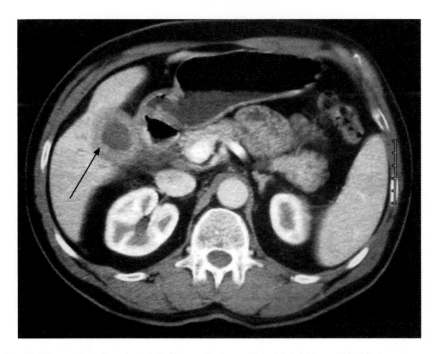

Fig. 5 CT scan showing chronic inflammatory reaction mimicking gallbladder cancer (arrow).

SURGERY FOR GALLBLADDER CANCER

The stage of the disease dictates the approach and the outcome. Patients with carcinoma confined to the mucosa of the gallbladder may be successfully treated by cholecystectomy alone.[54] However, an aggressive surgical approach is required for tumour invading into or beyond the muscularis of the gallbladder wall. These patients should all be treated by liver resection and *en bloc* lymphadenectomy (Figure 6).

97

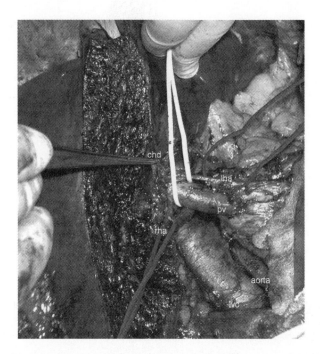

Fig. 6 Radical lymphadenectomy for the treatment of gallbladder carcinoma.

The extent of the liver resection is determined by the degree of invasion of the liver and the surgeon's desire for radicality. For tumours with early muscularis invasion, radical cholecystectomy with resection of the gallbladder bed to yield a centimetre-thick block of hepatic tissue is probably sufficient. For tumours invading beyond the muscularis, a formal segment IVb and V liver resection is indicated as a minimum requirement. For cases with more extensive hepatic involvement or encroachment upon hilar structures, right trisectionectomy (extended right hemihepatectomy) and caudate lobectomy is indicated.

Because of the risk of early nodal spread, radical lymphadenectomy should be performed in all cases. This should include all nodal sites in the hepatoduodenal ligament, retropancreatic, coeliac and para-aortic nodes as described for hilar tumours. This lymphadenectomy is most easily accomplished by excising the extrahepatic biliary tree below the hepatic duct confluence *en bloc* with the gallbladder, liver and associated neural and lymphatic tissue from the hepatoduodenal ligament. The alternative is to dissect out and preserve the bile duct; however, this is less radical and runs the risk of devascularising the bile duct, with subsequent ischaemic stricturing. If the cystic duct is involved with tumour then excision of the entire extrahepatic biliary tree is mandatory.

INCIDENTAL GALLBLADDER CARCINOMA

Incidental gallbladder carcinoma discovered at, or following, routine cholecystectomy merits special consideration. These cases fall into one of four groups:

1. Obvious carcinoma at laparoscopy. These cases should be abandoned *without intraoperative biopsy* and referred immediately to a specialist centre for evaluation.

2. The 'difficult cholecystectomy' for an abnormal, thick-walled gallbladder, presumed to be inflammatory but subsequently proven to be carcinoma on histology. These cases inevitably develop widespread peritoneal disease and port-site recurrence. Early repeat surgery with liver resection, lymphadenectomy and port-site resection is often advocated. However, the long-term results are poor; restaging with laparoscopy is essential prior to resection.

3. Incidental finding of early gallbladder carcinoma in a gallbladder removed intact at routine cholecystectomy. If there is only mucosal invasion, cholecystectomy may be all that is required. For tumours with involvement of the muscularis, further segmental hepatic resection, lymphadenectomy and port-site excision may be necessary.

4. Incidental finding of early carcinoma in a gallbladder inadvertently opened intraoperatively. Even in early disease confined to the mucosa, peritoneal seeding and port-site recurrence become highly likely. Patients should be laparoscoped and if clear treated according to the depth of gallbladder wall invasion.

NON-SURGICAL TREATMENT

As with cholangiocarcinoma, many patients are very elderly or frail and present with advanced disease. For these cases, early palliative care referral is the most humane and appropriate management. For fit patients with inoperable disease, chemotherapy may be considered; however, this has a minimal effect on the outcome of the disease.

There is no role at present for adjuvant or neoadjuvant chemotherapy. Although newer agents such as gemcitabine have shown some promise, there is little evidence that they improve the overall median survival. Radiotherapy may be useful for the palliation of bone metastases, but is otherwise ineffective.

INTRAHEPATIC CHOLANGIOCARCINOMA

This condition is subject to the same aetiology and pathology as hilar cholangiocarcinoma. Small peripherally placed tumours are the easiest to deal with as they are usually amenable to either segmental resection or hemihepatectomy. Unfortunately, these tumours often have few symptoms and therefore late presentation is common, when more extensive resections are required. Although tumours with hepatic vein or inferior vena cava invasion may still be technically operable in experienced hands, their long-term outlook is bleak. Centrally placed lesions are frequently inoperable due to bilateral involvement of portal structures above the hilum. The role of radical lymphadenectomy is less clear-cut than with hilar tumours, since there is little value in performing a radical extrahepatic lymphadenectomy unless the intrahepatic lymphatics draining the tumour are also resected. With this logic, the minimum resection should be hemihepatectomy. Many Japanese and South Korean centres have adopted this approach and have reported 20–30% 5-year survival rates. Caudate lobectomy is not routinely practised.

CONCLUSIONS

Cholangiocarcinoma is a major surgical challenge. Recent advances in operative techniques and perioperative management have led to high resectability rates and improved survival data even in patients with locally advanced disease. Patients with intrahepatic, hilar and gallbladder cholangiocarcinomas should all be assessed in specialist hepatobiliary units. In operable cases an aggressive surgical approach is warranted combining hepatic resection with regional lymphadenectomy. Conservative bile duct resections cannot be supported as part of modern surgical practice for this condition.

Key points for clinical practice

- There is a fourfold rise in the incidence of cholangiocarcinoma over the last few decades. Intrahepatic cholangiocarcinoma now accounts for more deaths than hepatoma in the UK.

- Recently, with aggressive surgical approach, higher resection rates with good median survival have been reported.

- The medical and surgical treatment of ulcerative colitis does not appear to influence the subsequent development of biliary tract cancer.

- Biopsy of the suspected tumour is contraindicated in operable disease because of the high risk of needle track and peritoneal seeding.

- Radical surgery remains the only means of possible cure in patients with cholangiocarcinoma.

- The role of radiotherapy and chemotherapy in the treatment of cholangiocarcinoma remains limited.

References

1. Sako S, Seitzinger GL, Garside E. Carcinoma of the extrahepatic bile ducts: Review of the literature and report of six cases. *Surgery* 1957; **41**: 416.
2. Taylor-Robinson SD, Toledano MB, Arora S *et al*. Increase in mortality rates from intrahepatic cholangiocarcinoma in England and Wales 1968–98. *Gut* 2001; **48**: 754–755.
3. Brown G, Myers N. The hepatic ducts. A surgical approach for resection of tumour. *Aust NZ J Surg* 1954; **23**: 308–312.
4. Edmondson HA, Steiner PE. Primary carcinoma of the liver. A study of 100 cases among 48,900 necropsies. *Cancer* 1954; **7**: 462–503.
5. Klatskin G. Adenocarcinoma of the hepatic duct at its bifurcation within the porta hepatis. *Am J Med* 1965; **38**: 241–256.
6. Iwasaki Y, Ohto M, Todoroki T *et al*. Treatment of carcinoma of the biliary system. *Surg Gynecol Obstet* 1977; **144**: 219–224.

7. Launois B, Campion JP, Brisset P *et al*. Carcinoma of the hepatic hilus: surgical treatment and the case for resection. *Ann Surg* 1979; **190**: 151–157.

8. Bismuth H, Corlette MB. Intrahepatic cholangioenteric anastomosis in carcinoma of the hilus of the liver. *Surg Gynecol Obstet* 1975; **140**: 170–178.

9. Bismuth H, Nakache R, Diamond T. Management strategies in resection for hilar cholangiocarcinoma. *Ann Surg* 1992; **215**: 31–38.

10. Lodge JPA, Ammori BJ. Aggressive surgery for hilar cholangiocarcinoma: Is it worthwhile? *Gut* 1999; **44(Suppl)**: A49.

11. Nimura Y, Hayakawa N, Kamiya J *et al*. Hepatic segmentectomy with caudate lobe resection for bile duct carcinoma of the hepatic hilus. *World J Surg* 1990; **14**: 535–544.

12. Pichlmayr R, Weimann A, Klempnauer J *et al*. Surgical treatment in proximal bile duct cancer. A single centre experience. *Ann Surg* 1996; **224**: 628–638.

13. Sugiura Y, Nakamura S, Iida S *et al*. Extensive resection of the bile ducts combined with liver resection for cancer of the main hepatic duct junction: a cooperative study of the Keio bile duct cancer study group. *Surgery* 1994; **115**: 445–451.

14. Jarnagin W, Fong Y, DeMatteo R *et al*. Staging, resectability, and outcome in 225 patients with hilar cholangiocarcinoma. *Ann Surg* 2001; **234**: 507–519.

15. Kitagawa Y, Nagino M, Kamiya J, et al. Lymph node metastasis from hilar cholangiocarcinoma: audit of 110 patients who underwent regional and paraaortic node dissection. *Ann Surg* 2001; **233**: 385–392.

16. Kosuge T, Yamamoto J, Shimada K *et al*. Improved surgical results for hilar cholangiocarcinoma with procedures including major hepatic resection. *Ann Surg* 1999; **230**: 663–671.

17. Kosuge T, Yamamoto J, Shimada K *et al*. Improved surgical results for hilar cholangiocarcinoma with procedures including major hepatic resection. *Ann Surg* 1999; **230**: 663–671.

18. Launois B, Terblanche J, Lakehal M *et al*. Proximal bile duct cancer: high resectability rate and five year survival. *Ann Surg* 1999; **230**: 266–275.

19. Lodge JPA, Ammori BJ, Miller GV *et al*. Surgery for hilar cholangiocarcinoma: early results. *Dig Surg* 1999; **16 (Suppl 1)**: 71.

20. Meyer CG, Penn I, James L. Liver transplantation for cholangiocarcinoma: results in 207 patients. *Transplantation* 2000; **69**: 1633–1637.

21. Longmire WP Jr, Mcarthur MS,Bastounis EA *et al*. Carcinoma of extrahepatic biliary tract. *Ann Surg* 1973; **178**: 333.

22. Ross AP, Braaasch JW, Warren KW. Carcinoma of proximal bile ducts. *Surg Gynecol Obstet* 1973; **136**: 923.

23. Todani T, Tabuchi K, Watanabe Y *et al*. Carcinoma arising in the wall of congenital bile duct cysts. *Cancer* 1979; **44**: 1134.

24. Voyles CR, Smadja C, Shands WC *et al*. Carcinoma in choledochal cysts: age related incidence. *Arch Surg* 1963; **118**: 986.

25. Bloustein PA. Association of carcinoma with congenital cystic conditions of liver and bile ducts. *Am J Gastroenterol* 1977; **67**: 40.

26. Dayton MT, Longmire WP Jr, Tompkins RK. Caroli's disease: a premalignant condition? *Am J Surg* 1983; **145**: 41.

27. Black K, Hanna SS, Langer B *et al*. Management of carcinoma of the extrahepatic bile ducts. *Can J Surg* 1978; **21**: 542.

28. Koo J, Ho J, Wong J *et al*. Mucoepidermoid carcinoma of the bile duct. *Ann Surg* 1982; **196**: 140.

29. Braasch JW. Carcinoma of the bile ducts. *Surg Clin North Am* 1973; **53**: 1217.

30. Iemoto Y, Kondo J, Fukamachi S. Biliary cystadenocarcinoma with peritoneal carcinomatosis. *Cancer* 1982; **48**: 1664.

31. Farris FB, Faust BF. Granular cell tumours of biliary ducts. *Arch Pathol Lab Med* 1979; **103**: 510.

32. Kuwayti K, Baggenstoss AH, Stauffler MH *et al*. Carcinoma of major intrahepatic and extrahepatic bile ducts exclusive of papilla of vater. *Surg Gynecol Obstet* 1953; **104**: 357.

33. Sons HU,Borchard F. Carcinoma of extrahepatic bile ducts: a post-mortem study of 65 cases and review of literature. *J Surg Oncol* 1987; **34**: 6.

34. International Union Against Cancer (UICC). *TNM Classification of Malignant Tumours*, 5th edn. New York: Wiley-Liss, 1997.

35. Burke EC, Jarnagin WR, Hochwald SN *et al*. Hilar cholangiocarcinoma: patterns of spread, the importance of hepatic resection for curative operation, and a presurgical clinical staging system. *Ann Surg* 1998; **228**: 385–394.

36. Neuhaus P, Jonas S, Bechstein WO *et al*. Extended resections for hilar cholangiocarcinoma. *Ann Surg* 1999; **230**: 808–818.

37. van Delden OM, de Wit LT, van Dijkum EJMN *et al*. Value of laparoscopic ultrasonography in staging of proximal bile duct tumours. *J Ultrasound Med* 1997; **16**: 7–12.

38. Vollmer CM, Drebin JA, Middleton WD *et al*. Utility of staging laparoscopy in subsets of peripancreatic and biliary malignancies. *Ann Surg* 2002; **235**: 1–7.

39. Gores GJ. Early detection and treatment of cholangiocarcinoma. *Curr Treat Options Gastroenterol* 2003; **6**: 105–112.

40. Makuuchi M, Thai BL, Takayasu K *et al*. Preoperative portal embolisation to increase safety of major hepatectomy for hilar bile duct carcinoma: a preliminary report. *Surgery* 1990; **107**: 521–527.

41. Nagino M, Nimura Y, Kamiya J *et al*. Right or left trisegment portal vein embolization before hepatic trisegmentectomy for hilar bile duct carcinoma. *Surgery* 1995; **117**: 677–681.

42. Tsukada K, Yoshida K, Aono T *et al*. Major hepatectomy and pancreatoduodenectomy for advanced carcinoma of the biliary tract. *Br J Surg* 1994; **81**: 108–110.

43. Miyazaki M, Ito H, Nakagawa K *et al*. Parenchyma-preserving hepatectomy in the surgical treatment of hilar cholangiocarcinoma. *J Am Coll Surg* 1999; **189**: 575–583.

44. Mizumoto R, Kawarada Y, Suzuki H. Surgical treatment of hilar carcinoma of the bile duct. *Surg Gynecol Obstet* 1986; **162**: 153–159.

45. Tsao JI, Nimura M, Kamiya J *et al*. Management of hilar cholangiocarcinoma: comparison of an American and a Japanese experience. *Ann Surg* 2000; **232**: 166–174.

46. Oberfield RA, Rossi RL. The role of chemotherapy in the treatment of bile duct carcinoma. *World J Surg* 1988; **12**: 105–108

47. Harder J, Blum HE. Cholangiocarcinoma. *Schweiz Rondsch Med Prax* 2002; **91**: 1352–1356.

48. Piehler JM, Crichlow RW. Primary carcinoma of gallbladder. *Surg Gynecol Obstet* 1978; **147**: 929.

49. Carty NJ, Johnson CD. Carcinoma of the gallbladder: a survey of cases in Wessex 1982–1989. *J R Coll Surg Edinb* 1991; **36**: 238–241.

50. Grobmyer SR, Lieberman MD, Daly JM. Gallbladder cancer in the twentieth century: Single Institution's Experience. *World J Surg* 2003; **28**: 47–49.

51. Noshiro H, Chijiiwak K, Yamaguchi K, Shimizu S, Sugitani A, Tanaka M. Factors affecting surgical outcome for gallbladder carcinoma. *Hepatogastroenterology* 2003; **50**: 939–944.

52. Mancuso TF, Brennan MJ: Epidemiological consideration of cancer of the gallbladder, bile duct and salivary glands in rubber industry. *J Occup Med* 1970; **12**: 333.

53. Nevin JE, Moran TJ, Kay S, King R. Carcinoma of gallbladder. *Cancer* 1976; **37**: 141–148.

Colin D. Johnson

8

Oral intake and enteral feeding in acute pancreatitis

Many surgeons believe that the management of acute pancreatitis should start from the concept of 'pancreatic rest'. Based on a simple understanding of pancreatic physiology and a belief that further stimulation of the pancreas during an attack of pancreatitis would exacerbate the inflammatory process by releasing more enzymes, traditional teaching has been that it is necessary to avoid all oral intake to prevent any inappropriate stimulation of pancreatic enzyme production. This concept is now known to be completely wrong.

First, although early events of acute pancreatitis probably do include enzyme activation, we now know that pancreatic enzyme synthesis is virtually abolished early in the course of acute pancreatitis.[1,2] There is therefore no need to avoid stimuli that might release cholecystokinin from the intestine. Second, many patients with acute pancreatitis have a relatively mild attack that resolves rapidly and spontaneously. There is now wide clinical experience that such patients require no special manipulation of oral intake other than withholding food during the period of pain and anorexia. Third, our understanding of the pathophysiology of severe acute pancreatitis includes the appreciation of the role of the gut mucosa in preventing endotoxin absorption. During the systemic inflammatory response that leads to organ failure, the integrity or otherwise of the mucosal barrier is a major determinant of outcome. Rather than resting the gut, it may be necessary to supply it with nutrients in order to maintain the integrity of this mucosal barrier.

MILD ACUTE PANCREATITIS

NASOGASTRIC DRAINAGE

Some textbooks still advocate the placement of a nasogastric tube for all patients with acute pancreatitis. This is unnecessary in patients with mild

Mr Colin D. Johnson MChir FRCS, Reader in Surgery, University Surgical Unit, F Level Centre Block (816), Southampton General Hospital, Southampton SO16 6YD, UK

disease. The only indication for nasogastric aspiration should be persistent nausea or vomiting in a patient with severe disease.

Patients with mild acute pancreatitis have pain but rarely have persistent nausea. No benefit is obtained by nasogastric aspiration. Three randomised trials showed no benefit for the use of a nasogastric tube in mild acute pancreatitis.[3-5] These studies also showed clearly that in patients with mild pancreatitis a nasogastric tube is uncomfortable to the patient, and does not affect the duration of pain, time to bowel opening, or duration of hospital stay.

ORAL INTAKE

If nasogastric intubation is unnecessary in mild acute pancreatitis, what should be the policy regarding oral intake? Clinical experience shows that it is not necessary to apply any restriction of fluid intake in these patients. Some years ago we abandoned the policy of restricting oral fluids. This followed the observation that patients with episodes of recurrent acute pancreatitis could safely manage their own acute attacks at home, by avoiding food, but continuing oral liquids. The appreciation of the role of gut mucosal barrier in severe acute pancreatitis and the growing evidence of the safety of enteral nutrition (see below) led us to conclude that oral intake of fluid would be safe in patients with mild disease. Our policy therefore is to allow free oral fluids in these patients.

FLUID MANAGEMENT IN MILD ACUTE PANCREATITIS

Immediately after diagnosis of acute pancreatitis we place an intravenous line for fluid resuscitation. Supplemental oxygen is also given until the initial severity has been determined. In the absence of any sign of organ failure, or other feature predicting a severe attack, oxygen supplements are discontinued and intravenous fluids are maintained for 24–48 hours. During this time the patient is fasted until an ultrasound scan has been obtained on the morning after admission. Following this, free oral fluids are allowed, including drinks such as tea or coffee. Typically during the first 24 hours, the patient is anorexic and oral fluid intake will be less than normal. On the second or third day, as the inflammation and pain settle, appetite returns and full oral fluid intake is resumed.

We have observed no complications or disadvantages with this regimen for patients with mild acute pancreatitis, and it appears that there is no value in restricting oral fluid intake other than for the requirements of imaging investigations or before general anaesthetic procedures.

Key point 1

- In mild acute pancreatitis nasogastric intubation and drainage is not necessary. Free oral fluid intake is safe in these patients.

SEVERE ACUTE PANCREATITIS

THE ROLE OF THE GUT

In severe acute pancreatitis there is a substantial systemic inflammatory response, which is now accepted as the basis of early organ failure. Nearly half the patients have evidence of organ failure at the time of admission.[6,7] The progression of the systemic inflammatory response syndrome (SIRS) to organ failure is believed to depend on a 'second hit' that leads to over-stimulation of an already-primed immune system. In acute pancreatitis the pancreatic inflammation is the 'first hit' and it is believed that absorption of endotoxin from the intestine provides the 'second hit' that over-stimulates the already-primed immune system.

Absorption of endotoxin undoubtedly occurs in severe acute pancreatitis. Exley et al.[7] showed that endotoxaemia was much more frequent in severe acute pancreatitis than in mild pancreatitis. The absorbed endotoxin stimulates release of tumour necrosis factor (TNF) from circulating monocytes in a phasic pulsatile manner that makes the detection of elevated TNF levels rather difficult. However, following combination of TNF with its cell surface receptor, the TNF/receptor complex is shed from the cell and this soluble TNF receptor (sTNFR) can be measured relatively easily. De Beaux et al.[8] demonstrated high levels of sTNFR in patients with severe pancreatitis. The most likely stimulus for this process is endotoxin absorbed from the gut.

MUCOSAL PERMEABILITY

Patients with predicted severe acute pancreatitis studied during the first few days of the attack demonstrate increased absorption from the gut of experimental markers. These macromolecules are normally not absorbed, but may diffuse out of the gut when the mucosa is abnormally permeable. Ammori et al.[9] showed that intestinal permeability was increased in severe acute pancreatitis but not in mild disease, and also that intestinal permeability correlated with endotoxin absorption rather than bacterial translocation.[10] In a subsequent paper they also showed that these changes correlated with a marker of intestinal mucosal ischaemia, lending support to the concept of ischaemic injury leading to absorption of endotoxin.[11]

The integrity of the mucosal barrier depends on a number of factors. Obviously an adequate blood supply is important to allow sufficient oxygen delivery to maintain the metabolism of the gut mucosa cells. Two other mechanisms also play a role: gastrointestinal hormones and the presence of nutrients in the lumen (Fig. 1).

Gastrointestinal mucosa is under the constant trophic influence of a number of hormones, including gastrin and cholecystokinin (CCK). These hormones are necessary to maintain normal division and growth of mucosal cells. The widespread mucosal atrophy seen in patients who receive long-term parenteral nutrition is thought to be due in part to the absence of hormone release normally triggered by ingestion of food.

However, the most important determinant of mucosal viability is the presence of luminal nutrients. Mucosal cells derive almost all their nutrient requirements from the gut lumen, rather than from the blood stream. Mucosal

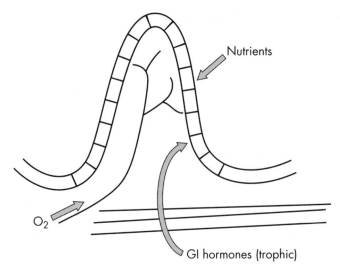

Fig. 1 What maintains healthy gut?

atrophy occurs in any part of the intestine deprived of normal luminal content, which is the major factor in the enteric mucosal atrophy of patients receiving parenteral nutrition,[12,13] and in the colonic mucosal atrophy in patients who have a proximal diverting stoma (diversion colitis).[14,15]

Thus there is clearly a theoretical justification for attempts to maintain delivery of nutrients to the gut in patients with severe acute pancreatitis, in order to prevent loss of mucosal integrity, and the consequent absorption of endotoxin.

Key point 2

- The integrity of the gut mucosa is of crucial importance in severe acute pancreatitis. General measures to maintain the perfusion and oxygenation of the gut are clearly of great importance. All patients require adequate fluid resuscitation and oxygen supplements.

Key point 3

- Theoretical evidence to support nutrient supply to the gut is sufficient justification for studies to determine the practicality and safety of enteral feeding to prevent complications in severe acute pancreatitis.

EARLY ENTERAL NUTRITION TO PREVENT COMPLICATIONS

Some early studies investigated the possibility of enteral feeding in patients with mild acute pancreatitis. These demonstrated the absence of any harmful effects in these patients. However, patients with mild pancreatitis respond rapidly to simple measures, without complication. There is no justification for additional enteral feeding in these patients.

In contrast, patients with severe acute pancreatitis might benefit substantially from enteral nutrition. Such patients may be anorexic or nauseated, and will have difficulty in drinking significant amounts of nutrient fluids. There may be duodenal ileus as a consequence of peripancreatic inflammation. These patients are most likely to benefit from an intervention designed to maintain mucosal integrity and so reduce the absorption of endotoxin from the gut.

The first clinical trials of enteral feeding in severe acute pancreatitis were all concerned with the comparison of enteral against parenteral feeding. Most made an attempt to provide isocaloric feeding to the two patient groups. This was a reasonable trial design, which sought to examine the effect of the route of nutritional supplementation, while ensuring that patients in the treatment and control groups all received a nutrient supplement.

These trials[16–19] are consistent in showing the safety of enteral nutrition. There were very few feeding-related complications in the enterally fed patients – mostly diarrhoea. Catheter-related sepsis was the main complication of parenteral nutrition. The use of enteral nutrition appears to be associated with fewer complications of pancreatitis (Table 1), and although there was no difference in hospital stay, enterally fed patients had fewer operations and fewer ITU admissions (Table 2). All authors concluded that the enteral route should be preferred to parenteral feeding early in the treatment of acute pancreatitis for reasons of fewer treatment-related complications, fewer septic complications, lower cost, more rapid return of intestinal function or more rapid resolution of markers of the inflammatory response.

However, the findings of these trials can be interpreted to suggest that while enteral feeding may be safe early in acute pancreatitis, the differences observed may arise because parenteral feeding is associated with more complications, particularly related to infection. Powell et al.[20] therefore compared early enteral

Table 1. Complications of pancreatitis in patients with predicted severe attack randomised to either enteral nutrition (EN) or parenteral nutrition (PN)

Study	Complication	EN	PN
Kalfarentzos et al.[17]	Pancreatic complication	2/18	7/20
	Septic	5/18	10/20
Windsor et al.[19]	Systemic inflammatory response syndrome	2/16	10/18
	Multiple organ failure	0	5/18
Gupta et al.[16]	ITU admission	0	5/18
	Organ failure	0/8	6/9
Olah et al.[18]	Necrosis	12/41	16/48
	Sepsis	5/41	13/48
	Multiple organ failure	2/41	5/48

Table 2. Clinical outcome in predicted severe acute pancreatitis (combined data from four studies[8,16,18,19])

	EN (n=83)	PN (n=95)
Hospital stay (days) (mean values from 3 studies)	7, 12.5, 40	10, 15, 39
Mean ITU stay (days) (one study)	11	12
Patients with: Multiple organ failure	2	10
Operation	8	18
Death	3	8

feeding with no nutritional supplements. They found no difference in markers of the inflammatory response or clinical outcome between the enterally fed and control groups. However, this study was small, and further data from a larger number of patients are required before a beneficial effect of early enteral nutrition can be excluded.

Key point 4

- In severe acute pancreatitis early enteral nutrition is safe, although the benefits of this approach remain unproven. Early parenteral nutrition may be harmful.

NUTRITIONAL SUPPORT AFTER THE EARLY PHASE

The above discussion relates to enteral nutrition designed as a means of protecting the gut mucosa and preventing absorption of endotoxin. The rationale for early enteral nutrition is that it might reduce the severity of acute pancreatitis. In patients with established severe pancreatitis it is necessary to provide nutritional support for the body's metabolic needs. In these patients it is feasible to provide at least some of the calories by the enteral route, although there may be difficulties associated with ileus in those who are severely ill.[21] Consideration of prolonged nutritional support is beyond the scope of this chapter. However, it is believed that in acute pancreatitis, in common with many other critical illnesses, administration of at least some calories by the enteral route is beneficial, not only for maintaining the gut mucosal barrier but also to improve the metabolic use of the nutrients provided.

ROUTE OF ADMINISTRATION

In the management of acute pancreatitis it is often assumed that the enteral nutrients should be delivered to the jejunum, although this assumption is based on theoretical considerations only. As we have seen above, it is not necessary to avoid nutrients in the duodenum, from fear of stimulating release of CCK. In acute pancreatitis the gland is unresponsive to hormonal stimulation, so the passage of nutrients through the duodenum is unlikely to cause any harm.

The frequent observation of duodenal oedema and duodenal ileus secondary to peripancreatic inflammation has prompted the belief that enteral nutrients should be delivered by nasojejunal tube, to ensure that they reach the absorptive mucosa. However, the advice to place a nasojejunal tube ignores the practical difficulty that duodenal oedema will also impede the passage of the tube. In practice, even after successful placement of a nasojejunal tube, the tube will often be displaced back into the stomach, with no ill effect.

These observations led the Glasgow group to explore the feasibility of nasogastric administration.[22] They found that this was possible in approximately 80% of patients with severe acute pancreatitis. The early administration of enteral feeding was particularly favourable to successful use of the nasogastric route.

Key point 5

- If enteral feeding is to be used in the first week of acute pancreatitis, it should be started early, and it is usually possible to achieve by the nasogastric route.

CONCLUSIONS

Patients with acute pancreatitis do not require 'pancreatic rest'. On the contrary, there is potential benefit from maintaining nutrient supply to the gut. There is no justification for the use of a nasogastric tube in patients with mild acute pancreatitis. These patients can be allowed free intake of oral fluids until their appetite returns.

In severe acute pancreatitis early enteral nutrition during the first week may be considered as a means of supporting the gut mucosa, with the rationale that this may reduce endotoxin absorption and minimise the risk of complications. The evidence suggests that such early enteral nutrition is safe, but there is insufficient evidence at present that early enteral nutrition confers an advantage over no nutrition. Early parenteral nutrition should be avoided.

In the later stages of the disease nutritional support of metabolic requirements is essential. If possible, this should be delivered by the enteral route, for metabolic reasons. However, supplementation with parenteral feeding may be necessary if intestinal absorption is inadequate.

Key points for clinical practice

- In mild acute pancreatitis nasogastric intubation and drainage is not necessary. Free oral fluid intake is safe in these patients.

- The integrity of the gut mucosa is of crucial importance in severe acute pancreatitis. General measures to maintain the perfusion and oxygenation of the gut are clearly of great importance. All patients require adequate fluid resuscitation and oxygen supplements.

- Theoretical evidence to support nutrient supply to the gut is sufficient justification for studies to determine the practicality and safety of enteral feeding to prevent complications in severe acute pancreatitis.

- In severe acute pancreatitis early enteral nutrition is safe, although the benefits of this approach remain unproven. Early parenteral nutrition may be harmful.

- If enteral feeding is to be used in the first week of acute pancreatitis, it should be started early, and it is usually possible to achieve by the nasogastric route.

References

1. Iovanna JL, Keim V, Michel R, Dagorn JC. Pancreatic gene expression is altered during acute experimental pancreatitis in the rat. *Am J Physiol* 1991; **261**: G485–G489.
2. Niederau C et al. Pancreatic exocrine secretion in acute experimental pancreatitis. *Gastroenterology* 1990; **99**: 1120–1127.
3. Sarr MG, Sanfey H, Cameron JL. Prospective, randomized trial of nasogastric suction in patients with acute pancreatitis. *Surgery* 1986; **100**: 500–504.
4. Goff JS, Feinberg LE, Brugge WR. A randomized trial comparing cimetidine to nasogastric suction in acute pancreatitis. *Dig Dis Sci* 1982; **27**: 1085–1088.
5. Naeije R, Salingret E, Clumeck N, De Troyer A, Devis G. Is nasogastric suction necessary in acute pancreatitis? *BMJ* 1978; **ii**: 659–660.
6. Johnson CD et al. Double blind, randomised, placebo controlled study of a platelet activating factor antagonist, lexipafant, in the treatment and prevention of organ failure in predicted severe acute pancreatitis. *Gut* 2001; **48**: 62–69.
7. Exley AR, Leese T, Holliday MP, Swann RA, Cohen J. Endotoxaemia and serum tumour necrosis factor as prognostic markers in severe acute pancreatitis. *Gut* 1992; **33**: 1126–1128.
8. de Beaux AC, Goldie AS, Ross JA, Carter DC, Fearon KC. Serum concentrations of inflammatory mediators related to organ failure in patients with acute pancreatitis. *Br J Surg* 1996; **83**: 349–353.
9. Ammori BJ et al. Early increase in intestinal permeability in patients with severe acute pancreatitis: correlation with endotoxemia, organ failure, and mortality. *J Gastrointest Surg* 1999; **3**: 252–262.
10. Ammori BJ, Fitzgerald P, Hawkey P, McMahon MJ. The early increase in intestinal permeability and systemic endotoxin exposure in patients with severe acute pancreatitis is not associated with systemic bacterial translocation: molecular investigation of microbial DNA in the blood. *Pancreas* 2003; **26**: 18–22.
11. Rahman SH, Ammori BJ, Holmfield J, Larvin M, McMahon MJ. Intestinal hypoperfusion contributes to gut barrier failure in severe acute pancreatitis. *J Gastrointest Surg* 2003; **7**: 26–35.

12. Sasaki M, Fitzgerald AJ, Mandir N, Berlanga-Acosta J, Goodlad RA. Keratinocyte growth factor and epidermal growth factor can reverse the intestinal atrophy associated with elemental diets in mice. *Exp Physiol* 2003; **88**: 261–267.

13. Goodlad RA, Lee CY, Wright NA. Cell proliferation in the small intestine and colon of intravenously fed rats: effects of urogastrone–epidermal growth factor. *Cell Prolif* 1992; **25**: 393–404.

14. Whelan RL, Abramson D, Kim DS, Hashmi HF. Diversion colitis. A prospective study. *Surg Endosc* 1994; **8**: 19–24.

15. Roe AM, Warren BF, Brodribb AJ, Brown C. Diversion colitis and involution of the defunctioned anorectum. *Gut* 1993; **34**: 382–385.

16. Gupta R *et al*. A randomised clinical trial to assess the effect of total enteral and total parenteral nutritional support on metabolic, inflammatory and oxidative markers in patients with predicted severe acute pancreatitis (APACHE II $\geq$ 6). *Pancreatology* 2003; **3**: 406–413.

17. Kalfarentzos F, Kehagias J, Mead N, Kokkinis K, Gogos CA. Enteral nutrition is superior to parenteral nutrition in severe acute pancreatitis: results of a randomized prospective trial. *Br J Surg* 1997; **84**: 1665–1669.

18. Olah A *et al*. Early nasojejunal feeding in acute pancreatitis is associated with a lower complication rate. *Nutrition* 2002; **18**: 259–262.

19. Windsor AC *et al*. Compared with parenteral nutrition, enteral feeding attenuates the acute phase response and improves disease severity in acute pancreatitis. *Gut* 1998; **42**: 431–435.

20. Powell JJ, Murchison JT, Fearon KC, Ross JA, Siriwardena AK. Randomized controlled trial of the effect of early enteral nutrition on markers of the inflammatory response in predicted severe acute pancreatitis. *Br J Surg* 2000; **87**: 1375–1381.

21. Abou-Assi S, Craig K, O'Keefe SJ. Hypocaloric jejunal feeding is better than total parenteral nutrition in acute pancreatitis: results of a randomized comparative study. *Am J Gastroenterol* 2002; **97**: 2255–2262.

22. Eatock FC *et al*. Nasogastric feeding in severe acute pancreatitis may be practical and safe. *Int J Pancreatol* 2000; **28**: 23–29.

Åke Andrén-Sandberg

9

Treatment of pancreatic pseudocysts

A pseudocyst presents as a cystic cavity bound to the pancreas by inflammatory tissue.[1] Typically the wall of a pancreatic pseudocyst lacks an epithelial lining, and the cyst contains pancreatic juice or amylase-rich fluid.[2,3] Today the most widely used definitions make a difference between peripancreatic fluid collections, pseudocysts and pancreatic abscess, as in the Atlanta classification system for acute pancreatitis.[4] Description of the separate entity of acute fluid collections is important as it represents an earlier point in the development of acute pseudocysts and abscesses. Distinction between pseudocysts and acute fluid collections leads to a better understanding of the natural history of peripancreatic fluid collections and facilitates the treatment of these as two separate entities, even though they are a part of a continuous pathological process.

A pseudocyst is usually rich in pancreatic enzymes and is most often sterile. Formation of a pseudocyst by definition requires 4 or more weeks (some clinicians state 6) from the onset of acute pancreatitis.[5] In this regard, an acute pseudocyst is a fluid collection that arises in association with an episode of acute pancreatitis, is of more than 4 weeks' duration, and is surrounded by a defined wall. Fluid collections of less than 4 weeks' duration that lack a defined wall are more properly termed acute fluid collections. In contrast, chronic pseudocysts have a well-defined wall, but arise in patients with chronic pancreatitis and lack an antecedent episode of acute pancreatitis.

It is important to note that in the classification the terms 'acute' and 'chronic' refer to the pancreatitis behind the pseudocyst and not to the presentation of the pseudocyst itself. This means that an acute pseudocyst may have been known for months, whereas a chronic pseudocyst in the next patient has been documented for only a week or two.

Prof. Åke Andrén-Sandberg MD PhD, Department of Gastrointestinal Surgery, Sentralsjukehuset i Rogaland, 4069 Stavanger, Norway

Bacteria may be present or not in a pseudocyst culture. However, a pseudocyst is defined as a fluid collection without clinical signs of infection. The term 'infected pseudocyst' is a less well-chosen term as it has no exact definition. Moreover, it is probably from a biological point of view impossible to find a border between this infected fluid collection and an abscess. On the other hand, most positive cultures from pseudocysts without clinical signs of infection are of no clinical significance and probably represent contamination during the culture procedure. When obvious pus is present, the lesion is of course more correctly termed a pancreatic abscess.[4]

Key point 1

- By definition, a pseudocyst must be present for at least 4 weeks. 'Acute' and 'chronic' pseudocysts refer to the nature of the preceding pancreatitis, not the duration of the cyst.

INCIDENCE

Pseudocysts were once considered to be an unusual complication of pancreatitis. As recently as 1968, Becker and colleagues[6] wrote: 'The experience (with pseudocysts) in most large surgical clinics is limited to relatively few patients'. Some earlier studies, based on upper gastrointestinal series, reported an extremely low incidence (1.6–4.5%) of pseudocyst formation, regardless of the cause (0.5–1 per 100 000 adults per year).[7-13]

INCIDENCE OF PSEUDOCYSTS AFTER ACUTE PANCREATITIS

The estimated incidence of peripancreatic fluid collections after acute pancreatitis is dependent both on how a pseudocyst is defined and on how it should be looked for. The incidence has increased with the advent of ultrasonography and computed tomography (CT). However, some authors still favour the terms pancreatic and peripancreatic fluid collections, which now encompass two separate entities such as acute fluid collection and acute pseudocyst.[5] Others have used the term pseudocyst without any explanation,[14-16] which makes it very difficult to evaluate what they have found. Altogether, there is, however, agreement that significant fluid collections develop in 30–60% of cases of acute pancreatitis.[4] Many of these acute fluid collections resolve without formation of a pseudocyst.

Key point 2

- Acute fluid collections are common after a severe episode of acute pancreatitis. Most resolve without formation of a pseudocyst.

INCIDENCE OF PSEUDOCYSTS IN CHRONIC PANCREATITIS

Pseudocysts in chronic pancreatitis have a higher incidence compared with acute pancreatitis. Incidence figures of 20–40% have been reported in the literature.[17-19] However, there is a lack of precise data based on long-term follow-up of patients with chronic pancreatitis – in contrast to acute pseudocysts, the patient with chronic pancreatitis may have 10, 20 or more years with the disease, which gives a high risk of developing pseudocysts at least once over a long period of sickness. Also, there must be a criterion concerning size regarding chronic pseudocysts: is it a pseudocyst if it is only seen at resection or in the microscope or must it be larger than 0.5, 1 or more centimetres in diameter? There are pathologists who advocate that microcysts are an integral part of the histologic picture of chronic pancreatitis, which makes the term pseudocyst merely a matter of definition of size – and maybe of the severity of the desmoplastic reaction and the duration of the disease.

NATURAL HISTORY

The widespread application of ultrasonography and CT has advanced our knowledge of the natural history of pancreatic pseudocysts. The quality of data about spontaneous resolution of acute pseudocysts varies from study to study, and when there is no precise definition of the pseudocyst and when alcohol is the major cause selection bias can occur that threatens the reliability of the results. The only documented mode of resolution is spontaneous rupture of a pancreatic pseudocyst into the adjacent organs.[20,21] The other supposed mechanisms are merely based on speculations rather than facts. Since resolution, when it does take place, seems to be complete within a few days, it may be unlikely that anterior transmural absorption is taking place in the absence of peritoneal signs of the development of ascites. A theoretical possibility is that in such cases drainage into the extrapancreatic retroperitoneal tissues as well as internal drainage through the pancreatic ductal system after clearance of a temporary obstruction of the duct may take place.[22]

RESOLUTION OF ACUTE PSEUDOCYSTS

Earlier studies suggest that spontaneous resolution of an acute pseudocyst occurred in 8–70% of patients,[20,23-26] i.e. the span of results is so wide that no conclusions can be drawn except that spontaneous resolution does occur. However, some important limitations are present in these studies. When diagnosis is based on clinical presentation, barium meal study or angiography, one can expect that acute fluid collections and real pancreatic pseudocysts are mixed in one group. The situation has not changed even with the advent of ultrasonography, as often there is no precise definition of the pseudocyst and in many earlier studies any fluid present in the lesser sac was regarded as a pseudocyst. Also, there is the possibility that the results of resolution of acute fluid collections and acute pseudocysts are presented together. Warshaw and Rattner[27] performed endoscopic retrograde cholangiopancreatography (ERCP) for patients with pancreatic pseudocysts. According to their findings, pancreatitis can be divided in acute, chronic and acute-on-chronic groups. A resolution rate of 21% was observed into the acute pancreatitis group, while no pseudocysts resolved in the other two groups.

When alcohol is the major cause of pancreatic pseudocysts, a 20–29% spontaneous resolution rate has been reported by other pancreatologists. Bourliere and colleagues[28] noted a similar 20% spontaneous resolution rate in pseudocysts with biliary pancreatitis as the major cause. Alcohol-related pancreatitis was present in only 4% of cases in their series. However, a recent prospective cohort study of a non-alcoholic population with acute pancreatitis revealed that 65% of acute pancreatic pseudocysts resolved spontaneously within 1 year.[29] This study used the Atlanta criteria for reliable diagnosis of acute pancreatic pseudocyst.

DURATION OF THE PSEUDOCYST *VERSUS* SIZE

Warshaw and Rattner[27] reported that no cyst that presented more than 6 weeks following an attack of acute pancreatitis resolved. On the other hand, the authors noted that the size of the cyst did not seem to affect the chance of resolution. Similarly, Bradley and colleagues[30] followed the natural history of pseudocysts in 93 patients, 31 of whom had acute pancreatitis and 62 had chronic disease. Spontaneous resolution occurred in 10 (42%) of 24 patients in whom a pseudocyst was present for less than 6 weeks. In contrast, of 13 pseudocysts that had been present for 7–12 weeks, only 1 (8%) resolved spontaneously. Spontaneous resolution did not occur in any of the remaining 12 patients followed for up to 18 weeks. The clear implication was that pseudocysts still present at 6 weeks are unlikely to resolve spontaneously.[30]

This conclusion was challenged by the results of more recent studies. In the series of Vitas and Sarr,[31] of 68 patients treated with expectant approach, overall resolution of the pseudocyst occurred in 57% of the 24 patients with satisfactory radiographic follow-up, and 38% resolved more than 6 months after diagnosis. O'Malley and colleagues[32] noted that pseudocysts larger than 4 cm resolved spontaneously at a mean of 3 months after diagnosis, although in one case resolution did not occur until 28 months. Maringhini and colleagues[29] found that within 1 year after diagnosis 65% of acute pseudocysts resolved. Pseudocysts less than 5 cm in size were more likely to resolve than larger ones. Gouyon and colleagues[33] observed a pseudocyst resolution rate of 26% in patients with chronic alcoholic pancreatitis. The median time to regression was 29 weeks (range 2–143) and an independent predictive factor of pseudocyst resolution or asymptomatic course was size less than 4 cm.

The size was a major factor predicting pseudocyst resolution in the series of Aranha and colleagues.[34] The mean diameter of cystic lesions that resolved was 4±1 cm, compared with a diameter of 9±1 cm in those cysts that did not resolve, which was a significant difference. Only 4 of 26 pseudocysts greater than 6 cm in diameter at initial examination resolved. Several more studies also confirmed that cysts less than 4 cm in diameter could resolve spontaneously.[34–37]

> **Key point 3**
>
> • Acute pseudocysts may resolve spontaneously, irrespective of size or duration. However, larger cysts are more likely to require intervention for symptoms.

RESOLUTION OF CHRONIC PSEUDOCYSTS

Aranha and colleagues[34] noted that patients with pancreatic calcifications and evidence of chronic pancreatitis had no resolution of their pancreatic pseudocyst. Warshaw and Rattner,[27] from their series of 42 patients with pancreatic pseudocysts, also concluded that evidence of chronic pancreatitis and pancreatic duct abnormality other than communication with the pseudocyst were criteria suggesting that a pseudocyst will not resolve spontaneously.

McConnell and colleagues[24] reported resolution rate in only 3% of cases with chronic pancreatic pseudocysts. Bourliere and Sarles[28] reviewed 77 consecutive patients with pseudocysts of the pancreas associated with chronic pancreatitis. Ultrasonography and/or CT showed that 9% resolved spontaneously. The mean diameter of chronic pancreatic pseudocysts that resolved was 3 cm.[28] Gouyon and colleagues[33] retrospectively studied the factors predicting the outcome of pseudocysts complicating alcoholic chronic pancreatitis. The patients were included if the presence of at least one of the following criteria was documented: calcifications; pancreatic duct anomalies at least moderate according to the International Cambridge Classification; histologic diagnosis of chronic pancreatitis. The pseudocyst resolution rate was 26% in their group of 90 cases.

RISK FOR COMPLICATIONS IN UNTREATED PANCREATIC PSEUDOCYSTS

It is difficult to interpret the current literature because patients whose pseudocyst follows acute or chronic pancreatitis are grouped together. Furthermore, papers on the natural history of pancreatic pseudocyst, due to their retrospective approach, may have some methodologic bias, such as selection bias,[30,31] an elevated number of dropouts,[30] or no regular imaging and clinical follow-up.[30,31,38]

In the series of Bradley and colleagues,[30] the incidence of complications correlated directly with the length of time the pseudocyst was present: 20% of patients with early pseudocyst (<6 weeks) had a complication, as opposed to 46% with cysts that were 7–12 weeks old and 75% of those with cysts present (beyond 13 weeks. Of particular interest is the observation that each of the seven deaths (12%) occurred as a direct result of the pseudocyst and that their complications developed an average of 13.5 weeks after the presumed initial development of the pseudocyst.

More recently, Yeo and colleagues[38] in Baltimore used serial CT to observe the natural history of pancreatic pseudocysts in 75 patients; their findings challenge the conclusion of Bradley and colleagues[30] that delay is at best fruitless and at worst hazardous. Thirty-six patients who were asymptomatic were managed without operation and were observed for a mean of 1 year. Of these, 60% had complete resolution of the pseudocyst and 40% had pseudocysts that remained stable or decreased in size. Only 1 patient of the 36 treated expectantly, i.e. without operation, developed a complication from the pseudocyst, in the form of a transient intracystic haemorrhage.

Vitas and Sarr[31] reported 68 patients initially treated selectively with a non-operative, expectant approach. Severe, life-threatening complications in this group followed-up for a mean of 46 months occurred in only 6 patients (9%), including intracystic haemorrhage in 3, perforation in 2 and cyst infection in 1. Nineteen patients (28%) eventually underwent elective operation directed at either the pseudocyst or other complications related to pancreatitis.

Maringhini and colleagues[29] analysed the natural history of 83 non-alcoholic patients with fluid collections and/or pseudocysts in which chronic pancreatitis was accurately excluded. In the first 6 weeks of follow-up spontaneous disappearance was observed in 12 (15%) and complications in 19 (23%) of 83 patients. The complications observed were pain in 12 patients, infection in 4, fistula in 2, and rupture in 1. Only 2 patients died. After the first 6 weeks of follow up, the pseudocyst spontaneously disappeared in 31 and complications occurred in 14 of 48 patients. Eleven of the patients with complications had pain, while 3 presented fistulae.

ASYMPTOMATIC *VERSUS* SYMPTOMATIC PSEUDOCYSTS

Bradley and colleagues[30] found 41% of patients to have complications in the non-operative treatment group. In contrast, two other studies reported complication rates from 3%[38] to 9%.[31] In patients managed without operation and observed for a mean of 1 and 3.5 years, respectively. These results may represent different study populations and selection bias. In their prospective study Bradley and colleagues[30] aimed to explore the natural history of the pseudocyst. They excluded from the study 11 patients with acute pancreatitis who underwent urgent exploration and drainage because of a suspected intra-abdominal catastrophe or the appearance of superimposed sepsis. Patients with chronic symptoms and pseudocyst were excluded only when they underwent elective drainage primarily due to a pre-study bias on the part of the surgical investigator. Thus their report contains a mixed series of symptomatic and asymptomatic pseudocysts. In contrast, in the studies with a low complication rate, non-operative management was reserved only for those patients who had asymptomatic pseudocysts and were able to tolerate oral intake. Moreover, they continued with a non-operative approach only if the patient had no enlargement or complications of the pseudocyst. These studies represent the success of patient selection for non-operative approach rather than the real natural course of pancreatic pseudocysts.

Key point 4

- In the absence of symptoms, it is safe to manage acute or chronic pseudocysts without intervention.

INDICATIONS FOR AND OPTIONS FOR INTERVENTION

The indications for pseudocyst drainage, whether performed by radiologic, endoscopic, or surgical means, remain basically unchanged. Symptomatic pseudocysts, infected pseudocysts (i.e. pancreatic abscesses) and enlarging pseudocysts affecting the function of adjacent organs unequivocally require drainage. The necessity of draining pseudocysts based strictly on size has been questioned,[38,39] but many authorities recommend that pseudocysts larger than 6 cm in diameter should be drained once their wall has 'matured'.[40]

Surgery has remained the standard for drainage of pseudocysts against which new methods have been compared – but this must now be seriously questioned as so few of these procedures are performed today. Surgical operations usually consist of open or laparoscopic gastropseudocystostomy, duodenopseudocystostomy, Roux-en-Y-jejunopseudocystostomy or resection. These operative procedures carry a 10–30% morbidity rate, a 1–5% mortality rate, and a 10–20% rate of recurrence;[41–43] thus endoscopic drainage[44–51] and percutaneous techniques[53–57] in many respects compare favourably with this surgical 'standard'. However, these newer techniques are reported mainly from referral centres, and recurrence rates tend to be higher than after surgical treatment.

Controversy exists concerning which of these techniques should be offered to the patient as initial therapy.

Key point 5

- Good results are reported for non-surgical intervention. However, open surgical drainage to the stomach or small bowel remains safe appropriate treatment, especially after failure of other interventions.

Three options exist for the surgical management of pancreatic pseudocysts: excision, external drainage and internal drainage. Surgery, which traditionally was the major treatment approach for pancreatic pseudocysts, has been challenged by the newer endoscopic techniques. Given the low complication and mortality rates and the high success rate of endoscopic drainage when compared with surgery, surgical intervention should be reserved only for certain cases. Addition of endoscopic ultrasonography for endoscopic drainage is a new development and may decrease the risks associated with endoscopic drainage.

Resolution rates after surgical and non-surgical methods are similar, but clinical and technical aspects may mandate either method. Each patient requires an individual, multidisciplinary approach, thereby obtaining optimal treatment outcome.

However, all these options – especially in the light of economic incentives for treatment – must be balanced against the natural history of pancreatic pseudocysts. The possibility to treat may not be an indication to treat *per se*. This means that little has changed concerning the indication for treatment of pancreatic pseudocysts despite the new options, but the treatment can be better tailored to the individual patient. The choice of mode of treatment will be influenced by the availability of appropriate expertise.

A management plan for pancreatic pseudocysts is given in Table 1.

Table 1 Management plan for pancreatic pseudocysts

- Exclude a neoplastic cyst (neoplasia is more likely if there is no acute or chronic pancreatitis)
- If possible, allow the pseudocyst time to mature
- Identify and treat pseudoaneurysms
- Evaluate for the presence of portal hypertension and gastric varices
- Determine whether the pseudocyst is in close apposition to the gastric or duodenal wall
- Optional: Perform pancreatography to determine if there is a communication to the pancreatic duct
- Use a method of treatment where local expertise is available:
  - percutaneous technique
  - endoscopic technique
  - surgical drainage
  - resection

Key points for clinical practice

- By definition, a pseudocyst must be present for at least 4 weeks. 'Acute' and 'chronic' pseudocysts refer to the nature of the preceding pancreatitis, not the duration of the cyst.

- Acute fluid collections are common after a severe episode of acute pancreatitis. Most resolve without formation of a pseudocyst.

- Acute pseudocysts may resolve spontaneously, irrespective of size or duration. However, larger cysts are more likely to require intervention for symptoms.

- In the absence of symptoms, it is safe to manage acute or chronic pseudocysts without intervention.

- Good results are reported for non-surgical intervention. However, open surgical drainage to the stomach or small bowel remains safe appropriate treatment, especially after failure of other interventions.

References

1. Klöppel G. Pseudocysts and other non-neoplastic cysts of the pancreas. *Semin Diagn Pathol* 2000; **17**: 7–15.
2. Richter HM. Natural history of pancreatic pseudocysts. In: Howard J, Idezuki Y, Ihse I, Prinz R, eds. Surgical Diseases of the Pancreas. Baltimore: Williams and Wilkins, 1998: 417–421.
3. Breslin N, Wallace MB. Diagnosis and fine needle aspiration of pancreatic pseudocysts: the role of endoscopic ultrasound. *Gastrointest Endosc Clin N Am* 2002; **12**: 781–790.
4. Bradley EL. A clinically based classification system for acute pancreatitis. *Arch Surg* 1993; **128**: 586–590.

5. Bradley EL, Gonzalez AC, Clements JL. Acute pancreatic pseudocysts: incidence and implications. *Ann Surg* 1976; **184**: 734–737.
6. Becker WF, Pratt HS, Ganji H. Pseudocysts of the pancreas. *Surg Gynecol Obstet* 1968; **127**: 744–747.
7. Rosenberg IK, Kahn JA, Walt AJ. Surgical experience with pancreatic pseudocysts. *Am J Surg* 1969; **117**: 11–17.
8. Trapnell J. Management of the complications of acute pancreatitis. *Ann R Coll Surg Engl* 1971; **49**: 361–372.
9. Elechi EN, Callender CO, Leffall LD, Kurtz LH. The treatment of pancreatic pseudocysts by external drainage. *Surg Gynecol Obstet* 1979; **148**: 707–710.
10. Bodker A, Kjaergaard J, Schmidt A, Tilma A. Pancreatic pseudocysts. A follow-up study. *Ann Surg* 1981; **194**: 80–84.
11. Shetty AN. Pseudocysts of the pancreas: an overview. *South Med J* 1980; **73**: 1239–1242.
12. Sandy JT, Taylor RH, Christensen RM, Scudamore C, Leckie P. Pancreatic pseudocyst. Changing concepts in management. *Am J Surg* 1981; **141**: 574–576.
13. Wade JW. Twenty-five year experience with pancreatic pseudocysts. Are we making progress? *Am J Surg* 1985; **149**: 705–708.
14. O'Malley VP, Cannon JP, Postier RG. Pancreatic pseudocysts: cause, therapy, and results. *Am J Surg* 1985; **150**: 680–682.
15. London NJ, Neoptolemos JP, Lavelle J, Bailey I, James D. Serial computed tomography scanning in acute pancreatitis: a prospective study. *Gut* 1989; **30**: 397–403.
16. Kourtesis G, Wilson SE, Williams RA. The clinical significance of fluid collections in acute pancreatitis. *Am J Surg* 1990; **56**: 796–799.
17. Barthet M, Bugallo M, Moreira LS, Bastid C, Sastre B, Sahel J. Management of cysts and pseudocysts complicating chronic pancreatitis. A retrospective study of 143 patients. *Gastroenterol Clin Biol* 1993; **17**: 270–276.
18. Ammann RW, Akovbiantz A, Largiader F, Schueler G. Course and outcome of chronic pancreatitis. Longitudinal study of a mixed medical-surgical series of 245 patients. *Gastroenterology* 1984; **86** (5 Pt 1): 820–828.
19. Elliott DW. Pancreatic pseudocysts. *Surg Clin North Am* 1975; **55**: 339–362.
20. Sankaran S, Walt AJ. The natural and unnatural history of pancreatic pseudocysts. *Br J Surg* 1975; **62**: 37–44.
21. Hanna WA. Rupture of pancreatic cysts. *Br J Surg* 1960; **47**: 495.
22. Bradley EL, Clements LJ. Spontaneous resolution of pancreatic pseudocysts: implications for timing of operative intervention. *Am J Surg* 1975; **129**: 23–28.
23. Agha FP. Spontaneous resolution of acute pancreatic pseudocysts. *Surg Gynecol Obstet* 1984; **158**: 22–26.
24. McConnell DB, Gregory JR, Sasaki TM, Vetto RM. Pancreatic pseudocyst. *Am J Surg* 1982; **143**: 599–601.
25. Pollack EW, Michas CA, Wolfman EF. Pancreatic pseudocyst: management in fifty-four patients. *Am J Surg* 1978; **135**: 199–201.
26. Czaja AJ, Fisher M, Marin GA. Spontaneous resolution of pancreatic masses (pseudocysts?) – development and disappearance after acute alcoholic pancreatitis. *Arch Intern Med* 1975; **135**: 558–562.
27. Warshaw AL, Rattner DW. Timing of surgical drainage for pancreatic pseudocyst. Clinical and chemical criteria. *Ann Surg* 1985; **202**: 720–724.
28. Bourliere M, Sarles H. Pancreatic cysts and pseudocysts associated with acute and chronic pancreatitis. *Dig Dis Sci* 1989; **34**: 343–348.
29. Maringhini A, Uomo G, Patti R, Rabitti P, Termini A, Cavallera A, Dardanoni G, Manes G, Ciambra M, Laccetti M, Biffarella P, Pagliaro L. Pseudocysts in acute nonalcoholic pancreatitis: incidence and natural history. *Dig Dis Sci* 1999; **44**: 1669–1673.
30. Bradley E, Clements J, Gonzales AC. The natural history of pancreatic pseudocysts: a unified concept of management. *Am J Surg* 1979; **137**: 135–141.
31. Vitas GJ, Sarr MG. Selected management of pancreatic pseudocysts: operative versus expectant management. *Surgery* 1992; **111**: 123–130.
32. O'Malley VP, Cannon JP, Postier RG. Pancreatic pseudocysts: cause, therapy, and results. *Am J Surg* 1985; **150**: 680–682.

33. Gouyon B, Levy P, Ruszniewski P, Zins M, Hammel P, Vilgrain V, Sauvanet A, Belghiti J, Bernades P. Predictive factors in the outcome of pseudocysts complicating alcoholic chronic pancreatitis. *Gut* 1997; **41**: 821–825.

34. Aranha GV, Prinz RA, Esguerra AC, Greenlee HB. The nature and course of cystic pancreatic lesions diagnosed by ultrasound. *Arch Surg* 1983; **118**: 486–488.

35. Andersson R, Janzon M, Sundberg I, Bengmark S. Management of pancreatic pseudocysts. *Br J Surg* 1989; **76**: 550–552.

36. Ravelo HR, Alderlete JS. Analysis of forty-five patients with pseudocysts of the pancreas treated surgically. *Surg Gyn Obstet* 1979; **148**: 735–738.

37. Beebe DS, Bubrick MP, Onstad GR, Hitchcock CR. Management of pancreatic pseudocysts. *Surg Gynecol Obstet* 1984; **159**: 562–564.

38. Yeo CJ, Bastidas JA, Lynch-Nyhan A, Fishman EK, Zinner MJ, Cameron JL. The natural history of pancreatic pseudocysts documented by computed tomography. *Surg Gynecol Obstet* 1990; **170**: 411–417.

39. Warshaw AL. Pancreatic cysts and pseudocysts: new rules for a new game. *Br J Surg* 1989; **76**: 533–534.

40. Chak A. Endosonographic-guided therapy of pancreatic pseudocysts. *Gastrointest Endosc* 2000; **52** suppl: S23–S27.

41. Kohler H, Schafmayer A, Ludtke FE, Lepsien G, Peiper JH. Surgical treatment of pancreatic pseudocysts. *Br J Surg* 1987; **74**: 813–815.

42. Moran B, Rew DA, Johnson CD. Pancreatic pseudocysts should be treated by surgical drainage. *Ann R Coll Surg Engl* 1994; **76**: 54–58.

43. Williams KJ, Fabian TC. Pancreatic pseudocysts: recommendations for operative and nonoperative management. *Am Surg* 1992; **58**: 199–205.

44. Binmoeller KF, Seifert H, Walther A, Soehendra N. Transpapillary and transmural drainage of pancreatic pseudocysts. *Gastrointest Endosc* 1995; **42**: 219–224.

45. Smits ME, Rauws EAJ, Tytgat GNJ, Huibregtse K. The efficacy of endoscopic treatment of pancreatic pseudocysts. *Gastrointest Endosc* 1995; **42**: 202–207.

46. Cremer M, Deviere J, Engelholm L. Endoscopic management of cysts and pseudocysts in chronic pancreatitis: long term follow-up after 7 years of experience. *Gastrointest Endosc* 1989; **35**: 1–9.

47. Sahel J. Endoscopic drainage of pancreatic cysts. *Endoscopy* 1991; **23**: 181–184.

48. Huibregtse K, Schneider B, Vrij AA, Tytgat GNJ. Endoscopic pancreatic drainage in chronic pancreatitis. *Gastrointest Endosc* 1988; **34**: 9–15.

49. Grimm H, Meyer WH, Nahm Vch, Soehendra N. New modalities for treating chronic pancreatitis. *Endoscopy* 1989; **21**: 70–4.

50. Kozarek RA, Ball TJ, Patterson DJ, Freeny PC, Ryan JA, Traverso LW. Endoscopic transpapillary therapy for disrupted pancreatic duct and peripancreatic fluid collections. *Gastroenterology* 1991; **100**: 1362–1370.

51. Barthet M, Sahel J, Bodiou-Bertel C, Bernard JP. Endoscopic transpapillary drainage of pancreatic pseudocysts. *Gastrointest Endosc* 1995; **42**: 208–213.

52. Catalano MF, Geenen JE, Schmalz MJ, Johnson GK, Dean RS, Hogan WJ. Treatment of pancreatic pseudocysts with ductal communication by transpapillary pancreatic duct endoprosthesis. *Gastrointest Endosc* 1995; **42**: 214–218.

53. Gerzof SG, Johnson WC, Robbins AH, Spechler SJ, Nabseth DC. Percutaneous drainage of infected pancreatic pseudocysts. *Arch Surg* 1984; **119**: 888–893.

54. vanSonnenberg E, Wittich GR, Casola G, Stauffer AE, Polansky AD, Coons HG, Cabera OA, Gerver PS. Complicated pancreatic inflammatory disease: diagnostic and therapeutic role of interventional radiology. *Radiology* 1985; **155**: 335–340.

55. Freeny PC, Lewis GP, Traverso LW, Ryan JA. Infected pancreatic fluid collections: percutaneous catheter drainage. *Radiology* 1988; **167**: 435–441.

56. vanSonnenberg E, Wittich GR, Casola G, Brannigan TC, Karnel F, Stabile BE, Varney RR, Christensen RR. Percutaneous drainage of infected and noninfected pancreatic pseudocysts: experience in 101 cases. *Radiology* 1989; **170**: 757–761.

57. Freeny PC. Percutaneous management of pancreatic fluid collections. *Baillière's Clin Gastroenterol* 1992; **6**: 259–272.

Christopher P. Gandy   Roger M. Kipling
Robin H. Kennedy

10

Laparoscopic colorectal surgery

The laparoscopic technique is widely practised and regarded as the gold standard technique for cholecystectomy and fundoplication but has yet to gain widespread acceptance for colorectal surgery. The term minimally invasive surgery has been coined, which embodies the rationale for these procedures, i.e. minimal tissue damage to gain access to the surgical field without compromising exposure.

In our unit minimally invasive surgery is not practised as a subspeciality but rather as a general philosophy to surgery, with preoperative optimisation of patients and the use of laparoscopic procedures. Importantly, we also use an enhanced recovery programme, as advocated by Kehlet,[1,2] to minimise the perioperative stress response and optimise patient recovery, leading to earlier discharge and resumption of normal activities.

The nomenclature of laparoscopic colorectal surgery has evolved over the last 10 years. True laparoscopic colorectal resections are those where all aspects of the operation proceed laparoscopically, for example abdominoperineal excisions where the specimen is removed through the perineum. Hand-assisted laparoscopic surgery is practised with a hand introduced to the abdomen through a specially designed port (Lap Disc from Ethicon Endo-surgery Inc. or GelPort from Applied Medical), which prevents loss of the pneumoperitoneum and allows manipulation of the tissues.[3] The most widely used technique is laparoscopically assisted resection, where laparoscopic colon or rectal resection

Mr Christopher P. Gandy, Specialist Registrar in General Surgery, Department of General Surgery, Yeovil District Hospital, Higher Kingston, Yeovil, Somerset BA21 4AT, UK

Dr Roger M. Kipling, FRCA, Consultant Anaesthetist, Department of Anaesthesia, Yeovil District Hospital, Higher Kingston, Yeovil, Somerset BA21 4AT, UK

Mr Robin H. Kennedy, FRCS, Consultant Surgeon, Department of General Surgery, Yeovil District Hospital, Higher Kingston, Yeovil, Somerset BA21 4AT, UK (for correspondence)

proceeds as normal with an extracorporeal component to allow specimen retrieval and in some cases assistance with the anastomosis.[4] The feasibility of remote controlled surgical robots has also been tested;[5] however, the technology is currently prohibitively expensive and its application unclear.

The conversion rate from laparoscopic to open surgery varies considerably between authors and its definition is controversial.[6] Some authors believe that any incision greater than 5 cm for specimen retrieval or anastomosis should be regarded as a conversion. We define conversion as an inability to complete the intra-abdominal resection laparoscopically; this usually, but not always, requires a larger incision than required for specimen retrieval.

RATIONALE FOR LAPAROSCOPIC SURGERY

Conventional surgery often involves the use of large incisions to gain access to the surgical field. Laparoscopic surgery has shown us that these incisions can be more traumatic than the actual procedure and contribute to adverse metabolic responses seen in the perioperative period. Reports of surgical stress have revealed that cortisol levels are higher and revert to normal more slowly after open procedures.[7] Research on immune and inflammatory responses in laparoscopic surgery is conflicting; however, some investigators have shown less attenuation of the immune response[8] and a dampened inflammatory response.[9,10]

Laparotomy incisions, unlike laparoscopic ports, lose large volumes of fluid and heat to the atmosphere, resulting in dehydration and hypothermia. The pain from these incisions is a major contributor to postoperative morbidity. Early complications such as wound infections and dehiscence, later complications in the form of adhesions and incisional hernias, are all relatively common after laparotomy compared with laparoscopic procedures.[11,12]

Although the incisions used for laparoscopic surgery are small (< 1.5 cm), access is not compromised once surgeons have become familiar with the techniques. The laparoscope can be moved easily from one port to another and magnification affords a superior view of the operative field, particularly in inaccessible areas such as the pelvis.[13]

Although of secondary importance to safe surgery, cosmetic results are far superior after laparoscopic procedures.[14]

DISADVANTAGES OF LAPAROSCOPIC SURGERY

Operating from a monitor reduces the three-dimensional perception of stereoscopic vision, and this has to be overcome, in part, by moving in and out of the area of interest with the laparoscope (optic flow). There is also a reduction in the tactile feedback from tissues, which can be a problem, for example when trying to palpate a small colorectal tumour. For this reason the technique of endoscopically marking tumour sites with India ink has been advocated.[15]

Free blood from excessive bleeding absorbs light and degrades the laparoscopic picture. This may be a cause for open conversion, although this is rare in our practice because good views allow more accurate haemostasis with considerably reduced blood loss. This is borne out in the results of laparoscopic colectomy, where blood loss is considerably less than in the open equivalent.[16,17]

There is no doubt that laparoscopic surgery is more time-consuming during the learning curve, but it is likely that operating times will approximate to those of open surgery with increased experience.

Initially there were concerns that laparoscopic procedures would prove more expensive than the open equivalent.[18] Direct costs in the form of equipment, stapling devices, disposables and increased theatre time are, however, offset by shorter hospital stays and lower out-of-hospital costs such as convalescence and wound care.[19] Recent detailed analyses of open and laparoscopic colorectal surgery have shown a cost benefit for the laparoscopic approach.[19] Even these studies have failed to include indirect costs, such as the expense to the patient and family through time off work. We have to await the results of detailed randomised studies, which contain robust health economics and quality of life analysis, before we will know the true cost benefit of laparoscopic colorectal procedures.

Finally specimen extraction can be a problem. Although 85–90% of resections can be completed laparoscopically, a 4–5 cm incision is still required for specimen extraction in laparoscopically assisted procedures, and on occasions when large tumours are present this incision is lengthened. A retrieval bag may also be used to reduce incision size as well as resealable plastic wound protectors that allow immediate recreation of the pneumoperitoneum for further laparoscopic inspection.

SURGICAL INSTRUMENTS FOR LAPAROSCOPIC SURGERY

Laparoscopic surgery employs rigid endoscopes, which contain the widely used glass rod and lens systems. The solid quartz rods within the laparoscope use the principle of total internal reflection to transmit the image to the camera. Light is delivered to the tissues through a separate internal system. The diameter of these instruments ranges from 2 mm to the most commonly used 10 mm endoscopes, the latter being more durable and allowing more light delivery. The end of the laparoscope may be angled up to 45° to allow views over the 'horizon', although the same effect may be produced by digital image manipulation in certain systems. Modern cameras fitted to the external end of the laparoscope use charge-coupled devices (CCDs), consisting of a series of minute light-sensitive capacitors that turn light energy into an electrical charge, forming pixels. These are processed in the camera control box and transmitted to the monitor as a picture. Cameras may comprise a single CCD chip that senses the image in greyscale, the microprocessors within the camera control box estimating the colour and displaying it on the monitor. Three-chip cameras that sense the image in green, red and blue are able to provide true colour, which in combination with digital enhancements provides excellent-quality images.

A whole industry has developed to provide equipment for laparoscopic surgery, including ports, laparoscopic instruments and adjuncts in surgery. Some of these have been adapted from open surgery whereas others have been developed specifically for the new technology. Stapling devices, clips and suture materials have all been adapted for the laparoscopic approach whereas the harmonic scalpel is an example of an instrument developed for laparoscopic surgery. This device vibrates at 55 kHz, vaporising tissue and sealing vessels.[20] Together with bipolar cutting diathermy, the harmonic scalpel has transformed our ability to dissect laparoscopically where the absence of blood is so important.

Laparoscopic surgery is usually performed with a pneumoperitoneum, although gasless procedures may be performed using abdominal wall lifting devices.[21] Either an open or Veress needle technique is used to produce the pneumoperitoneum. The Veress needle is inserted blindly, using loss of resistance as a guide to placement within the abdominal cavity. The open or Hasson technique utilises a blunt-tipped port that is placed under direct vision through a small incision in the peritoneum. Ports utilising an optical blunt tip trocar have also been developed for visualisation of tissues during port insertion (Endopath from Ethicon Endo-surgery or Visiport from Autosuture/Tyco). Once a pneumoperitoneum has been established, further ports can be placed, guided by the laparoscope. No firm data exist favouring one technique over another, although some authorities believe an open approach to be safer.[22] When adhesions are likely, we use a remote insufflation technique, the Veress needle and initial port inserted away from scars, using simultaneous fascial countertraction for safety.

PHYSIOLOGICAL CONSEQUENCES OF LAPAROSCOPIC SURGERY AND ANAESTHETIC CONSIDERATIONS

Although some laparoscopic procedures may be performed without muscle relaxation, colorectal laparoscopic surgery requires general anaesthesia, muscle relaxants, endotracheal intubation and ventilation. Carbon dioxide (CO_2) is used for the pneumoperitoneum and is supplied via an insufflator that can be set to provide a constant intra-abdominal pressure, usually between 10 and 15 cmH$_2$O. Both the CO_2 and the intra-abdominal pressure have physiological consequences that may require consideration when selecting patients for laparoscopic procedures and during anaesthesia. The CO_2 is cheap and non-inflammable, and any residual gas is rapidly absorbed into blood, where it is buffered and expired in the lungs. During procedures longer than 60 minutes, there is a demonstrable increase in end-tidal CO_2 and hypercarbia may be observed during the initial recovery period. This can be corrected during surgery by hyperventilation or removing the pneumoperitoneum for a short period to allow recovery. Hypercarbia stimulates catecholamine release, which can result in tachyarrhythmias, increased vascular resistance and myocardial dysfunction; however, this is rarely a problem in practice.

CO_2 embolism occurs when veins under low pressure are opened, allowing CO_2 to enter the circulation. This rare complication has been reported with fatal consequences mainly after laparoscopic cholecystectomy, but may be possible with all procedures.[23]

A pneumoperitoneum results in increased intra-abdominal pressure, which can compress the inferior vena cava, reducing venous return from the lower limbs. This theoretically predisposes to deep vein thrombosis and thromboembolic disease – a complication rarely seen in our practice. Decreased venous return reduces cardiac output, which may be a problem when using high intra-abdominal pressures (> 20 cmH$_2$O), in prolonged procedures or in patients with pre-existing heart disease. Reduced venous return stimulates a vasoconstrictor reflex, and the subsequent hypertension may require treatment in patients at risk. Renal perfusion is also reduced with a pneumoperitoneum and intraoperative oligouria is observed, which may have implications for patients with pre-existing renal impairment.

Stretching of the peritoneum during production of a pneumoperitoneum may be a cause of postoperative pain and can result in vasovagal activity and bradycardia. Diaphragmatic splinting occurs particularly in the morbidly obese, but may also be a problem in patients with lung disease; this may require the use of a positive end-expiratory pressure to prevent basal collapse during ventilation. These physiological changes may be further compounded by the patient's position, which may need to be considerably head down when performing rectal or sigmoid laparoscopic resections.

The difficulties occasionally encountered when anaesthetising patients during laparoscopic procedures are preferable to managing the respiratory complications associated with large abdominal incisions; indeed, studies of lung function have shown less postoperative compromise with laparoscopic procedures.[24] Patients unsuitable for the laparoscopic approach because of comorbidity are equally unlikely to be suitable for an open procedure, and we rarely advocate an open procedure in preference to the laparoscopic approach in this situation.

TRAINING

To date there is no formalised accreditation process for laparoscopic colorectal surgery in the UK; however, it is recommended that surgeons undertaking this surgery should be appropriately trained and experienced in both open and laparoscopic colorectal surgery and that their results should be carefully audited.[25,26] The National Institute for Clinical Excellence (NICE) has recommended that for colorectal cancer, laparoscopic resections should only be performed in the context of a randomised clinical trial.[27]

Training units such as minimal access therapy training units (MATTU) have introduced basic and advanced laparoscopic courses, and it is likely that formalised structured training programmes for advanced laparoscopic surgery (such as colorectal surgery) will be introduced. A priority of the Association of Coloproctology of Great Britain and Ireland for 2003 is to achieve adequate training resources to develop laparoscopic colorectal surgery in the UK.

Key point 1

- A carefully structured training programme is necessary to achieve good outcomes in laparoscopic colorectal surgery.

THE SCOPE OF LAPAROSCOPIC COLORECTAL SURGERY

Virtually all elective intra-abdominal colorectal surgery can be performed laparoscopically. To date there are relatively few centres worldwide that have a large experience but a wide range of procedures has been reported for both malignancy and benign disease. Benign conditions treated in this way include diverticular disease,[28] including reversal of Hartmann's procedure,[29] inflammatory bowel disease with reports of ileocaecal resections for Crohn's disease,[30] subtotal colectomy for ulcerative colitis[31] and even restorative proctocolectomy for ulcerative colitis or familial adenomatous polyposis (FAP).[32] Rectal prolapse[7] and rectocele repair[33] have also been undertaken laparoscopically.

For colorectal cancer staging, laparoscopy is useful in the management of patients with locally recurrent disease who are considered for further resections.[34] For primary disease, we use laparoscopic resection as the mainstay of surgical management. Outside the setting of a randomised trial we begin with open procedures in only 2–4% of patients. Occasionally laparoscopy will be undertaken prior to embarking on aggressive preoperative chemo-radiotherapy regimes in order to ensure that incurable peritoneal or hepatic disease has not been missed by preoperative imaging.

There are no absolute contraindications to the laparoscopic technique, but occasionally dense adhesions[35] or excessive obesity[36] make surgery more difficult, complications more likely and conversion necessary. For cancer resections, conversion is higher with rectal than colonic tumours,[6] and for benign disease, diverticular disease associated with abscesses has higher conversion rates.[35] For these difficult procedures, we believe it is inappropriate to cause complications that would not be encountered in open surgery merely to proceed laparoscopically. For surgeons learning these procedures, good case selection is important to minimise complications and conversions.

Key point 2

- For surgeons learning these procedures, good case selection is important to minimise complications and conversions – avoiding patients with morbid obesity, multiple adhesions, advanced or rectal tumours.

LAPAROSCOPIC APPENDICECTOMY

Laparoscopic appendicectomy was first described by Semm[37] in 1983, but over 20 years later it is still not widely practised in the UK.

Although there are many techniques described, we place the patient in a Lloyd Davis position and insert three ports: a 10 or 12 mm infraumbilical port for the camera, a 5 mm left iliac fossa port and a 5 or 10 mm suprapubic port. The abdominal cavity is inspected, and if pelvic pathology is identified then the hips can be flexed to allow greater pelvic access or manipulation of the cervix. If appendicular pathology is demonstrated, the patient is positioned head-down with left lateral tilt. The appendix is mobilised, taking any associated adhesions, and held at the tip. The mesoappendix is dissected from the appendix in a plane close to the serosal surface where tiny arteries enter the appendix. These are controlled with diathermy, although ligaclips can be used.

The appendix base is ligated with two endoloops and divided. The stump mucosa is ablated with diathermy and the appendix is removed through the umbilical port. Any intra-abdominal collections are drained as for open procedures and antibiotic therapy is tailored to the individual patient.

The results of laparoscopic appendicectomy have been the subject of a Cochrane review.[38] The conclusions are that laparoscopic appendicectomy takes longer and theatre costs are higher. However pain scores are reduced, as is hospital stay and return to normal activity is faster. As appendicectomy is performed in combination with diagnostic laparoscopy the negative appendicectomy rate is reduced and the proportion of positive diagnoses increased. Superficial wound infection rates are halved with the laparoscopic approach although the incidence of intra-abdominal abscesses is possibly increased. However, one large randomised trial found that, when controlling for perforated or gangrenous appendices, there were no significant differences in intra-abdominal abscess formation.[39]

The fate of a normal appendix has also been defined – it is safe to remove it just as in open surgery, but it is also safe to leave: in one study there was only a 1% incidence of subsequent appendicitis after 4 years of follow-up.[40]

We find laparoscopy in suspected appendicitis a particularly useful procedure in women of childbearing age, where there is a high incidence of other pelvic pathology and visualisation of the pelvis is far superior.

Key point 3

• Diagnostic laparoscopy in suspected appendicitis is particularly useful in women of childbearing age and laparoscopic appendicectomy will facilitate rapid recovery.

LAPAROSCOPIC COLORECTAL RESECTION

It is possible to perform any elective open colorectal resection laparoscopically, with 85–90% of planned colorectal resections being completed this way. In malignancy, preoperative staging, oncological principles and adjuvant therapy apply as for open surgery. Since the tactile facility is decreased, it is important that synchronous tumours have been excluded and that small lesions or polyps are localised carefully using barium enema or by marking endoscopically with India ink.[15] Resections are based on the major lymphovascular pedicles, with resection margins and anastomoses performed using the principles learned from open surgery. Involvement of other organs by T4 tumour is managed with *en bloc* resection of the involved structure; however, some surgeons regard adjacent organ involvement as a relative contraindication to the laparoscopic approach. Laparoscopic colectomy for benign conditions follows the same principles as for malignancy. We generally modify the extent of vascular resection in diverticular disease by preserving the inferior mesenteric artery and the superior rectal artery,[41] in an attempt to decrease the risk of anastomotic complications.

Laparoscopic colectomy: surgical technique

Patients are placed in a Lloyd Davis position with the hips fully extended and knees slightly flexed, allowing the surgeon or assistant to stand between the legs. A Trendelenburg position with lateral tilt is often used, which permits gravitational retraction of the small bowel and omentum. Laparoscopic colonic mobilisation is usually undertaken within the retroperitoneal plane in a medial-to-lateral direction, unlike open surgery, where mobilisation begins at the peritoneal reflection. This difference in approach has been adopted to maintain fixation of the colon until the retroperitoneal dissection is complete. Early ligation of vascular pedicles is undertaken to allow access, but may also confer an oncological advantage.[42]

For right-sided resections the surgeon stands between the legs, the vascular pedicles are divided and the dissection proceeds laterally in the retroperitoneum. The caecum is mobilised at its pole in a cranial direction to expose the ureter and gonadal vessels; lastly the lateral peritoneal attachment is divided. For left-sided or rectal tumours the inferior mesenteric artery (IMA) is identified running in the base of the sigmoid mesentery. This is approached from the right side and the peritoneum overlying the vessel is incised. A plane between the mesentery and the retroperitoneum is entered beneath the IMA to expose the ureter. This plane is developed to the proximal and lateral extent of the resection and into the mesorectal plane for anterior resections. Again the lateral peritoneal reflection is divided as the last stage of mobilisation. For anterior resection the mesorectum is dissected, applying the principles of total mesorectal excision.

Specimen retrieval and anastomoses are performed through small transverse muscle-splitting incisions: a supraumbilical incision for right-sided resections and a left iliac fossa or Pfannenstiel incision for left-sided or rectal resections. Anastomoses are usually performed extracorporeally for right-sided resections but with a double-staple technique for left-sided or rectal resections.

Results of laparoscopic colectomy

Currently operative times are longer for laparoscopic colorectal resections than for the equivalent open procedure, although Lacy et al.[16] have reported differences of only 20 minutes for colonic resections. These differences will decrease with increasing experience and are likely to reach equivalence. It is accepted that the conversion rate for laparoscopic colectomy runs at less than 10%, but it is slightly higher for rectal surgery.[43] Unfortunately some patients converted from laparoscopic to open surgery may fare badly, with higher complication rates and slower recovery than for the corresponding open procedure[44] – possibly reflecting the patients' underlying condition rather than the conversion per se.

Postoperative pain and analgesia requirements are significantly lower for laparoscopic resections.[17,45] Recovery of bowel function is also more rapid, with faster resolution of postoperative ileus,[46] which is reflected in earlier oral intake[47] and defecation.[17] These functional improvements all facilitate earlier discharge,[45,47] with discharge day brought forward considerably within fast-track or enhanced recovery programmes.[16] Kehlet has reported median postoperative stays of 3 days for both open and laparoscopic resections.[1,2]

Key point 5

- Single-centre randomised studies demonstrate significant improvements in short-term outcome when comparing laparoscopic with open colorectal resection.

In our experience blood loss at laparoscopic resections is negligible. Over the last 3 years our median blood loss has been nil, with less than 10% of patients losing more than 100 ml. Similar results are reported by others for both malignant[47] and benign[28] disease. Hospital complications are consistently reduced in all studies and anastomotic dehiscence rates seem similar to open procedures.[16,28] Like open anterior resection with total mesorectal excision (TME), the laparoscopic approach seems to have higher leak rates than resections above the peritoneal reflection, but again there seems to be equity between the open and laparoscopic approaches.[48,49]

Quality of life studies in laparoscopic colorectal cancer surgery have to date shown modest advantages favouring laparoscopic resections on short-term follow-up.[4,50,51] Studies in benign disease show long-term advantages for laparoscopic resections beyond 3 years.[52] More sensitive cancer specific quality of life questionnaires such as EORTC QLQ-30 may provide a more accurate reflection of this outcome measure.[53]

Oncological outcome in laparoscopic colorectal resections

The first reports of laparoscopic resections for colorectal cancer were published in 1991.[54] The development of new skills, extra expense, increased operating times and concerns regarding its oncological safety, particularly with the early reports of port-site recurrence, have hampered its development. As a result, uptake has been limited, accounting for only 1–2% of colorectal resections within the UK.

Oncological results confirm that tumour clearance is comparable to that with open procedures,[17,55] and this holds true for rectal cancer.[56] Lymph node status is important as this not only influences prognosis but also determines the need for adjuvant chemotherapy. Lymph node yields following laparoscopic resections are similar to those following open procedures, with numbers adequate to stage the disease.[14,16] Local and distant recurrence rates are also similar to those for open procedures, with no difference in the patterns of recurrence.[57,58] Advanced disease can be a challenge laparoscopically; however, there are no differences in the patterns or frequency of recurrence when compared with open resections.[59,60]

For rectal cancer the introduction of total mesorectal excision (TME) has reduced local recurrence rates to less than 7% in open surgery.[61] Poulin et al.[62]

reported similar low levels of recurrence for laparoscopic TME (4.3% at 2.5-year follow-up). Laparoscopic abdominoperineal excision of the rectum (APER) achieves similar local recurrence rates to the open equivalent;[13] however, both approaches yield higher recurrence rates than sphincter-conserving surgery.

To date there have been no randomised trials reporting 5-year survival; however, there are a number of observational and cohort studies with 3-year[63] and 5-year[57] follow-up in which results match those of open surgery.

The most exciting study of survival to date comes from Lacy's work in Barcelona. This trial of surgery in colonic or rectosigmoid tumours randomised over 200 patients to laparoscopic-assisted colectomy or open colectomy. With a median follow up of 43 months, it showed that cancer-related survival was significantly higher in the laparoscopic group, the difference being due to improved outcomes in stage III disease.[16] These results need to be confirmed in further randomised studies, but if consistent will provide added impetus to the further development of laparoscopic colorectal cancer surgery.

Key point 6

- To date only one randomised study has reported on cancer-related survival nearly 4 years following laparoscopic colectomy – this revealed improved cancer-related survival for the laparoscopic group.

Finally the question of port-site recurrences, which blighted the early years of laparoscopic colorectal surgery, has been addressed. Port-site recurrence in current practice seems to be no more common than wound recurrence after open resections, and accounts for less than 1% of all recurrences.[64] In our practice there have been no port-site recurrences in over 180 colorectal cancer resections since 1994.

SUMMARY AND CONCLUSIONS

A laparoscopic approach is feasible for a wide variety of colorectal procedures. Unlike laparoscopic cholecystectomy, it has yet to become the gold standard, but it is gaining acceptance. To date clear advantages have been demonstrated for the laparoscopic approach in terms of decreased blood loss, faster postoperative recovery and return of bowel function, decreased pain and hospital stay, and improved rehabilitation. Improved quality of life has been shown in the short term but the question of cost efficiency needs detailed studies.

For colorectal cancer, oncological results are at least as good as those of open surgery and there is the tantalising prospect of a survival benefit if further research confirms Lacy's results. There are a number of large multicentre randomised trials, including the CLASICC trial from the UK, whose results are eagerly awaited.

The use of a multimodal approach to rehabilitation in colorectal surgery significantly enhances postoperative recovery. It is only by applying such a programme in laparoscopic colorectal surgery, to optimise quality and speed of recovery, that the full potential of this technique will be realised.

ACKNOWLEDGEMENTS

Mr RH Kennedy received funding from the NHS Executive South West; the views expressed in this chapter are those of the authors and not necessarily those of the NHS Executive South West.

Key points for clinical practice

- A carefully structured training programme is necessary to achieve good outcomes in laparoscopic colorectal surgery.

- For surgeons learning these procedures, good case selection is important to minimise complications and conversions – avoiding patients with morbid obesity, multiple adhesions, advanced or rectal tumours.

- Diagnostic laparoscopy in suspected appendicitis is particularly useful in women of childbearing age and laparoscopic appendicectomy will facilitate rapid recovery.

- Laparoscopic colorectal resections are possible in 85–90% of elective patients.

- Single-centre randomised studies demonstrate significant improvements in short-term outcome when comparing laparoscopic with open colorectal resection.

- To date only one randomised study has reported on cancer-related survival nearly 4 years following laparoscopic colectomy – this revealed improved cancer-related survival for the laparoscopic group.

References

1. Basse L, Hjort Jakobsen D, Billesbolle P, Werner M, Kehlet H. A clinical pathway to accelerate recovery after colonic resection. *Ann Surg* 2000; **232**: 51–57.
2. Bardram L, Funch-Jensen P, Kehlet H. Rapid rehabilitation in elderly patients after laparoscopic colonic resection. *Br J Surg* 2000; **87**: 1540–1545.
3. Nakajima K, Lee SW, Cocilovo C *et al.* Hand-assisted laparoscopic colorectal surgery using GelPort. *Surg Endosc* 2003; 102–105.
4. Psaila J, Bulley SH, Ewings P, Sheffield JP, Kennedy RH. Outcome following laparoscopic resection for colorectal cancer. *Br J Surg* 1998; **85**: 662–664.
5. Vibert E, Denet C, Gayet B. Major digestive surgery using a remote-controlled robot: the next revolution. *Arch Surg* 2003; **138**: 1002–1006.
6. Gervaz P, Pikarsky A, Utech M *et al.* Converted laparoscopic colorectal surgery. *Surg Endosc* 2001; **15**: 827–832.
7. Solomon MJ, Young CJ, Eyers AA, Roberts RA. Randomized clinical trial of laparoscopic versus open abdominal rectopexy for rectal prolapse. *Br J Surg* 2002; **89**: 35–39.
8. Whelan RL, Franklin M, Holubar SD *et al.* Postoperative cell mediated immune response is better preserved after laparoscopic vs open colorectal resection in humans. *Surg Endosc* 2003; **17**: 972–978.

9. Delgado S, Lacy AM, Filella X *et al*. Acute phase response in laparoscopic and open colectomy in colon cancer: randomized study. *Dis Colon Rectum* 2001; **44**: 638–646.

10. Braga M, Vignali A, Gianotti L *et al*. Laparoscopic versus open colorectal surgery: a randomized trial on short-term outcome. *Ann Surg* 2002; **236**: 759–766; discussion 767.

11. Martz J, Marcello P, Braveman J *et al*. Does laparoscopic colectomy prevent small-bowel obstruction? A long-term analysis. *Dis Colon Rectum* 2001; **44**: A27–A59.

12. Lumley J, Stitz R, Stevenson A, Fielding G, Luck A. Laparoscopic colorectal surgery for cancer: intermediate to long-term outcomes. *Dis Colon Rectum* 2002; **45**: 867–872; discussion 872–875.

13. Fleshman JW, Wexner SD, Anvari M *et al*. Laparoscopic vs. open abdominoperineal resection for cancer. *Dis Colon Rectum* 1999; **42**: 930–939.

14. Baker RP, White EE, Titu L, Duthie GS, Lee PW, Monson JR. Does laparoscopic abdominoperineal resection of the rectum compromise long-term survival? *Dis Colon Rectum* 2002; **45**: 1481–1485.

15. Fu KI, Fujii T, Kato S *et al*. A new endoscopic tattooing technique for identifying the location of colonic lesions during laparoscopic surgery: a comparison with the conventional technique. *Endoscopy* 2001; **33**: 687–691.

16. Lacy AM, Garcia-Valdecasas JC, Delgado S *et al*. Laparoscopy-assisted colectomy versus open colectomy for treatment of non-metastatic colon cancer: a randomised trial. *Lancet* 2002; **359**: 2224–2229.

17. Milsom JW, Bohm B, Hammerhofer KA, Fazio V, Steiger E, Elson P. A prospective, randomized trial comparing laparoscopic versus conventional techniques in colorectal cancer surgery: a preliminary report. *J Am Coll Surg* 1998; **187**: 46–54; discussion 54–55.

18. Philipson BM, Bokey EL, Moore JW, Chapuis PH, Bagge E. Cost of open versus laparoscopically assisted right hemicolectomy for cancer. *World J Surg* 1997; **21**: 214–217.

19. Delaney CP, Kiran RP, Senagore AJ, Brady K, Fazio VW. Case-matched comparison of clinical and financial outcome after laparoscopic or open colorectal surgery. *Ann Surg* 2003; **238**: 67–72.

20. Msika S, Deroide G, Kianmanesh R *et al*. Harmonic scalpel in laparoscopic colorectal surgery. *Dis Colon Rectum* 2001; **44**: 432–436.

21. Jiang JK, Chen WS, Yang SH, Lin TC, Lin JK. Gasless laparoscopy-assisted colorectal surgery. *Surg Endosc* 2001; **15**: 1093–1097.

22. Merlin TL, Hiller JE, Maddern GJ, Jamieson GG, Brown AR, Kolbe A. Systematic review of the safety and effectiveness of methods used to establish pneumoperitoneum in laparoscopic surgery. *Br J Surg* 2003; **90**: 668–679.

23. O'Sullivan DC, Micali S, Averch TD *et al*. Factors involved in gas embolism after laparoscopic injury to inferior vena cava. *J Endourol* 1998; **12**: 149–154.

24. Schwenk W, Bohm B, Witt C, Junghans T, Grundel K, Muller JM. Pulmonary function following laparoscopic or conventional colorectal resection: a randomized controlled evaluation. *Arch Surg* 1999; **134**: 6–12; discussion 13.

25. ASGBI. 1998 Consensus Statement, Association of Surgeons of Great Britain and Ireland and Association of Coloproctologists of Great Britain and Ireland.

26. Association of Coloproctology of Great Britain and Ireland. 1996 Guidelines for the Management of Colorectal Cancer, The Royal Collage of Surgeons of England.

27. Technology Appraisal Guidance No. 17. 2000 Guidance on the use of laparoscopic surgery in colorectal cancer, National Institute of Clinical Excellence.

28. Dwivedi A, Chahin F, Agrawal S *et al*. Laparoscopic colectomy vs. open colectomy for sigmoid diverticular disease. *Dis Colon Rectum* 2002; **45**: 1309–1314; discussion 1314–1305.

29. Sosa JL, Sleeman D, Puente I, McKenney MG, Hartmann R. Laparoscopic-assisted colostomy closure after Hartmann's procedure. *Dis Colon Rectum* 1994; **37**: 149–152.

30. Shore G, Gonzalez QH, Bondora A, Vickers SM. Laparoscopic vs conventional ileocolectomy for primary Crohn disease. *Arch Surg* 2003; **138**: 76–79.

31. Dunker MS, Bemelman WA, Slors JF, van Hogezand RA, Ringers J, Gouma DJ. Laparoscopic-assisted vs open colectomy for severe acute colitis in patients with inflammatory bowel disease (IBD): a retrospective study in 42 patients. *Surg Endosc* 2000; **14**: 911–914.

32. Kienle P, Weitz J, Benner A, Herfarth C, Schmidt J. Laparoscopically assisted colectomy

and ileoanal pouch procedure with and without protective ileostomy. *Surg Endosc* 2003 ; **17**: 716–720.

33. Lyons TL, Winer WK. Laparoscopic rectocele repair using polyglactin mesh. *J Am Assoc Gynecol Laparosc* 1997; **4**: 381–384.

34. Metcalfe MS, Close JS, Iswariah H, Morrison C, Wemyss-Holden SA, Maddern GJ. The value of laparoscopic staging for patients with colorectal metastases. *Arch Surg* 2003; **138**: 770–772.

35. Le Moine MC, Fabre JM, Vacher C, Navarro F, Picot MC, Domergue J. Factors and consequences of conversion in laparoscopic sigmoidectomy for diverticular disease. *Br J Surg* 2003; **90**: 232–236.

36. Senagore AJ, Delaney CP, Madboulay K, Brady KM, Fazio CV. Laparoscopic colectomy in obese and nonobese patients. *J Gastrointest Surg* 2003; **7**: 558–561.

37. Semm K. Endoscopic appendectomy. *Endoscopy* 1983; **15**: 59–64.

38. Sauerland S, Lefering R, Neugebauer E. 2003 Laparoscopic versus open surgery for suspected appendicitis (Cochrane Review). In: The Cochrane Library. Chichester, UK John Wiley & Sons, Ltd., 2003.

39. Pedersen AG, Petersen OB, Wara P, Ronning H, Qvist N, Laurberg S. Randomized clinical trial of laparoscopic versus open appendicectomy. *Br J Surg* 2001; **88**: 200–205.

40. van den Broek WT, Bijnen AB, de Ruiter P, Gouma DJ. A normal appendix found during diagnostic laparoscopy should not be removed. *Br J Surg* 2001; **88**: 251–254.

41. Ignjatovic D, Bergamaschi R. Preserving the superior rectal artery in laparoscopic anterior resection for complete rectal prolapse. *Acta Chir Iugosl* 2002; **49**: 25–26.

42. Turnbull RB, Jr. Current concepts in cancer. Cancer of the GI tract: colon, rectum, anus. The no-touch isolation technique of resection. *JAMA* 1975; **231**: 1181–1182.

43. Perniceni T, Burdy G, Gayet B, Dubois F, Boudet MJ, Levard H. [Results of elective segmental colectomy done with laparoscopy for complicated diverticulosis]. *Gastroenterol Clin Biol* 2000; **24**: 189–192.

44. Marusch F, Gastinger I, Schneider C *et al*. Importance of conversion for results obtained with laparoscopic colorectal surgery. *Dis Colon Rectum* 2001; **44**: 207–214; discussion 214–206.

45. Stage JG, Schulze S, Moller P *et al*. Prospective randomized study of laparoscopic versus open colonic resection for adenocarcinoma. *Br J Surg* 1997; **84**: 391–396.

46. Chen HH, Wexner SD, Iroatulam AJ *et al*. Laparoscopic colectomy compares favorably with colectomy by laparotomy for reduction of postoperative ileus. *Dis Colon Rectum* 2000; **43**: 61–65.

47. Lacy AM, Garcia-Valdecasas JC, Pique JM *et al*. Short-term outcome analysis of a randomized study comparing laparoscopic vs open colectomy for colon cancer. *Surg Endosc* 1995; **9**: 1101–1105.

48. Morino M, Parini U, Giraudo G, Salval M, Brachet Contul R, Garrone C. Laparoscopic total mesorectal excision: a consecutive series of 100 patients. *Ann Surg* 2003; **237**: 335–342.

49. Zhou ZG, Wang Z, Yu YY *et al*. Laparoscopic total mesorectal excision of low rectal cancer with preservation of anal sphincter: a report of 82 cases. *World J Gastroenterol* 2003; **9**: 1477–1481.

50. Schwenk W, Bohm B, Muller JM. Postoperative pain and fatigue after laparoscopic or conventional colorectal resections. A prospective randomized trial. *Surg Endosc* 1998; **12**: 1131–1136.

51. Weeks JC, Nelson H, Gelber S, Sargent D, Schroeder G. Short-term quality-of-life outcomes following laparoscopic-assisted colectomy vs open colectomy for colon cancer: a randomized trial. *JAMA* 2002; **287**: 321–328.

52. Thaler K, Dinnewitzer A, Mascha E *et al*. Long-term outcome and health-related quality of life after laparoscopic and open colectomy for benign disease. *Surg Endosc* 2003;

53. Osoba D, Aarsonson N, Zee B, Spingers M, Velde A. Modification of the EORTC QLQ-30 (version2.0) based on content validity and reliability testing in large samples of patients with cancer. The Study Group on Quality of Life of the EORTC and Symptom Control and Quality of Life Committees of the NCI of Canada Trials Group. *Qual Life Res* 1997; **6**: 103–108.

54. Fowler DL, White SA. Laparoscopy-assisted sigmoid resection. *Surg Laparosc Endosc* 1991; **1**: 183–188.

55. Korolija D, Tadic S, Simic D. Extent of oncological resection in laparoscopic vs. open colorectal surgery: meta-analysis. *Langenbecks Arch Surg* 2003; **387**: 366–371.

56. Schwandner O, Schiedeck TH, Killaitis C, Bruch HP. A case–control-study comparing laparoscopic versus open surgery for rectosigmoidal and rectal cancer. *Int J Colorectal Dis* 1999; **14**: 158–163.

57. Champault GG, Barrat C, Raselli R, Elizalde A, Catheline JM. Laparoscopic versus open surgery for colorectal carcinoma: a prospective clinical trial involving 157 cases with a mean follow-up of 5 years. *Surg Laparosc Endosc Percutan Tech* 2002; **12**: 88–95.

58. Patankar SK, Larach SW, Ferrara A *et al*. Prospective comparison of laparoscopic vs. open resections for colorectal adenocarcinoma over a ten-year period. *Dis Colon Rectum* 2003; **46**: 601–611.

59. Franklin ME, Kazantsev GB, Abrego D, Diaz EJ, Balli J, Glass JL. Laparoscopic surgery for stage III colon cancer: long-term follow-up. *Surg Endosc* 2000; **14**: 612–616.

60. Yamamoto S, Watanabe M, Hasegawa H, Kitajima M. Oncologic outcome of laparoscopic versus open surgery for advanced colorectal cancer. *Hepatogastroenterology* 2001; **48**): 1248–1251.

61. Heald RJ, Moran BJ, Ryall RD, Sexton R, MacFarlane JK. Rectal cancer: the Basingstoke experience of total mesorectal excision, 1978–1997. *Arch Surg* 1998; **133**: 894–899.

62. Poulin EC, Schlachta CM, Gregoire R, Seshadri P, Cadeddu MO, Mamazza J. Local recurrence and survival after laparoscopic mesorectal resection for rectal adenocarcinoma. *Surg Endosc* 2002; **16**: 989–995.

63. Fleshman JW, Nelson H, Peters WR *et al*. Early results of laparoscopic surgery for colorectal cancer. Retrospective analysis of 372 patients treated by Clinical Outcomes of Surgical Therapy (COST) Study Group. *Dis Colon Rectum* 1996; **39**: S53–S58.

64. Silecchia G, Perrotta N, Giraudo G *et al*. Abdominal wall recurrences after colorectal resection for cancer: results of the Italian registry of laparoscopic colorectal surgery. *Dis Colon Rectum* 2002; **45**: 1172–1177; discussion 1177.

Ian G. Finlay

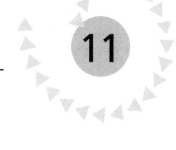

11

Lower gastrointestinal bleeding

Bleeding from the lower gastrointestinal tract (LGIT) is a relatively common cause of emergency admission to hospital. In the USA it has been estimated to occur in 20 people per 100 000 of the population per annum[1] and accounts for approximately 0.7% of emergency surgical admissions.[2] At Glasgow Royal Infirmary approximately 70 patients are admitted each year with a primary complaint of LGIT bleeding, suggesting a similar incidence in the UK.

In most cases LGIT bleeding proves to be a minor, self-limiting event. Consequently, the reported overall mortality rates are low, ranging from only 2–4%.[1,2] A small number of patients, however, present with life-threatening haemorrhage and pose both a diagnostic and therapeutic challenge. In one of the few prospective studies to be reported,[3] less than half of patients admitted as an emergency with suspected LGIT haemorrhage subsequently proved to have had a significant bleed (defined as a fall in haemoglobin or cardiovascular compromise). Of those who did, however, 29% had further bleeding within 2 years and 12% required surgery.[3] The present overview seeks to determine the current evidence and best practice in the management of LGIT bleeding. It is limited, however, by the fact that there are few prospective or randomised trials and the patient populations that have been studied (invariably retrospectively) are not homogeneous.

PRESENTING CLINICAL FEATURES AND AETIOLOGY

In a retrospective study from the Massachussets General Hospital it was noted that although the majority of patients with LGIT bleeding present with a history of passing either maroon or red blood per rectum, syncope or orthostatic hypotension was the first presentation in over 30% of patients. Irrespective of the mode of presentation, the first clinical priority is to identify

Mr Ian G. Finlay Consultant Colorectal Surgeon, Department of Coloproctology, Lister Surgical Unit, Glasgow Royal Infirmary, 16 Alexandra Parade, Glasgow G31 2ER, UK

the small number of patients who have had a life-threatening bleed, since the management of these patients differs from the majority who have had a small bleed. The recognised criteria of tachycardia, hypotension and a low central venous pressure are helpful in identifying the big bleed. Systemic effects from bleeding, however, are a function of both the volume and the rate of blood loss. This interaction between volume and rate is especially important in LGIT bleeding since patients often have persistent rather than rapid haemorrhage, leading to large-volume blood transfusions over several days. In these patients optimising the timing for surgery may be difficult and requires clinical experience. We have known, however, for over 25 years, that patients who have continued bleeding, hypotension, an increased prothrombin time, confusion or unstable comorbidity are at significantly higher risk of recurrent bleeding, surgery and death than those patients who do not have these features.[4]

Consequently, these factors help to predict those at higher risk.

Key point 1

- Patients with signs of continued bleeding or hypotension are at greatest risk of fatal outcome.

IDENTIFICATION OF THE CAUSE OF LGIT BLEEDING

Causes of LGIT bleeding are listed in Table 1.

Table 1 Causes of LGIT bleeding

	Collected published series (n = 912 patients)	Glasgow Royal Infirmary 2001 (n = 70 patients)
Diverticular disease	33%	39%
Colitis (IBD and ischaemic)	18%	21%
Neoplasm	11%	3%
Angiodysplasia	6%	1%
Anorectal	6%	19%
Unknown	27%	12%
Miscellaneous causes	—	5%

RED CELL SCAN

It is vitally important, if a patient with severe LGIT bleeding requires surgery, that the exact site of bleeding should be identified. Until recently, technetium-labelled red cell scintigraphy was the principal investigative tool for this purpose.[5] It has the advantage of being non-invasive but requires the patient to be bleeding at a rate greater than 0.1 ml/min if the source is to be identified. In a compiled series of 1523 patients the median accuracy was only 44% (range 26–78%) while the false-positive rate was 22% (range 6–59%). These disappointing figures and the availability of alternative options probably explain why the technique is now infrequently used in the investigation of

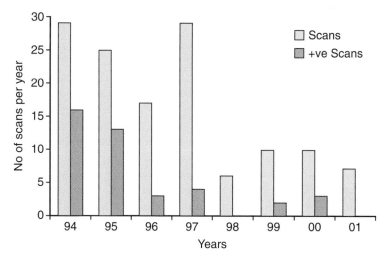

Fig. 1 The number of technetium labelled red cell scans performed at Glasgow Royal Infirmary 1994–2001.

significant LGIT bleeding.[6] At Glasgow Royal Infirmary, for example, the number of red cell scans performed for the investigation of bleeding reduced from approximately 30 per year to only 5 in 2001 (Fig. 1). Despite this trend, it has been suggested that red cell scanning remains useful since it screens out 'non-significant bleeders', thereby increasing the diagnostic yield of angiography by a factor of 2.4.

ANGIOGRAPHY

Angiography is the investigation of choice for patients who are bleeding at a rate of at least 1 ml/min. Although according to the published literature the overall sensitivity of angiography in identifying the bleeding source is only 46% (range 27–77) it has the advantage that there are no false positives and multiple bleeding sites may be detected. Angiography also offers the therapeutic option of embolisation of the bleeding vessel.[7] In early reports, however, the technique was associated with a risk of intestinal ischaemia.[8] For this reason, it has been suggested that the risks of angiography outweigh any benefit. The advent of superselective angiography with microcoil embolisation has largely eliminated these risks, in addition to reducing the need for surgery[9,10,11] Success rates of over 80% have been reported in several studies, with few complications. Availability of the technique is limited by the need for appropriate radiology facilities and a skilled interventional radiologist.

In an astonishing study from Duke University, heparin provocation was used to enhance the diagnostic rate for angiography.[12] Sixteen patients who had received between 6 and 69 units of blood and in whom angiography had been negative were given heparin at the time of a repeat angiogram. The bleeding source was identified in 6 patients; 5 of these were successfully embolised. This apparently 'courageous' action emphasises how important it is to identify the exact site of bleeding as steps may then be taken to control it.

Key point 2

- Angiography is helpful in localising the source of rapid bleeding.

COLONOSCOPY

There is increasing interest in the role of colonoscopy as both a diagnostic and a therapeutic tool in the management of acute LGIT bleeding with a spectrum of opinion with regard to the value of the technique.[13,14,15] This varies from the view that 'urgent colonoscopy has emerged as the initial diagnostic and main therapeutic tool in the evaluation and treatment of colonic bleeding'[13] to the view that 'urgent colonoscopy fails to affect management in LGIT bleeding'.[15] How can we be presented with such diametrically opposed opinions? Perhaps it is because these reports describe dissimilar patient populations with different causes and intensities of bleeding. It has certainly been the author's anecdotal experience that colonoscopy is unhelpful (indeed impossible) in patients with substantial haemorrhage but that colonoscopy increases the diagnostic yield for 'small bleeds'. It is of interest to note, for example, that since the advent of colonoscopy the percentage of patients with LGIT bleeding found to have bled from inflammatory bowel disease and ischaemic colitis has increased when compared with reports from 20 years ago.

Turning to the published evidence, in a meta-analysis of 1751 patients from 14 studies the overall accuracy of urgent colonoscopy was found to be 69% (range 40–90%).[16] Further, colonoscopy offers the opportunity to stop bleeding using band ligation,[17,18] injection of epinephrine or electrocoagulation.[19] The number of patients reported to have been treated by these techniques, however, remains small, and although the early results are promising, longer follow-up is required to determine the re-bleeding rate. It has also been suggested that early colonoscopy significantly reduces hospital stay[20] and costs,[21] predominantly by improving diagnostic yield rather than due to the use of therapeutic intervention.[20] The exact timing of the colonoscopy, however, has been shown not be important in coming to a definitive diagnosis.[22] This may explain why in some studies relatively few bleeding patients have been found to be suitable for a colonoscopic haemostasis technique.[15]

Stigmata of significant haemorrhage

In the management of upper gastrointestinal haemorrhage, clinicians have been aware for more than two decades of the importance of stigmata of recent/significant haemorrhage in the management of peptic ulcer,[23] since these appearances identify patients at risk of continued bleeding. The concept of stigmata of significant haemorrhage (SSH) has now been applied to LGIT bleeding[24] as a consequence of the use of colonoscopy; these include visualisation of active bleeding, a visible vessel and/or adherent clot (Fig. 2). Several studies have shown that patients with LGIT bleeding who have SSH will have more bleeding episodes and lower haemoglobin levels, will require more transfusions and are more likely to need surgical intervention than patients who do not exhibit these signs.

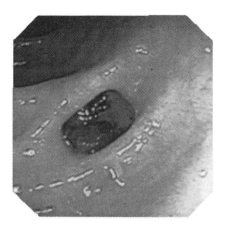

Fig. 2 A colonic diverticulum identified at colonoscopy showing stigmata of recent haemorrhage: clot over a visible vessel (the latter subsequently revealed by washing).

Perhaps the most exciting aspect of the use of urgent colonoscopy in the management of LGIT bleeding arises from a report that suggests that it reduces the need for surgery in these high-risk patients. In a prospective, sequential study performed at the University of California,[25] 121 patients with bleeding from a single cause (diverticular disease) underwent colonoscopy within 12 hours of admission to hospital. In the first 73 patients the colonoscopy was restricted to identifying the diagnosis. No haemostasis techniques were employed, but stigmata of recent haemorrhage (active bleeding, visible vessels and adherent clot) were identified in 17 patients (23%); 6 subsequently required open surgery. In the second group of 48 patients the colonoscopy was supplemented with therapeutic intervention. Ten patients (21%) had stigmata of recent haemorrhage but none required surgery. This provides the best evidence to date that therapeutic colonoscopy may be able to reduce the need for urgent surgery.

Key point 3

- Colonoscopy is the mainstay of accurate localisation, and may provide the opportunity for endoscopic therapy.

Key point 4

- Stigmata of significant haemorrhage may help to identify patients for surgical or endoscopic treatment.

NEW TECHNIQUES

Despite the use of the techniques described above, there will remain a minority of patients who have persistent LGIT bleeding sufficient to necessitate repeat blood transfusion, but in whom no definite bleeding source can be found. With the increasing use of colonoscopy, at least two-thirds of these patients will prove to have bleeding from the small bowel.[26] In these patients the use of push enteroscopy and capsule endoscopy has been advocated.[27,28] In a small study comparing the two techniques, capsule endoscopy identified significantly more bleeding sites within the small bowel than push enteroscopy and was preferred by the patients.[26] These would appear to be promising techniques, but at present they are research tools limited to only a few centres.

There have also been encouraging reports of the use of helical computed tomographic (CT) scanning in locating the source of LGIT bleeding. The site of bleeding is identified by observing the following features: hyperdensity of the peribowel fat, contrast enhancement of the bowel wall and/or vascular extravasation of the contrast medium. In one study the technique correctly identified the source of bleeding in 73% of patients, including sites in the small bowel.[29] Given that CT is a non-invasive investigation, it merits further evaluation.

ANGIODYSPLASIA

Angiodysplasia or vascular ectasia producing chronic obstruction to the submucosal veins used to be considered a common cause of severe LGIT bleeding especially in the elderly.[30] As a consequence of the frequent use of colonoscopy in the investigation of LGIT, it is now recognised that angiodysplasia is an uncommon cause of LGIT bleeding. In a colonoscopic screening programme of 964 normal individuals over the age of 50 years, angiodysplasia was identified in only 8 subjects (0.83%).[31] Of these, 6 were found in the right side of the colon and 2 in the left. In 3 patients the lesions were multiple. None of these patients bled during a 5-year follow-up. It is also recognised that angiodysplasia will be present in the small bowel in at least 20% of patients who have lesions in the large bowel.

Angiodysplasia is especially amenable to colonoscopic therapeutic intervention, including diathermy and adrenaline injection. Consequently few patients now need surgery. Those who do will frequently be found to be bleeding from the small bowel.

The only prospective randomised trial of the management of patients with LGIT bleeding was conducted in patients bleeding from colonic angiodysplasia who were randomised to receive either progestogen/oestrogen or placebo. Unfortunately there was no difference in the re-bleeding rates.[32]

SURGERY

Few patients with LGIT bleeding now require surgery. Although, historically, approximately 10–15% of patients underwent surgery,[2] this has reduced to less than 5%, predominantly due to the impact of therapeutic angiography and colonoscopy. At Glasgow Royal Infirmary, for example, only 2–3% of patients per annum have required surgery since 1999.

The single most important step to be undertaken prior to any operation is for the surgeon to attempt to identify the exact bleeding site using the techniques described above. When this is known, an appropriate segmental resection should be performed. On the basis of collected series from the published literature (Table 2), this will achieve a re-bleeding rate of only 8% but a mortality rate of 15%.

Table 2 Mortality and re-bleeding rates after 'directed' or 'non-directed' surgery (collected series, n = 384 patients)

	Patients re-bleeding (%)	Mortality (%)
Segmental resection (directed)	8	15
Segmental resection (blind)	54	39
Total colectomy	2	15

Key points for clinical practice

• Few patients now require surgery, but if operation is needed then accurate preoperative localisation of the bleeding is important to allow segmental resection.

Difficulty only arises for the surgeon when the exact site of bleeding has not been identified before the operation. It is then important to have a methodical approach to identifying the bleeding source during and immediately prior to surgery. This should include performing an upper gastrointestinal endoscopy and a fibreoptic examination of the anorectum to exclude haemorrhoidal bleeding. The author is aware of at least one patient who has had a 'pan-proctocolectomy' performed for severe haemorrhoidal bleeding. It is also important for the surgeon to be aware that in the era of preoperative angiography and colonoscopy, there is a high probability that occult bleeding will prove to be from the small bowel.[33] Consequently, an attempt should be made to view both the small and large bowel at laparotomy using intraoperative colonoscopy and/or push enteroscopy after on-table colonic lavage. This may require the judicious use of enterotomies. If the bleeding source is identified, a limited resection may be performed. The surgeon must be alert to the possibility of multiple bleeding sites, particularly in the small bowel.

If, after an exhaustive search, no bleeding source is found then a colectomy and end-ileostomy should be performed. This may be expected to lead to a re-bleeding rate of only 2%, although the mortality rate remains high at 15%. It is very important not to perform a 'blind segmental' resection in this situation, since, according to the published literature, the mortality rate will be 39% and the risk of re-bleeding 54%.

A management protocol is summarised in the algorithm given in Figure 3.

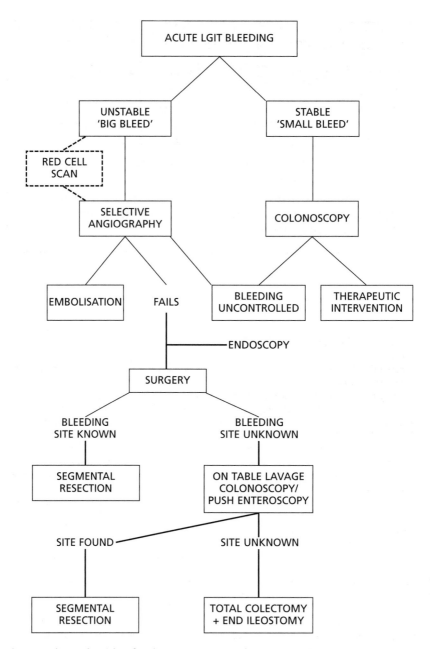

Fig. 3 Author's algorithm for the management of patients with lower gastrointestinal haemorrhage.

Key points for clinical practice

- Patients with signs of continued bleeding or hypotension are at greatest risk of fatal outcome.

- Angiography is helpful in localising the source of rapid bleeding.

- Colonoscopy is the mainstay of accurate localisation, and may provide the opportunity for endoscopic therapy.

- Stigmata of significant haemorrhage may help to identify patients for surgical or endoscopic treatment.

- Few patients now require surgery, but if operation is needed then accurate preoperative localisation of the bleeding is important to allow segmental resection.

References

1. Longstreth GF. Epidemiology and outcome of patients hospitalized with acute lower gastrointestinal haemorrhage: a population based study. *Am J Gastroenterol* 1997; **92**: 419–424.
2. Vernava III AM, Moore BA, Longo WE, Johnson FE, Lower gastrointestinal bleeding. *Dis Colon Rectum* 1997; **40**: 846–858.
3. Bramley PN, Masson JW, McKnight G *et al. Scand J Gastroenterol* 1996; **31**: 764–769.
4. Kollef MW, O'Brian JD, Zuckerman GR, Shannon W. BLEED: a classification tool to predict outcomes in patients with acute upper and lower gastrointestinal haemorrhage. *Crit Care Med* 1997; **25**: 1125–1132.
5. Dolezal J, Vizd'a J, Bures J. Detection of acute gastrointestinal bleeding by means of technetium-99m in vivo labelled red blood cells. *Nucl Med Rev* 2002; **5**: 151–154.
6. Levy R, Barto W, Gani J. Retrospective study of the utility of nuclear scintigraphic-lab red cell scanning for lower gastrointestinal bleeding. *ANZ J Surgery* 2003; **73**: 205–209.
7. Luchtefeld MA, Senagore AJ, Szomstein M *et al.* Evaluation of transarterial embolization for lower gastrointestinal bleeding. *Dis Colon Rectum* 2000; **43**: 532–534.
8. Rosenkrantz H, Bookstein JJ, Bosen RJ *et al.* Post embolic colonic infarction. *Radiology* 1982; **142**: 47–57.
9. Nicholson AA, Ettles DF, Hartley JE *et al.* Transcatheter coil embolotherapy. *Gut* 1998; **43**: 4–5.
10. Gordon RL, Ahl KL, Kerlan RK *et al.* Selective arterial embolization for the control of lower gastrointestinal bleeding. *Am J Surg* 1997; **174**: 24–28.
11. Funaki B, Kostelic JK, Lorenz J *et al.* Superselective microcoil embolization of colonic haemorrhage. *Am J Radiol* 2001; **177**: 829–836.
12. Ryan JM, Key SM, Dumbleton SA, Smith TP. Non localised lower gastrointestinal bleeding: provocative bleeding studies with heparin. *J Vasc Inter Radiol* 2001; **12**: 1273–1277.
13. Beejay U, Marcon NE. Endoscopic treatment of lower gastrointestinal bleeding. *Curr Opin Gastroenterol* 2002; **18**: 87–93.
14. Dell'Abate P, Del Rio P, Soliani P, Sianesi M. Value and limits of emergency colonoscopy in cases of severe lower gastrointestinal haemorrhage. *Chir Ital* 2002; **54**: 123–126.
15. Angtuaca TL, Reddy SK, Drapkin S, Harrell LE, Howden CW. The utility of urgent colonoscopy in the evaluation of acute lower gastrointestinal tract bleeding: a 2 year experience from a single centre. *Am J Gastroenterol* 2001; **96**: 1782–1785.
16. Zuckerman GR and Prakash C. Acute lower gastrointestinal bleeding: clinical presentation and diagnosis. *Gastrointestinal Endoscopy* 1998; **48**: 606–617.
17. Witte JT. Band ligation for colonic bleeding. *Gastrointest Endosc* 2000; **52**: 762–765.

18. Farrell JJ, Graeme-Cook F, Kelsey PB. Treatment of bleeding colonic diverticula by endoscopic band ligation: an *in-vivo* and *ex-vivo* pilot study. *Endoscopy* 2003; **35**: 823–829.
19. Bloomfield RS, Rockey DC, Shetzline MA. Endoscopic therapy of acute diverticular haemorrhage. *Am J Gastroenterol* 2001; **96**: 2367–2372.
20. Strate LL, Syngal S. Timing of colonoscopy: impact on length of hospital stay. *Am J Gastroenterol* 2003; **98**: 317–322.
21. Machicado GA, Jensen DM. Acute and chronic management of lower gastrointestinal bleeding: cost-effective approaches. *Gastroenterologist* 1997; **5**: 189–201.
22. Smoot RL, Gostout CJ, Rajan E, Pardi DS *et al.* Is early colonoscopy after admission for acute diverticular bleeding needed? *Am J Gastroenterol* 2003; **98**: 1996–1999.
23. Forrest JA, Finlayson ND, Shearman DJ. Endoscopy in gastrointestinal bleeding. *Lancet* 1974; **2**: 394–397.
24. Foutch PG. Diverticular bleeding: are nonsteroidal anti-inflammatory drugs risk factors for haemorrhage and can colonoscopy predict outcome for patients. *Am J Gastroenterol* 1995; **90**: 1779–1784.
25. Jenson DM, Machicado GA, Jutabha R, Kovacs TO. Urgent colonoscopy for the diagnosis and treatment of severe diverticular disease. *N Engl J Med* 2000; **342**: 78–82.
26. Mylonaki M, Fritscher-Ravens A, Swain P. Wireless capsule endosopy: a comparison with push enteroscopy in patients with gastroscopy and colonoscopy negative bleeding. *Gut* 2003; **52**: 1122–1126.
27. Lewis B, Goldfarb N. Review article: The advent of capsule endoscopy. *Aliment Pharmacol Therapeut* 2003; **17**: 1085–1096.
28. Van Gossum A, Hittelet A, Schmit A, Francois E. A prospective comparative study of push and wireless-capsule endoteroscopy in patients with obscure digestive bleeding. *Acta Gastroenterol Belg* 2003; **66**: 199–205.
29. Ernst O, Bulois P, Saint-Drenant S *et al.* Helical CT in acute lower gastrointestinal bleeding. *Eur Radiol* 2003; **13**: 114–117.
30. Boley SJ, Sammartano R, Adams A *et al.* On the nature and aetiology of vascular ectasias of the colon. Gastroenterology 1997; **72**: 650–659
31. Foutch PG, Rex DK, Leiberman DA. Prevalence and natural history of colonic andiodysplasia among healthy asymptomatic people. *Am J Gastroenterol* 1995; **90**: 564–567.
32. Junquera F, Feu F, Papo M, Videla S *et al.* A multi centre, randomised, clinical trial of hormonal therapy in the prevention of rebleeding from gastrointestinal angiodysplasia. *Gastroenterology* 2001; **121**: 1073-1079.
33. Zaman A, Sheppard B, Katon RM. Total peroral intraoperative enteroscopy for obscure GI bleeding using a dedicated push enteroscope: diagnostic yield and patient outcome. *Gastrointest Endosc* 1999; **50**: 506–510.

Robert B. Galland

12

Extra-anatomic bypass for leg ischaemia

Extra-anatomic bypasses are grafts that occupy a significantly different anatomic route to the arteries that they replace. Their development is described in detail elsewhere.[1] In 1952 Freeman and Leeds first described a femorofemoral bypass using superficial femoral artery as the conduit. In 1958 McCaughan used Dacron from the left external iliac to the right profunda femoris artery. The fact that upper limb arteries could be used to revascularise the lower limb was first demonstrated by Lewis in 1959. Femorofemoral and axillofemoral bypasses became established in the early 1960s. In 1962 Shaw and Baue first described the use of an obturator bypass to avoid sepsis localised to a groin.

This chapter will concentrate on the commonest extra-anatomic bypasses, namely femorofemoral crossover and axillofemoral grafts. The obturator bypass will also be described. Other extra-anatomic bypasses include carotid–subclavian, axillary–axillary, spleno–renal and crossover femoro-popliteal bypasses. These will not be considered further.

When originally described, femorofemoral and axillofemoral bypasses tended to be used for unfit patients for whom aortofemoral bypass (AFBG) would be too dangerous, or in the presence of a 'hostile' abdomen. AFBG for aortoiliac occlusive disease has a 30-day mortality rate of approximately 3%.[2] In recent years there has been a trend away from AFBG to the less-invasive extra-anatomic bypasses even in fit individuals.[3] Following AFBG there can be sexual dysfunction in men. Failure to ejaculate occurs as a result of damage to the pre-aortic sympathectic plexus and failure of erection due to reduced internal iliac artery perfusion. Extra-anatomic bypasses avoid these problems. Differences in patient selection explains some of the wide variation in results in different series of extra-anatomic bypass. Figure 1 shows an algorithm for management of aortoiliac occlusive disease and the role of femorofemoral and axillofemoral bypasses.

Mr Robert B. Galland MD FRCS, Consultant Surgeon, Royal Berkshire Hospital, London Road, Reading, Berkshire RG1 5AN, UK

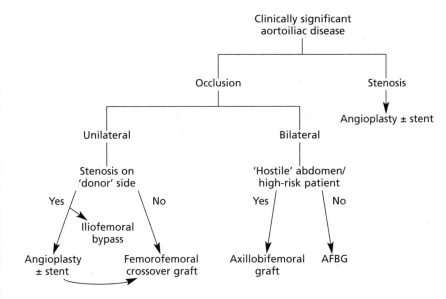

Fig. 1 Algorithm for the management of aortoiliac disease. AFBG, aortofemoral bifurcation graft.

Key point 1

- There is an increasing trend towards less-invasive procedures in managing aortoiliac disease.

HAEMODYNAMICS AND GRAFT CONFIGURATION

Concerns about a 'steal' phenomenon in the donor limb of a femorofemoral bypass resulting in significant clinical problems have proved largely unfounded. Should a 'steal' occur it is almost always due to unmasking pre-existing 'donor'-side disease. Even if there is a stenosis in the donor artery, usually no steal is experienced, as the ankle brachial pressure index will fall in both limbs. A pressure fall has been demonstrated in about 80% of femorofemoral crossover graft donor limbs, but this is rarely clinically important.[4] However, in the presence of superficial femoral artery occlusion and donor artery stenosis there is little improvement in leg blood flow in response to exercise. Early reports of axillofemoral bypasses suggested that flow rates and patency were greater in axillobifemoral compared with axillounifemoral grafts. However, the evidence is conflicting and there seems little advantage in carrying out a bifemoral anastomosis if only one leg is symptomatic.

Several different ways of constructing the bypass have been described. For femorofemoral crossover grafts there is a 'lazy S' configuration, whereby the donor end of the graft is directed proximally and the recipient distally, and the 'bucket handle' configuration, where both ends are directed distally. For axillofemoral bypasses configurations include an axillounifemoral graft, with a crossover graft taken either from the common femoral or from the graft itself, and an axillofemoral crossover, with another graft taken from the cross to the ipsilateral groin. There is no evidence that any one configuration is any better than another in terms of patency. It is reasonable to tailor the graft configuration to the anatomic needs of the patient.

Key point 2

- Graft configuration for extra-anatomic bypass is unimportant.

FEMOROFEMORAL BYPASS

TECHNIQUE

The operation is usually carried out under general anaesthetic, but local or regional anaesthesia are reasonable alternatives. The femoral arteries are exposed through groin incisions. The graft is usually tunnelled subcutaneously; however, it can be placed beneath the external oblique aponeurosis or in the preperitoneal plane if necessary. The common femoral artery is usually the donor artery. Assessment of the donor artery by two-plane angiography, duplex or pressure studies is important to exclude an asymptomatic stenosis. The recipient artery can be either the common femoral or profunda femoris. Dacron or polytetrafluoroethylene (PTFE), 8 mm diameter, are the usual graft materials, but with increasing concern regarding infection, particularly methicillin-resistant *Staphylococcus aureus* (MRSA), the long saphenous vein (LSV) is an option that should be considered. Although the operating time required is longer, as the vein needs to be harvested, short-term patency and morbidity rates seem no worse using LSV than using a synthetic graft.[5] Careful wound closure to obliterate dead space may reduce seroma formation. Drains are not necessary. All operations involving arterial crossclamping are usually carried out with intravenous heparin having been given. Similarly, when using a synthetic graft, prophylactic antibiotics are mandatory. It is assumed that all patients will have risk factor modification and will be taking an antiplatelet agent and probably a statin.

Key point 3

- Consider autologous vein for femorofemoral bypass.

RESULTS

The commonest indication for the operation is intermittent claudication. Table 1 shows some typical results of femorofemoral crossover grafting. Most series include procedures performed some years ago. With modern anaesthesia and better patient selection, improved results are being seen in recent years.

Table 1 Typical series of femorofemoral crossover grafts; primary patency is shown

Authors	Year	n	Country	Patency (year, %) 1	3	5	6	10	Complications	Indication	Mortality rate (%)	Graft material	Comparison with other techniques
Rutherford et al.[6]	1987	60	USA			67				IC 55%	0	Not stated	Patency better than axillofemoral bypass
Perler et al.[7]	1991	50	USA		57	57			Major 8%, wound 6%	IC 45%	10	Synthetic	Patency worse than iliofemoral bypass
Harrington et al.[8]	1992	130	USA			57			Wound complications in 6.8%	IC 32%	6.2	Synthetic mainly	Patency worse than iliofemoral bypass
Ng et al.[9]	1993	156	UK				92		Early re-operation in 5.1%	IC 51%	1.3	Synthetic mainly	Patency better than iliofemoral bypass
Criado et al.[10]	1993	110	USA	83	71	60	51		Major 11%, minor 8%	IC 56%	4.5	Synthetic mainly	
Schneider et al.[11]	1994	91	USA		60					IC 25%	8	Synthetic mainly	Patency worse than AFBG
Berce et al.[12]	1996	211	Australia	96		72		64		IC all	0	Synthetic	
Nazzal et al.[13]	1998	68	USA	92	82	82				IC 25%	2.9	Synthetic 88%	Patency similar to iliofemoral bypass
Lau et al.[14]	2000	61	China	86		79	71		Minor 16%	IC 15%	7	Synthetic	
Whatling et al.[15]	2000	87	UK			90+			Minor wound complications in 5%	IC mainly	0	Synthetic	Patency better than PTA and stenting
Pai et al.[5]	2003	161	UK	71						IC 41%	8.1	Synthetic 76%	

AFBG, aortofemoral bifurcation graft; PTA, percutaneous transluminal angioplasty; IC, intermittent claudication. Mortality rate is either 30-day or before discharge from hospital.

The procedure can also be used for bypass of a single limb occlusion of an AFBG. Patency rates at 5 years have been reported that are only slightly worse than those described for claudication.[16] Widening indications include limb revascularisation following aortouniiliac endovascular abdominal aortic aneurysm (AAA) repair.[17]

Morbidity and mortality

To a large extent this will depend upon the original indication for the procedure. Significant systemic morbidity and mortality, occurring mainly in those patients having the procedure for critical limb ischaemia, are largely cardiac-related. Specific early complications related to the operation involve minor wound complications in about 5% of cases.

The incidence of late complications is difficult to determine. Graft infection and anastomotic false aneurysms are the problems likely to lead to further surgical intervention. If groin infection involving a synthetic graft occurs, the options are debridement and covering the graft with a sartorius flap, removal of the graft and a further femorofemoral bypass using a vein graft or an obturator bypass. Debridement with a sartorius flap results in about half of the grafts being saved.[18]

Patency

Graft patency depends upon such factors as quality of the inflow and outflow vessels and indication for procedure. Graft occlusion within 30 days occurs in approximately 1–2% cases.[6,10,11] Schneider et al.[11] described an early occlusion rate of 2%, which was not significantly different to the results following AFBG. Table 1 shows a range of 1-year primary patency of 71–96% and 3-year patency of 60–90%. Graft failures are more likely to be due to progression of outflow disease than inflow disease.[19] Secondary patency is slightly higher. Berce et al.,[12] operating only on patients with claudication, found secondary patency rates of 98%, 89% and 87% at 1, 5 and 10 years respectively. Similarly, Harrington et al.,[8] where only approximately one-third of patients had claudication, described a 5-year secondary patency rate of 65%. Patients presenting with acute ischaemia do less well than those presenting with chronic ischaemia. Harrington et al. reported a 46% primary patency at 1 year in patients presenting with acute ischaemia compared with 76.6% in those with chronic ischaemia.

Superficial femoral occlusion in the recipient limb is probably a determinant of graft patency. Rutherford et al.[6] showed that 5 year primary patency rates were 79% and 53% for patent and occluded superficial femoral arteries respectively. Secondary patency rates were 95% and 67%. Those series that show that distal disease does not influence patency have tended to carry out simultaneous distal reconstruction.[10] Multilevel reconstruction seems to achieve similar results to femorofemoral crossover alone in the absence of distal disease.[20]

Limb salvage and patient survival

Both of these will depend upon the original indication for operation. Limb salvage following operation for critical ischaemia has been reported as 88% at 3 years[11] and 64% at 5 years.[10] The 5-year limb salvage rate when the initial indication was claudication is more than 90%. Berce et al.[12] found that of major amputations (2% of initial population) in patients having femorofemoral crossover grafts for claudication, two were in the inflow limb and three in the outflow limb.[12] This was at an average follow up of 5½ years.

The 5-year survival rate of patients following femorofemoral crossover graft is of the order of 80%.[9,13]

Patency compared with other techniques

Generally, patency following femorofemoral crossover grafting is less good than after AFBG, similar to iliofemoral bypass and better than percutaneous transluminal angioplasty and stenting.

Schneider et al.[11] described a 3-year primary patency of 85% for AFBG compared with 60% for femorofemoral crossover grafts.[11] They identified that patients undergoing crossover grafting were older and less fit than those having an AFBG. When just looking at the low-risk patients the 3-year primary patency rate was 87% versus 61% respectively. They concluded that this was due to inadequate inflow. If significant iliac stenosis is identified on the donor site then PTA with or without stenting should be carried out. Perler and Williams[21] found a 3-year patency rate of 72% in patients undergoing PTA with or without stenting compared with 80% for patients who required no inflow procedure. This difference was not statistically significant.

When comparing femorofemoral crossover grafts with iliofemoral grafting, there seems little difference. Harrington et al.[8] did find a 5-year primary patency rate of 75% in iliofemoral grafts compared with 57% in femorofemoral crossover grafts. However, excluding patients with acute ischaemia, the patency rate in both groups of patients was 73%. Nazzal et al.[13] described primary patency of 92.4%, 81.7% and 81.7% for femorofemoral crossover grafting and 83.9%, 68.1% and 61.3% for iliofemoral grafting at 1, 3 and 5 years respectively. These differences were not significant. Ng et al.[9] found femorofemoral crossover grafting to be superior to iliofemoral grafting. The 6-year primary patency rate was 92% compared with 75%, the operative mortality rate was 1.3% versus 6% and the 30-day re-operation rate was 5.1% compared with 11%. This was despite similar patient populations in the two groups of patients.

Finally, iliac angioplasty and stenting might seem to be an attractive endovascular alternative to femorofemoral crossover grafting. However, although the results of PTA and stenting of iliac stenoses are good, the results of PTA for occlusions are poor. For stenting of iliac stenoses there is minimal morbidity and mortality, a technical success rate of nearly 100% and a 4-year patency rate of 77%.[22] On the other hand, mortality and significant morbidity occur in 0.1% and approximately 10% respectively, following stenting of iliac occlusions where the indication is claudication and 4.7% and 20% in cases of critical ischaemia.[23] The 4-year patency rate based on 'intention to treat' is about 50%.[22] We compared 51 patients with unilateral iliac occlusion who underwent angioplasty and stenting with 87 patients with similar lesions undergoing crossover grafting.[15] All of the major complications (mainly thromboembolic) were in the patients who underwent stenting. Following successful stent insertion, the 6-month patency rate was only 78%; based on 'intention to treat', the patency rate was 52%. This was statistically significantly worse than patency following crossover grafting.

> **Key point 4**
>
> • Relatively poor early results in the literature for extra-anatomic bypass are largely due to the fact that the procedures were initially used for high-risk patients with critical ischaemia.

AXILLOFEMORAL BYPASS

The majority of surgeons tend to undertake an axillobifemoral rather than a unifemoral bypass. There seems to be no advantage in doing this if only one lower limb is ischaemic. Where unifemoral and bifemoral grafts have been compared, no differences have emerged. Mohan *et al.*[24] described 80% primary and 91% secondary patency rates at 3 years for bifemoral grafting compared with 80% and 89% respectively for unifemoral grafting. These differences were not statistically significant. The 30-day mortality rate was also similar in the two groups.

TECHNIQUE

The operation is usually performed under light general anaesthesia, but local anaesthesia is feasible. The patient lies supine with the donor arm abducted to 90°. The right arm is usually used as, theoretically at least, there is a lower risk of occlusive disease on the right than the left. Bilateral brachial artery pressures and auscultation for bruits are generally sufficient in assessing donor arteries. However, duplex scanning may be needed if there is any doubt. A transverse incision is made beneath the middle third of the clavicle. Fibres of the pectoralis major are split and the clavipectoral fascia divided. The pectoralis minor may need to be divided (either for access or to prevent compression of the graft). The axillary vein lies anteroinferior to the artery and tributaries must be divided so that the vein can be mobilised. The brachial plexus lies above and behind the artery. The first or second part of the axillary artery is usually used. The anastomosis should be as proximal as possible on the artery where there is likely to be less motion when the arm moves. Externally supported 8 mm PTFE or Dacron are generally used. No advantage has been shown for one graft material over another. It is convenient to use a preformed Y-shaped bypass. The graft is tunnelled into position subcutaneously down to the groin or groins. An anterior axillary line is preferable to placing the graft in the mid-axillary line as this allows the patient to sleep on that side without graft compression. The femoral anastomosis or anastomoses are completed end-to-side. No drains are required.

RESULTS

Whereas the commonest indication for femorofemoral crossover grafting is claudication, the majority of patients undergoing axillofemoral grafting have critical ischaemia (Table 2). This needs to be remembered when interpreting results. Axillobifemoral grafts are also used when an infected aortic graft (for aneurysmal or occlusive disease) has to be removed.

Table 2 Typical results of series comprising mainly or only axillobifemoral grafts; all grafts were synthetic; primary patency is described

Authors	Year	n	Country	Patency (year, %)			Complications	Indication	Mortality rate (%)	Comparison with other techniques
				1	3	5				
Donaldson et al.[25]	1986	100	USA		54			IC 19%	8	
Rutherford et al.[6]	1987	27	USA			62		IC 19%	11	
Naylor et al.[26]	1990	38	UK	74	71	68		IC 0%	11	
Harris et al.[27]	1990	76	USA	93	85	85	Major or minor morbidity in 29%	a	4.5	
El-Massry et al.[28]	1993	79	USA			78	Minor wound only	IC 38%	5	No difference unifemoral or bifemoral
Mohan et al.[24]	1995	36	USA		80		Minor wound 6%	IC 0%	11	No difference unifemoral or bifemoral
Passman et al.[29]	1996	108	USA			74	Major in 9.2%	IC 20%	3.4	No difference in patency compared with AFBG
Jain et al.[30]	1998	59	USA	72				IC 10%	12	

AFBG, aortofemoral bifurcation graft; IC, intermittent claudication. Mortality rate is either 30-day or before discharge from hospital.
a 'Absolute' indications included graft infection, aortoenteric fistula and infected aneurysm in 26%; 'relative' indications in the remainder were high-risk patients and potential technical problems.

Morbidity and mortality

Major morbidity and mortality are generally related to myocardial ischaemia. Wound problems are usually minor. Given the different patient population, it is not surprising that the reported mortality rates are higher than those associated with femorofemoral crossover grafting.

Patency

The 30-day graft occlusion rate is approximately 5%.[24,26,28,29]

There is a range of 1-year primary patency rate of 72–93% and 3-year patency rates of 54–85% (Table 2). The indication for the procedure is a determinant of patency. El-Massry et al. described a 6-year primary patency rate of 80% if the patient had claudication, compared with 65% for critical ischaemia. In the presence of distal occlusive disease, patency of axillofemoral bypass is poor. The axillobifemoral primary patency rate at 5 years fell from 92% to 41% in the presence of superficial femoral artery occlusion.[6] In the same series no axillounifemoral bypass remained patent beyond 27 months if the superficial femoral artery was occluded.

Limb salvage and patient survival

In the majority of patients having axillofemoral bypass the indication for the operation will have been critical ischaemia. The 3-year limb salvage rate for this group of patients following axillofemoral grafting is 69–80%.[31]

Three year survival varies widely between 35% to 79%.[31]

Patency compared with other techniques.

Rutherford et al.[6] found axillofemoral grafts to be less durable than femorofemoral crossover grafts. More recently, however, it has been suggested that axillobifemoral grafts may be as good as AFBGs.[29] In a comparison of the two procedures, the choice of operation being made by surgeons' preference, 5-year primary patency and limb salvage rates were similar at 74% and 89% for axillobifemoral grafts compared with 80% and 79% for AFBG. Not surprisingly, in this series patients undergoing axillobifemoral grafts were older and had more cardiovascular and renal disease. The long-term survival was significantly less in this group. The axillobifemoral operation was more likely to be combined with a distal reconstruction than the AFBG.

Key point 5

- Patency after axillofemoral grafting may be as good as AFBG when patients and disease are comparable. Morbidity is lower with extra-anatomic bypass.

OBTURATOR BYPASS

This is a useful bypass when there is an ischaemic limb in the presence of a 'hostile' groin. The usual indication is infection, often involving a synthetic graft at the groin. Other indications include mycotic aneurysm, previous radiation, malignancy or crushing injuries to the groin. Any infected synthetic graft will need to be removed if infection is to be controlled. Long-term antibiotics will be required.

TECHNIQUE

The patient lies supine under general anaesthetic. The affected limb is externally rotated, abducted and flexed to relax the thigh muscles. The aorta or iliac vessels can be approached either transabdominally or through the retroperitoneum as felt appropriate. Using 8 mm externally supported Dacron or PTFE, the upper anastomosis can be made to the aorta, uninfected remaining limb of graft or iliac vessels. The obturator foramen is ringed by the sharp margins of the pubis and ischium. The obturator membrane is attached to the margin of the foramen. The avascular area of the membrane is identified (fibres of obturator internus may need to be separated) and divided. This avascular area lies medial to the obturator vessels and nerves. The graft is then tunnelled through the obturator foramen and passed deep to the pectineus, adductor longus and adductor brevis and superficial to the adductor magnus. The lower anastomosis can then be made end-to-side to the popliteal artery above or below the knee.

RESULTS

Although 30-day mortality rates of up to 16% have been reported, largely due to the original sepsis, patency can be quite good.[32] Of 55 procedures described by Nevelsteen et al.[33] the 3-year patency rates were 71% and 45% for above- and below-knee distal anastomoses respectively. Patency is higher in those patients having the operation for aneurysmal rather than occlusive disease.[34] Patel et al.[32] reported 12 patients having obturator bypass. Of the 10 survivors, 4 required early re-operation but all were infection-free at a mean follow up of 37 months.

Key point 6

- Patency after obturator bypass is good, and the procedure should be considered in the presence of a 'hostile' groin.

Key points for clinical practice

- There is an increasing trend towards less-invasive procedures in managing aortoiliac disease.
- Graft configuration for extra-anatomic bypass is unimportant.
- Consider autologous vein for femorofemoral bypass.

Key points for clinical practice (continued)

- Relatively poor early results in the literature for extra-anatomic bypass are largely due to the fact that the procedures were initially used for high-risk patients with critical ischaemia.

- Patency after axillofemoral grafting may be as good as AFBG when patients and disease are comparable. Morbidity is lower with extra-anatomic bypass.

- Patency after obturator bypass is good, and the procedure should be considered in the presence of a 'hostile' groin.

References

1. Rutherford RB, Baue AE. Extra-anatomic bypass. In: Rutherford RB (ed). *Vascular Surgery* Philadelphia: WB Saunders, 1989; 705–716.
2. Galland RB. Mortality following elective infrarenal aortic reconstruction: a Joint Vascular Research Group study. *Br J Surg* 1998; **85**: 633–636.
3. Whiteley MS, Ray-Chaudhuri SB, Galland RB. Changing patterns in aortoiliac reconstruction: a 7-year audit. *Br J Surg* 1996; **83**: 1367–1369.
4. Flanigan DP, Pratt DG, Goodreau JJ, Burnham SJ, Yao JS, Bergan JJ. Hemodynamic and angiographic guidelines in selection of patients for femorofemoral bypass. *Arch Surg* 1978; **113**: 1257–1262.
5. Pai M, Handa A, Hands L, Collin J. Femoro-femoral arterial bypass is an effective and durable treatment for symptomatic unilateral iliac artery occlusion. *Ann R Coll Surg Engl* 2003; **85**: 88–90.
6. Rutherford RB, Patt A, Pearce WH. Extra-anatomic bypass: a closer view. *J Vasc Surg* 1987; **6**: 437–446.
7. Perler BA, Burdick JF, Williams GM. Femoro-femoral or ileo-femoral bypass for unilateral inflow reconstruction? *Am J Surg* 1991; **161**: 426–430.
8. Harrington ME, Harrington EB, Haimov M, Schanzer H, Hacobson JH. Iliofemoral versus femorofemoral bypass: the case for an individualized approach. *J Vasc Surg* 1992; **16**: 841–854.
9. Ng RLH, Gillies TE, Davies AH, Baird RN, Horrocks M. Iliofemoral versus femorofemoral bypass: a 6-year audit. *Br J Surg* 1992; **79**: 1011–1013.
10. Criado E, Burnham SJ, Tinsley EA, Johnson G, Keagy BA. Femorofemoral bypass graft: Analysis of patency and factors influencing long-term outcome. *J Vasc Surg* 1993; **18**: 495–505.
11. Schneider JR, Bessi SR, Walsh DB, Zwolak RM, Cronenwett JL. Femorofemoral versus aortobifemoral bypass: outcome and hemodynamic results. *J Vasc Surg* 1994; **19**: 43–57.
12. Berce M, Sayers RD, Miller JH. Femorofemoral crossover grafts for claudication: a safe and reliable procedure. *Eur J Vasc Endovasc Surg* 1996; **12**: 437–441.
13. Nazzal MM, Hoballah JJ, Jacobovicz C et al. A comparative evaluation of femorofemoral crossover bypass and iliofemoral bypass for unilateral iliac artery occlusive disease. *Angiology* 1998; **49**: 259–265.
14. Lau H, Cheng SWK, Hui J. Eighteen-year experience with femoro-femoral bypass. *Aust NZ J Surg* 2000; **70**: 275–278.
15. Whatling PJ, Gibson M, Torrie EPH, Magee TR, Galland RB. Iliac occlusions: Stenting or crossover grafting? An examination of patency and cost. *Eur J Vasc Endovasc Surg* 2000; **20**: 36–40.
16. Nolan KD, Benjamin ME, Murphy TJ et al. Femorofemoral bypass for aortofemoral graft limb occlusion: a ten-year experience. *J Vasc Surg* 1994; **19**: 851–857.
17. Hinchliffe RJ, Alric P, Wenham PW, Hopkinson BR. Durability of femorofemoral bypass grafting after aortouniiliac endovascular aneurysm repair. *J Vasc Surg* 2003; **38**: 498–503.

18. Galland RB. Sartorius transposition in the management of synthetic graft infection. *Eur J Vasc Endovasc Surg* 2002; **23**: 175–177.
19. Criado E, Farber MA. Femorofemoral bypass: appropriate application based on factors affecting outcome. *Semin Vasc Surg* 1997; **10**: 34–41.
20. Dalman RL, Taylor LM, Moneta GL, Yeager RA, Porter JM. Simultaneous operative repair of multilevel lower extremity occlusive disease. *J Vasc Surg* 1991; **13**: 211–221.
21. Perler BA, Williams GM. Does donor iliac artery percutaneous transluminal angioplasty or stent placement influence the results of femorofemoral bypass? Analysis of 70 consecutive cases with long-term follow up. *J Vasc Surg* 1996; **24**: 363–370.
22. Bosch JL, Hunink MGM. Meta-analysis of the results of percutaneous transluminal angioplasty and stent placement for aortoiliac occlusive disease. *Radiology* 1997; **204**: 87–96.
23. Gaines PA, Moss JG, Kinsman R. Iliac angioplasty study. BIAS 2001. British Society of Interventional Radiology.
24. Mohan CR, Sharp WJ, Hoballah JJ *et al*. A comparative evaluation of externally supported polytetrafluoroethylene axillobifemoral and axillounifemoral bypass grafts. *J Vasc Surg* 1995; **21**: 801–809.
25. Donaldson MC, Louras JC, Bucknam CA. Axillofemoral bypass: a tool with a limited role. *J Vasc Surg* 1986; **3**: 757–763.
26. Naylor AR, Ah-See AK, Engeset J. Axillofemoral bypass as a limb salvage procedure in high risk patients with aortoiliac disease. *Br J Surg* 1990; **77**: 659–661.
27. Harris EJ, Taylor LM, McConnell DB, Moneta GL, Yeager RA, Porter JM. Clinical results of axillobifemoral bypass using externally supported polytetrafluoroethylene. *J Vasc Surg* 1990; **12**: 416–421.
28. El-Massry S, Saad E, Sauvage LR *et al*. Axillofemoral bypass with externally supported, knitted Dacron grafts: a follow-IP through twelve years. *J Vasc Surg* 1993; **17**: 107–115.
29. Passman MA, Taylor LM, Moneta GL *et al*. Comparison of axillofemoral and aortofemoral bypass for aortoiliac occlusive disease. *J Vasc Surg* 1996; **23**: 263–271.
30. Jain KM, O'Brien SP, Munn JS *et al*. Axillobifemoral bypass: elective versus emergent operation. *Ann Vasc Surg* 1998; **12**: 265–269.
31. Schneider JR, Golan JF. The role of extra anatomic bypass in the management of bilateral aortoiliac occlusive disease. *Semin Vasc Surg* 1994; **7**: 35–44.
32. Patel A, Taylor SM, Langan EM 3rd *et al*. Obturator bypass: a classic approach for the treatment of contemporary groin infection. *Am Surg* 2002; **68**: 653–659.
33. Nevelsteen A, Mees U, Deleersnijder J, Suy R. Obturator bypass: a sixteen year experience with 55 cases. *Ann Vasc Surg* 1987: **1**: 558–563.
34. Reddy DJ, Shin LH. Obturator bypass: technical considerations. *Semin Vasc Surg* 2000; **13**: 49–52.

Bareen Shah   William R. Fleming   John Lynn

13

Thyroid cancer

Ninety percent of cases of thyroid cancer are well differentiated and include papillary, follicular and Hürthle cell tumours. The remaining 10% are poorly differentiated, comprising anaplastic and medullary cancers and lymphoma. Thyroid cancer represents less than 1% of all cancers. In the UK there are 1000 new cases a year, with only 250 deaths.[1]

PREDISPOSING FACTORS

Follicular cancer is more prevalent in iodine-deficient areas; this may be due to a marginally raised thyroid-stimulating hormone (TSH). It is also associated with an increased incidence of anaplastic cancer. Papillary cancers account for 80% of tumours in iodine-replete areas.[2-4]

Ionising radiation is a potent initiator of papillary cancer; exposure under the age of 10 significantly increases the risk, which is at its greatest at the age of 4. Studies from Hiroshima and Chernobyl show that exposure over the age of 20 is not associated with an increased incidence of cancer. Children with thyroid cancer due to accidental radiation exposure usually have papillary, or a follicular variant of papillary cancer.

Forty years ago, radiotherapy given to treat benign head and neck conditions in childhood was a significant cause of thyroid cancer. The latency period is greater than 8 years, but the tendency to develop cancer falls with time, although never quite to the level of the normal population. Patients given external-beam radiation to the head and neck for lymphoma or scattered radiation for breast cancer are at an increased risk. Iodine-131 (^{131}I) treatment

Miss Bareen Shah FRCS, Consultant Surgeon, Ealing Hospital, London, UK

Mr William R. Fleming MBBS FRACS, Consultant Surgeon, Endocrine Surgery Unit, Austin Health, Heidelberg, Victoria, Australia

Mr John Lynn MS FRCS, Consultant Endocrine Surgeon, Imperial College of Medicine, Hammersmith Hospital NHS Trust, Du Cane Road, London W12 0HS, UK (for correspondence)

of thyrotoxicosis however, is not associated with a significant increase in thyroid cancer.[5]

Patients with Hashimoto's thyroiditis have a 70-fold increased risk of developing lymphoma.

GENETIC FEATURES

Most well-differentiated tumours are sporadic. Genetic surveillance is revealing that more of the supposedly sporadic, well-differentiated tumours in fact have a genetic basis. Studies have demonstrated gene rearrangement of the *RET* proto-oncogene in 50% of tumours.[6]

Patients with an inherited predisposition include:

- kindreds of papillary cancer with no associated extrathyroid tumours;

- Cowden syndrome – the association of well-differentiated thyroid cancer and breast cancer and curious multiple hamartomas – the defect is due to germline mutations in the tumour suppressor gene *PTEN*;[6]

- familial adenomatous polyposis coli is associated with germline mutations in the *APC* gene with significantly increased incidence of papillary cancer;[7]

- familial medullary thyroid cancers are in three forms: familial non-MEN and multiple endocrine neoplasia (MEN) types IIA and IIB, all of which are due to various mutations in the *RET* gene.[8,9]

EVALUATION FOR MALIGNANCY

The clinical features of malignancy include a painless, fixed, hard thyroid mass, hoarseness, dysphagia and isolated lymph node enlargement (sometimes called 'lateral aberrant thyroid'). Significant voice change with evidence of recurrent laryngeal nerve paresis is a strong indicator of malignancy; however, presentation due to secondary deposits is rare. The differential diagnosis of any thyroid mass includes cancer, multinodular goitre, thyroid adenoma, developmental neck cysts, thyroiditis, thyroid cysts and ectopic thyroid tissue. It should be remembered that benign disease is a far more common cause of a thyroid mass than malignancy.

Key point 1

- Any thyroid mass may be caused by cancer, but benign disease is much more likely. Suggestive clinical features are previous radiation exposure, family cancer syndrome, a fixed hard thyroid mass, hoarseness or dysphagia.

PATHOLOGY OF WELL-DIFFERENTIATED THYROID CANCER

PAPILLARY CANCER

Most thyroid cancers are less than 1 cm in diameter and are typically papillary. The primary tumour in papillary cancer can vary enormously in size from a microscopic deposit to lesions greater than 5 cm. Grossly, these lesions are solid, whitish and obviously invasive and 10% have a complete capsule.

The microscopic features of papillary cancer include the demonstration of true papillae, which occasionally occur in combination with follicles. Such lesions should be considered as papillary cancer since this is how they behave. The diagnosis of papillary cancer also depends on specific nuclear features. The presence of 'orphan Annie' nuclei is characteristic, but is an artefact of paraffin fixation and is not seen in frozen section material. Nuclear pseudo-inclusions are also characteristic and occur in frozen section as well as paraffin sections. Nuclear grooves are a diagnostic sign and occur in oval or spindle nuclei. In 50% of cases psammoma bodies are seen, which are diagnostic as they are rare in other thyroid lesions and clear in frozen-section preparation.[10]

Variants of the standard papillary cancer are as follows.

Papillary microcarcinoma

This is papillary carcinoma measuring 1 cm or less in diameter, which can have features of a classic small papillary carcinoma or may appear as an encapsulated sclerotic nodule of 4 mm in size. These so-called occult lesions are found in 4–36% of autopsy material. The incidence depends on the geographical area, and in part on the extent of thyroid dissection. Papillary microcarcinoma is extremely rare in childhood, but is associated with cervical node metastases in about one-third of cases. Distant metastases are extremely rare and the prognosis is excellent. These lesions may be multiple in nature and we have seen up to four or five separate lesions within a single thyroid.[10]

Encapsulated variant of papillary carcinoma

This is characterised by the presence of a tumour capsule like an adenoma, but with local invasion. It may be associated with nodal metastases, but distant metastases and death are rare. The microscopic features of this variant are the same as the conventional invasive type. There can be difficulty distinguishing this lesion from the hyperplastic nodule with central cystic degeneration and papillary or pseudopapillary fronds. The overall prognosis is excellent.[11]

The follicular variant of papillary cancer

This is a mixed lesion with a predominance of follicles over papillae. When these lesions metastasise, the nodes show well-developed papillary formations.[12]

Lindsay's tumour

This is a combination of the encapsulated variant and the follicular variant. It has the cytological features of the follicular variant of papillary cancer, with a very distinct capsule. It usually behaves in a very indolent fashion and has an excellent prognosis.[13]

The diffuse sclerosing variant

This is seen primarily in children and is a very unpleasant tumour. It is often misdiagnosed as Hashimoto's thyroiditis but is highly aggressive. The thyroid gland is freely permeated by tumour and there is a typical prominent lymphocytic infiltrate. The incidence of lymph node involvement is up to 100%, with a high incidence of distant metastases and a poor prognosis.[14]

Tall cell papillary cancer

This is an aggressive variant that occurs as a rapidly growing thyroid mass in the elderly, and represents 10% of papillary tumours. The diagnosis is made when at least 50% of the cells making up the tumour are narrow and elongated. The typical tall cell tumour is greater than 5 cm in size on presentation, has extracapsular and vascular invasion in 30% of cases, and a 5-year survival rate of less than 30%. We have recently seen tall cell variants less than 1 cm in size in young people. We believe that these are related to previous exposure to ionising radiation. We know of no evidence that these variants in the young group have a worse prognosis than that of standard small papillary cancers.[10,15]

The columnar variant

This is exceptionally rare and has only been recorded in men. All patients have died within 5 years of presentation. The histological features are extremely papillary, with tall columnar cells and nuclear stratification. Such patients need aggressive treatment but even when young have an extremely poor prognosis.[16]

Papillary cancer and its variants have extrathyroidal extension in approximately 25% of cases. Involvement of lymph nodes is extremely common, particularly in the young. Nodal metastases may undergo cystic changes. Even with huge metastases, the primary may be very small indeed and occasionally it is impossible to find.

FOLLICULAR CANCER

This is a malignant epithelial tumour with evidence of follicular cell differentiation without the features of papillary cancer. The lesion is usually solid, occurs predominantly in women, approximately 10 years later than papillary cancers. There are two types, based on the degree of invasiveness of the lesion.

Minimally invasive

This is a solid, encapsulated, fleshy tumour that looks very much like a simple thyroid adenoma. The capsule tends to be extremely thick and irregular when compared with that of a simple adenoma. There can be difficulty following fine-needle aspiration to distinguish traumatic capsular rupture from true foci of capsular invasion. Diagnosis is usually made on paraffin section as determining capsular invasion is very difficult at frozen section.

Widely invasive

This shows widespread infiltration of blood vessels, the capsule and adjacent thyroid tissue. It can on occasions have no capsule whatsoever. The structural features are variable, but there is always a follicular element. Follicular cancer does not invade lymphatics and spreads by the bloodstream to the lungs, bones and less frequently to the brain. Immunostaining for thyroglobulin is usually positive in this tumour.

HÜRTHLE CELL TUMOURS

The Hürthle cell variant, unlike other follicular cells, does not take up radioactive iodine. Hürthle cell tumours are defined by the presence of more than 75% of follicular cells having oncocytic features. The lesion occurs particularly in adult women and is usually solid, well vascularised and well encapsulated. The microscopic features can be follicular (most commonly), trabecular, solid or even papillary. The nuclei of the cells are very pleomorphic and have prominent nucleoli with bizarre isolated forms. The characteristic feature is the distinct granular acidophilic cytoplasm. The cells stain for thyroglobulin, but less so than normal follicular lesions. Hürthle cell carcinoma occurs at a mean age of 60 and is frequently associated with extrathyroidal extension with both lymph node and distant metastases. These lesions are high risk, with 5-year mortality rate ranging from 20% to 40%.[17]

FINE-NEEDLE ASPIRATION CYTOLOGY (FNAC) AND FINE-NEEDLE NON-ASPIRATION CYTOLOGY (FNNAC)

Fine-needle aspiration cytology (FNAC) or fine-needle non-aspiration cytology (FNNAC) should be performed on all significant thyroid nodules, preferably by a cytologist. FNNAC is valuable in the assessment of vascular lesions which have been found on FNAC. Important points for these techniques are shown in Table 1.

All solitary nodules should be viewed with suspicion, particularly in children, who have a high incidence of malignancy (25%) in solitary nodules, with early lymphatic spread. Palpable dominant nodules in multinodular goitre have only a slightly lower incidence of thyroid cancer than true solitary nodules. Palpable cystic lesions are often degenerating thyroid nodules with a risk of malignancy that is only a little less than true solid nodules. Clinically suspicious nodules should be regarded as malignant despite negative cytology, until histological diagnosis has been confirmed.

Misdiagnosis of thyroid cysts is possible if FNAC is not performed under ultrasound control. Invariably the fluid contents will give no hint of malignancy, but biopsy of a thickened cyst wall under ultrasound control often identifies thyroid cancer.

Cancer risk in retrosternal goitre varies from 2% to 40%, with an average of 8%. These may be very large and may be present for many years, so that a long history does not exclude malignancy.

Cytology may be benign, malignant or non-diagnostic. Accurate diagnoses can be made in colloid nodules and inflammatory thyroid disease (Hashimoto's, De Quervain's and tuberculosis). Papillary, medullary,

Table 1 Important aspects of FNAC technique

- Aspirate different sites of the nodule or multinodular goitre
- Aspirate obvious malignant nodules
- If the lesion is cystic, perform a biopsy of the cyst wall under ultrasound control
- If the cystic fluid is clear, send for PTH and culture
- Biopsy even if thyroid nodule is 'hot' on scanning, as these can be malignant.

anaplastic cancers and thyroid lymphomas are diagnosed with ease, but the diagnosis of follicular cancers is virtually impossible. If the pathology is bizarre, medullary cancer must be excluded by staining for calcitonin and serum calcitonin analysis. It is best to treat all suspicious cytology surgically.

Key point 2

- Regard suspicious nodules with negative cytology as cancer until proven benign.

Key point 3

- Remember that 25% of solitary nodules in children are malignant.

THE ROLE OF INTRAOPERATIVE FROZEN SECTION

The role of intraoperative frozen section is controversial as cytology is so accurate in making a preoperative diagnosis. Many centres no longer use frozen section for the following reasons:

- FNA can diagnose papillary cancer in 90% of cases.

- False-positive diagnosis may occur due to frozen section technique causing artefactual nuclear changes mimicking papillary cancer.

- Frozen section is of limited use in follicular lesions, where malignancy can only be confirmed by the demonstration of capsular or vascular invasion. Few centres have the facility for extensive sampling of the capsule.

- Distortion of tissue after FNAC or FNNAC produces difficulties in separating pseudocapsular and vascular invasion from true invasion.

If frozen section is not used, this may commit the patient to a second operation with all its inherent risks and inconvenience. Despite its failings, we feel that multiple sections of the capsule should be taken, which has enabled us to confirm a malignant diagnosis in up to 75% of follicular lesions, avoiding a second procedure. Intraoperative cytology correlates well with final pathology. In centres where such facilities do not exist, a pragmatic approach is to offer patients with large follicular lesions a total thyroidectomy, overtreating a number, but avoiding the risks of secondary surgery.

RISK STRATIFICATION IN THYROID CANCER

The development of a thyroid tumour staging system that aids management and prognosis in well-differentiated tumours has remained a challenge. Four schemes are widely used. These are the American Joint Committee on Cancer (AJCC) classification,[18] the AGES system developed by Hay at the Mayo Clinic in 1987,[19] the AMES system developed in 1988 by Cady and Rossi[20] and a modification of the AGES system developed in 1993 by the Mayo Clinic workers and designated MACIS. In all of these systems, age, size of tumour and extent of spread are the major prognostic independent variables. These can be summarised as follows: a female under 50 or a male under 40 with a tumour 4 cm or smaller limited to the thyroid has an excellent prognosis, while a woman over 50 or a man over 40 with a tumour larger than 5 cm with extrathyroidal spread or distant metastases has a poor prognosis. Between these extremes, prognosis varies according to independent prognostic variables. All systems overlook the small percentage of low-risk patients who die of papillary cancer. Many argue that all these systems help in prognosis after surgery but are of little value as an intraoperative guide.

SURGICAL RESECTION OF THE THYROID IN WELL-DIFFERENTIATED TUMOUR

There is worldwide debate about the appropriate extent of thyroid resection, but it is well established that, compared with lobectomy, total thyroidectomy in high-risk patients reduces local recurrence and mortality.[21]

Total thyroidectomy is more difficult to justify in low-risk tumours. There is evidence that recurrence is reduced by near-total or total thyroidectomy, but other studies have shown little or no improvement in results.[21] If total thyroidectomy, near-total thyroidectomy and lobectomy had identical complication rates, there would be little argument. In expert hands a true total thyroidectomy has a complication rate of 4%. When performed by an occasional thyroidectomist, however, temporary complication rates rise to 40% and permanent complications occur in 20%. The main problem is not damage to the recurrent laryngeal nerve, but permanent hypoparathyroidism. Recurrent nerve damage in expert hands should be less than 1%, but a rate of up to 10% is more common in occasional hands.

Key point 4

- In high-risk patients total thyroidectomy gives low rates of local recurrence and late mortality.

SURGICAL RESECTION OF THE LYMPH NODES

Well-differentiated thyroid cancer is unusual in that the presence of positive lymph nodes has little or no effect on prognosis.[22] Management is controversial. It is agreed only that removing the lymph nodes individually ('berry picking') is associated with an unacceptable recurrence rate compared with a thorough skeletonisation of vital structures.

When lymph nodes are involved in the central compartment, a clearance should be performed, and this should include the thymus and thyroid *en bloc*. Most workers concede that this reduces the risk of recurrence; however, the lower parathyroids are at great risk and may need transplantation.

If there is no central node involvement, the appropriate course of action is less clear. A prophylactic central dissection on clinically negative nodes reveals 50% or more microscopically positive lymph nodes. Some believe that clearance of these has no effect on prognosis and that the risk of hypoparathyroidism is so high that it is actually detrimental. If the primary tumour is high-grade then most agree to a prophylactic central neck dissection. Our own policy is that central neck dissection should always be performed as long as a low incidence of hypoparathyroidism can be achieved. One factor not considered by many workers is the difficulty of re-exploration for recurrent central compartment lymph node disease. In our view, this in itself justifies initial clearance in node-negative patients.

When lymph nodes are involved in the lateral compartment, a functional neck dissection including levels II–V is performed. There is rarely a role for radical neck dissection. If invasion occurs in aggressive tumours, a more radical approach is necessary, sacrificing involved structures.

When lateral compartment nodes are not involved, there is considerable controversy. Many would perform a frozen section of one or two nodes and, if negative, leave well alone. This is now the most common approach. Unlike the central compartment, where re-exploration is difficult, re-exploration of the lateral part of the neck is not so problematic and vital structures can be preserved with minimal morbidity.

Key point 5

- Lymph node sampling ('berry picking') is associated with a high rate of local recurrence. When nodes are involved, functional neck dissection should be performed.

REDUCING COMPLICATIONS IN TOTAL THYROIDECTOMY

Recurrent laryngeal nerves should be identified in all thyroidectomies as identification is known to reduce the incidence of nerve palsy. We routinely use dexamethasone 8 mg intraoperatively to reduce nerve oedema. We recently evaluated the use of a nerve stimulator for identification of the recurrent laryngeal nerve. This is particularly helpful in patients who have had previous surgery, and for confirming that the nerve remains intact at the conclusion of the operation. This indicates that any postoperative neuropraxia will recover.

There are three approaches to identify the recurrent laryngeal nerve all of which have advantages and disadvantages.

Inferior approach

This is our routine approach. The nerve is found low in the neck before it branches, which avoids damage to minor divisions, and is dissected cranially until it enters the larynx. It has a distinct blood vessel running on its surface. The relationship to the inferior thyroid artery is variable and this structure is not a reliable landmark. The nerve is non-recurrent in 1% of cases, usually on the right, but non-recurrence occurs on the left in situs inversus. The problem with dissecting a long segment of nerve is the risk of damage to the lower parathyroid. This approach is particularly useful at re-operation, where often the nerve can be found low in the neck in virgin territory.

Superior approach
This approach is difficult and involves taking down the superior pole of the thyroid and finding the nerve beneath the tough vascular ligament of Berry. In nodular enlargement of the upper pole, this approach can be extremely difficult, but may be aided by the use of the nerve stimulator.

Lateral approach
This approach is simply the inferior approach done at a higher level, seeking the nerve among the branches of the inferior thyroid artery after the middle thyroid vein has been divided. Its only advantage is that by leaving the areolar tissue around the lower part of the nerve, the lower parathyroid is less likely to be devascularised; however, the nerve may be divided several times and its branches are at risk. In our view, this approach has little to recommend it.

In difficult cases a combination of all aspects of the three techniques should be considered.

PRESERVATION OF THE PARATHYROIDS

The upper parathyroid is not usually problematic, as it lies behind the recurrent laryngeal nerve and will not be devascularised. The lower parathyroid, however, can vary considerably in position, but usually lies close to the lower pole of the thyroid or within the upper pole of the thymus. The main inferior thyroid artery should not be ligated but the small divisions of the artery should be ligated close to the capsule. If there is doubt about parathyroid viability, a frozen-section biopsy should be taken and the parathyroid should be autotransplanted as 1 mm fragments in a muscular pocket in the neck or forearm.

INDICATIONS FOR RE-OPERATION

Reoperative surgery should take place 2 or 3 days after initial operation, or left for at least 12 weeks to allow inflammatory response to settle. Re-operative surgery should be considered in the following situation:

- After lobectomy for a presumed benign tumour. This should be converted to a total thyroidectomy and the lymph nodes dealt with on their merits. Microinvasive follicular neoplasms do not need conversion to total thyroidectomy.

- If there are enlarged nodes in a papillary cancer patient that were not detected perioperatively, it is important to re-explore and clear them. This will make radioactive iodine ablation more successful.

- After a so-called previous total thyroidectomy when ultrasound or other modality demonstrates bulky residual thyroid, irrespective of the previous operative notes, re-operative surgery should be considered.

RADIOACTIVE IODINE (^{131}I) THERAPY

It is virtually impossible to remove all thyroid tissue even with the most meticulous attempt at total thyroidectomy. Preoperative imaging studies, such as computed tomography (CT), should be performed without iodine contrast. In low-risk patients ^{131}I therapy may represent overtreatment. In high-risk groups ^{131}I ablation is considered standard management because large residual thyroid beds with high uptake may obscure metastases, serum thyroglobulin (Tg) is a better marker of recurrence after ^{131}I ablation, and retrospective studies show a reduced incidence of tumour recurrence and death.[23] In very low-risk groups, particularly in microcarcinomas, surgery will effect a cure and radioactive iodine is unnecessary.

Our policy of ^{131}I management is similar to that of the Royal Marsden thyroid cancer clinic.[23] Low-risk, young patients with tumours 1 cm or smaller confined to the thyroid with negative lymph nodes and no distant spread are not treated with ^{131}I. The cancer-specific mortality rate is 1% at 30 years. This group should not be considered for re-operative surgery if a lobectomy was initially performed.

^{131}I therapy is limited to more aggressive tumours. If ^{131}I ablation is to be considered and limited surgery has been performed then re-operation should be done to maximise the effect of the ^{131}I. Four weeks after total or near-total thyroidectomy, having allowed the TSH to rise to 50 iu or more, an ablative dose of 3 GBq is given. This requires treatment as an inpatient. Diagnostic doses to assess the extent of any residual thyroid tissue or the presence of metastases should not be given, as they have two great disadvantages. First, they may cause blocking of uptake by the tumour, making a subsequent ablative dose of radioactive iodine less effective. Second, the doses will not always demonstrate persistent tumour, which is later very obvious from the post-thyroid scan. Dosimetry studies at the Royal Marsden have shown that 3 GBq ablates 70% of all thyroid remnants, delivering a mean radiation dose of 410 Gy. Post-treatment scans are obtained on the third day, and if the patient's activity falls to permitted levels, he or she is discharged with advice by the medical physicist regarding contact with other people. Several studies suggest that if there is a small remnant, lower doses than the traditional 150 mCi are as effective in the management. Low-dose treatment has been popular in the USA because of cost implications, and it is done as an outpatient. Thyroid replacement at this stage is tri-iodothyronine (T_3) 20 µg three times a day.[23]

After 4 months the thyroglobulin is measured and a repeat total-body scan is performed having stopped T_3 for at least 10 days 185 MBq of ^{131}I is used. If successful ablation is achieved after the first dose of ^{131}I treatment, the patient is converted to thyroxine (T_4), regular thyroglobulin estimations are performed and no further treatment is necessary. Lifetime follow-up is mandatory.[23]

If initial ablation is not successful, remnant ablation will need to be performed at 6- to 12-monthly intervals until ablation is complete. The definition of complete ablation is arbitrary. A negative scan with an undetectable thyroglobulin clearly represents total ablation. Patients with negative scans or little uptake, but detectable thyroglobulins, do not benefit from a further dose of ^{131}I. These patients should be watched and given further ablation therapy if there is a significant rise in the thyroglobulin. When the scan is clear and the thyroglobulin is undetectable, further scanning is unnecessary and thyroglobulin alone is used as a tumour marker. Patients with a negative scan and significantly high thyroglobulins should have ablation therapy, as often their post-therapy scan will highlight residual disease.

The management of patients with persistent disease following ^{131}I treatment is difficult. This arises due to incomplete tumour resection or aggressive disease. Wherever possible, the surgical option of excising residual tissue should be followed, as this aids subsequent ^{131}I therapy. When recurrence is suspected, re-staging is performed using ultrasound, CT, magnetic resonance imaging (MRI) or positron emission tomography (PET) scanning.

Key point 6

- Preoperative imaging such as CT should be performed without iodine-containing contrast.

Key point 7

- Diagnostic doses of ^{131}I should not be given before treatment, as they may block uptake by the tumour.

TSH SUPPRESSION

TSH suppression with thyroxine is an integral part of thyroid cancer management. Thyroxine therapy, which keeps the TSH at the lower end of the range, significantly reduces mortality and recurrence. The risk of osteoporosis in patients having long-term toxic doses of thyroxine is of concern.

THYROID LYMPHOMA

PRESENTATION

Thyroid lymphoma represents 5% of all thyroid malignancies. The incidence is rising due to the increase in rates of Hashimoto's thyroiditis, which increases the risk of lymphoma 70-fold. Thyroid lymphoma is often associated with a history of thyroxine replacement and may present with hypothyroidism. The absence of hypothyroidism should alert one to the possibility of anaplastic or medullary cancer. Over 50% of patients present under the age of 60 and the presentation is similar to anaplastic cancer without hypothyroidism. Recurrent laryngeal nerve palsy may be a feature.

PATHOLOGY

Most lymphomas are of diffuse histiocytic type and vary from intermediate- to high-grade. It is important to separate the low-grade B-cell lymphomas of the distinct group of MALTomas, which rarely disseminate. Staging is mandatory and total-body scanning is performed, with bone marrow biopsy. Extrathyroidal extension or metastases worsen prognosis. On ultrasound, the thyroid is usually hypoechoic and CT or MRI cannot separate simple Hashimoto's from lymphoma. FNAC or FNNAC can usually secure a tissue diagnosis. Rarely, a core or open biopsy is necessary.

STAGING

The staging of thyroid lymphoma shown in Table 2.

Table 2 Staging of thyroid lymphoma

IE	Localised to the thyroid
IIE	Thyroid gland involved and more than one lymph node on the same side of the diaphragm
IIIE	Disease on both sides of the diaphragm
IVE	Disseminated disease

MANAGEMENT

There is no role for thyroidectomy or radioactive iodine treatment for thyroid lymphoma; the primary treatment is external-beam radiation with chemotherapy. When disease is limited to the neck, external-beam therapy alone achieves similar results to radiation plus additional chemotherapy, provided that the mediastinum is irradiated. It is known that 30% of clinically localised tumours develop distant metastases, so adjuvant chemotherapy gives the security of systemic treatment. Most centres use radiation and chemotherapy in stage IE disease, with 5-year survival rates of 80%. Stages IIE and worse are treated similarly. Chemotherapy regimes vary, using cyclophosphamide, doxorubicin, vincrinstine and prednisolone.[24]

A different approach is used in low-grade B-cell MALT (mucosa-associated lymphoid tissue) lymphomas. These rarely spread outside the thyroid and are treated by external-beam radiation alone, with a 90% survival rate at 5 years.[24,25]

The temptation for a tracheostomy in an intubated patient with tracheal obstruction must be resisted at all costs. Urgent chemotherapy will almost always resolve the obstruction allowing extubation within 48 hours.

Key point 8

- In thyroid lymphoma, tracheal obstruction almost always responds rapidly to chemotherapy, and tracheostomy is rarely required.

MEDULLARY THYROID CANCER

GENETIC BACKGROUND

Medullary thyroid cancer counts for 5–10% of all thyroid cancers. Eighty percent are sporadic, typically presenting with solitary thyroid nodules with involved lymph nodes. In its familial form, medullary cancer can occur as a non-MEN form (FMTC) or as part of either multiple endocrine neoplasia (MEN) type IIA or IIB. Once the diagnosis of medullary cancer is suspected, all patients should be screened for mutations of the *RET* proto-oncogene to exclude familial disease. Twenty percent of patients initially diagnosed as sporadic cases are subsequently found to be familial. All patients should have possible associated endocrine abnormalities excluded. When a genetic defect is found, all family members should be screened.

PATHOLOGY

Medullary thyroid cancer originates in the parafollicular or C cells of the thyroid, which secrete calcitonin. Calcitonin's role in calcium metabolism is antagonistic to parathyroid hormone (PTH); it has a minimal effect in humans, but is crucial in animals. Medullary thyroid cancer may be preceded by an increased mass of C cells, called C-cell hyperplasia. This is a misnomer, however, as it is in fact pre-invasive cancer, borne out by the fact that lymph node metastases can occur with C-cell hyperplasia alone. True pre-invasive C-cell hyperplasia is present when there are at least 50 C cells per low-power field, or it is bilateral and extensive. These criteria separate it from the occasional C-cell nodules found in normal thyroid. The presence of bilateral thyroid disease with C-cell hyperplasia is highly suggestive of the familial form but is not diagnostic, as it can be found in sporadic disease.

Classically, the tumour consists of round, polygonal or spindle cells with islands of tumour separated by fibrous bands. The nuclei are elongated, with cytoplasmic nuclear inclusions, and amyloid is abundant and may calcify. Positive immunostaining for calcitonin is frequent, but its absence does not exclude the diagnosis of medullary cancer.

FAMILIAL FORMS OF MEDULLARY CANCER

Three familial forms of medullary thyroid cancer are known.[8]

Familial medullary thyroid cancer (FMTC)
This has an indolent course with no features of MEN and a very good prognosis; the mean age at diagnosis is over 40 years. There is a subgroup that in addition to their medullary cancer have corneal thickening but no MEN features.

Multiple endocrine neoplasia type IIA (MEN IIA)
These patients also have phaeochromocytomas (frequently bilateral), which may be extra-adrenal. Less common are hyperplastic parathyroid glands, often asymmetrically enlarged. Rare subgroups of patients have amyloid deposits in the skin of the upper back (cutaneous lichen amyloidosis). This is the only form of MEN IIA that has a specific phenotypic marker.

Multiple endocrine neoplasia type IIB (MEN IIB)
These patients have a typical phenotype in addition to their aggressive medullary cancer. They are Marfanoid, tall with high arched palates, have characteristic neuromas on their tongue and eyelids, but, unlike true Marfan's

syndrome patients, do not have cardiac lesions or ectopia lentis. Hyperpara-thyroidism is rare but phaeochromocytomas are common. These patients have severe gastrointestinal symptoms due to the increased number of ganglion cells in the gastrointestinal tract resulting in abdominal distension, and alternating diarrhoea and constipation. A stercoral perforation is not unusual.

All the familial cancers arise from mutations in chromosome 10. The specific initiating abnormality lies in the *RET* proto-oncogene segment for both MEN II and familial non-MEN thyroid cancer. Point mutations lie in either the extra- or intracellular domains of the *RET* proto-oncogene. Point mutations on extracellular domains 609, 611, 618 or 620 in exon 10 and 634 in exon 12 are found in the vast majority of MEN II and FMTC patients. MEN IIB patients have mutations in the intracellular domain 918 of exon 16.[26]

CLINICAL PRESENTATION

Medullary cancer is a great imitator, being protean in its histology and clinical presentation. In any bizarre presentation of a thyroid mass or histology, medullary cancer should be excluded.

Patients with either sporadic or familial disease may present simply with a lump in the neck or lymph node metastases. Rarely, a syndrome like Cushing's may be the mode of presentation. Presentation of a familial form as a phaeochromocytoma is rare but may occur, and all phaeochromocytomas should have medullary cancer excluded by making sure that calcitonin is undetectable. Odd phenotypes will alert the physician to the possibility of medullary cancer.

The lymph nodes in both sporadic and familial medullary carcinoma of the thyroid are, in our view, often badly managed. We would suggest that both familial and sporadic type should have total thyroidectomy with routine dissection of nodes in the central part of the neck and sampling of the jugular nodes. We feel that a modified neck dissection is indicated if metastatic lymph nodes are found during sampling. The dissection of the neck should be meticulous and there is no justification for any form of 'berry picking'. The major structures of the neck should be skeletonised and microdissection techniques should be encouraged.[27] All too often recurrent disease arises either in the central part of the neck or laterally, due to inadequate primary lymph node clearance. Thymectomy should also be regularly performed, as metastatic disease is often present.

In patients with recurrent disease, further surgical exploration should be considered, but it is rare in these patients to achieve an undetectable calcitonin. Despite this, the overall prognosis is still around 85% at 10 years.

The management of a persistently raised calcitonin following surgery is a difficult problem. There is little evidence that re-operating on patients with mildly elevated calcitonin improves survival. In patients who have raised calcitonins and negative scans, laparoscopy should be performed as 20% of these patients will have micrometastases on the liver.

MANAGEMENT OF MEDULLARY CANCER

In the management of medullary carcinoma of the thyroid treatment cannot include ablative radioactive iodine as medullary cancer arises from the C cell and will not respond. The ideal management of medullary cancer, either sporadic or familial, is diagnosis by fine-needle aspiration and calcitonin estimation preoperatively followed by total thyroidectomy. There is absolutely no role for a lesser procedure than total thyroidectomy. This is true even in sporadic cases where the disease may appear to be localised to one lobe of the thyroid. Over 20% of sporadic cancers have been shown to have intrathyroidal lymphatic spread. In addition, a significant percentage of patients initially labelled sporadic are later shown to be familial. In essence therefore, the sporadic case is diagnosed by the absence of the *RET* proto-oncogene mutation.

In children who are carriers of the gene abnormality total thyroidectomy will eventually be necessary. The problem is at what age to perform the surgery. The report by the European Multiple Endocrine Neoplasia (Euro MEN) study group[26] demonstrates that medullary thyroid cancer associated with any mutation in codon 634 of *RET* commonly appears before the age of 10 years and in children aged as young as 17 months. It also states that it is rarely metastatic before the age of 14. Once malignant transformation has taken place, nodal metastasis occurs on average 6.6 years later. It has been our policy for several years to operate on all children with MEN IIA by the age of 3 years and those with MEN IIB at 1 year. Such an aggressive approach at an early age has the advantage that central neck dissection is less likely to be necessary, and the risks of lateral lymph node involvement are remote.

Key point 9

- Medullary cancer should be considered when a thyroid mass or histology has bizarre features.

Key point 10

- Because of the high risk of nodal disease in medullary cancer, we favour total thyroidectomy with routine dissection of central and jugular nodes.

ANAPLASTIC THYROID CANCER
INCIDENCE

Anaplastic thyroid cancer is a lethal disease, with a prognosis measured in months. It represents 5% of thyroid cancers, occurs in the elderly and, in contradistinction to lymphoma, which it mimics, it is not associated with Hashimoto's thyroiditis and its concomitant hypothyroidism. The introduction of iodine supplementation to endemic goitre regions may be the cause of its falling incidence. Fifty percent of cases are associated with concurrent or previous differentiated thyroid cancers, but anaplastic cancer can arise *de novo*.

PRESENTATION AND PATHOLOGY

Anaplastic thyroid cancer presents as a rapidly growing mass strangulating the structures of the neck. Most tumours are larger than 5 cm and local invasion is usually evident. An accurate assessment of the extent of the invasion is essential to planning the advisability and the extent of surgery. Vocal fold paralysis, oesophageal invasion or Horner syndrome are signs that make a 'trial dissection' almost always doomed to failure. FNAC or FNNAC must be performed with immunocytochemistry, aiming to exclude lymphoma and medullary, tall cell papillary and metastatic cancers. Any evidence of distant spread to lungs or bones renders heroic surgery inappropriate.

Anaplastic cancers are usually spindle or giant cell tumours. Rarely, small cell tumours may occur, but these usually represent misdiagnosed small cell lymphoma, medullary or insular thyroid cancers. The possibility of a secondary deposit in the thyroid must always be considered. Important subgroups are those tumours with a small focus and anaplastic tumours confined to a well-differentiated cancer.

MANAGEMENT

The results of all therapies are poor. Initial treatment aims to maintain the integrity of the aero-digestive tract, with attention to hydration and nutrition. The extent of primary surgery is controversial. Patients rarely survive more than 2 years, and the aim is to optimise quality of life. In impending airway obstruction, a central thyroid resection with freeing of the trachea and possible tracheostomy should be performed. As much thyroid as is feasible is resected by a gentle 'trial dissection' with a low threshold to stop. Preoperative scans help plan resectability, as evidence of extensive invasion of the trachea, oesophagus or carotid means that attempts at total excision will be 'foolhardy' and surgery should be limited to debulking with or without tracheostomy. Rarely, patients present without extrathyroidal spread; these patients should be treated aggressively with a total thyroidectomy and a central neck dissection.

In addition to surgery, all patients are considered for external-beam radiation and chemotherapy. Doxorubicin is the most effective agent, with the distinct advantage of being a radiosensitizer. It is used to downstage in the neoadjuvant setting or is given postoperatively with radiotherapy. Such regimes still result in a median survival of less than 1 year. Survival for more than a year occurs in the subgroup where radical surgery for disease to the thyroid has been possible. These patients may do well – but beware a misdiagnosed lymphoma.[28]

There is possible hope for the future. Mutation of the *p53* gene is almost always present in anaplastic cancers, where it does not initiate, but enhances the transformed phenotype. In the future, enzyme inhibitors may prevent tumour growth. Anaplastic cancer is known to be initiated by mutations in the *RAS* proto-oncogene. Mucomycin blocks *RAS*: it acts by interfering with farnesylation of the RAS protein and thus with tumour growth.[29]

THYROID CANCER IN CHILDREN

The common causes of benign neck masses in children are congenital or inflammatory lesions. Malignant lesions include medullary carcinoma of the thyroid, sarcomas, lymphomas and differentiated thyroid cancers. Any thyroid mass in a child should be regarded as malignant until proven otherwise. Fifty percent of children with thyroid cancer have nodal metastases on presentation. Management is similar to that in adults, with a radical approach to the lymph nodes. The high incidence of multiple metastases in the central compartment makes parathyroid preservation difficult, and parathyroid transplantation may be necessary. The outcome is favourable even with extensive metastases, as these respond well to radioactive iodine.

THYROID CANCER IN PREGNANCY

Proven thyroid cancer in pregnancy creates a difficult problem. If low-risk and before 16 weeks, assessment with MRI and a total thyroidectomy is a safe plan. Thyroid replacement is controlled, and, after delivery and a shortened period of breastfeeding, ^{131}I is given in the normal manner. ^{131}I is completely contraindicated in pregnancy. Occasionally, it is necessary to perform a neck dissection and a total thyroidectomy simultaneously, and this is usually well tolerated by mother and child. Patients with low-grade tumours diagnosed at or about 20 weeks should wait for delivery, after which the tumour is treated on its merits.

There is a dilemma regarding high-grade tumours in the first trimester. Counselling should be obtained, and although surgery can usually occur without loss of the fetus, this cannot be guaranteed. ^{131}I is completely contraindicated, although some patients will opt for thyroxine alone until term and then have ^{131}I therapy; the possibility of termination and immediate ^{131}I must be entertained. Patients with medullary cancer in pregnancy should have surgery until 20 weeks. Patients presenting later than this should be considered for possible induction at 32 weeks, when the risk to the fetus is smaller, followed by standard surgery.

Key points for clinical practice

- Any thyroid mass may be caused by cancer, but benign disease is much more likely. Suggestive clinical features are previous radiation exposure, family cancer syndrome, a fixed hard thyroid mass, hoarseness or dysphagia.

- Regard suspicious nodules with negative cytology as cancer until proven benign.

- Remember that 25% of solitary nodules in children are malignant.

- In high-risk patients total thyroidectomy gives low rates of local recurrence and late mortality.

Key points for clinical practice (continued)

- Lymph node sampling ('berry picking') is associated with a high rate of local recurrence. When nodes are involved, functional neck dissection should be performed.

- Preoperative imaging such as CT should be performed without iodine-containing contrast.

- Diagnostic doses of ^{131}I should not be given before treatment, as they may block uptake by the tumour.

- In thyroid lymphoma, tracheal obstruction almost always responds rapidly to chemotherapy, and tracheostomy is rarely required.

- Medullary cancer should be considered when a thyroid mass or histology has bizarre features.

- Because of the high risk of nodal disease in medullary cancer, we favour total thyroidectomy with routine dissection of central and jugular nodes.

References

1. Coleman PM, Babb P, Damiecki P et al. *Cancer Survival Trends in England and Wales 1971–1995; Deprivations and NHS Region (Series SMPS No. 61)*. London: Stationery Office, 1999: 471–478.
2. Pacini F et al. Post-Chernobyl thyroid carcinoma in Belarus children and adolescents: comparison with naturally occurring thyroid carcinoma in Italy and France. *J Clin Endocrinol Metab* 1997; **82**: 3563.
3. Santoro M et al. Gene rearrangement and Chernobyl related thyroid cancers. *Br J Cancer* 2000; **82**: 315.
4. Nikiforov Y, Gnepp DR, Fagin JA. Thyroid lesions in children and adolescents after the Chernobyl disaster: implications for the study of radiation tumorigenesis. *J Clin Endocrinol Metab* 1996; **81**: 9.
5. Holm LE. Thyroid cancer after diagnostic and therapeutic use of radionuclides: a review of the association. In: Thomas G, Karaoglou A. Williams ED (eds). *Radiation and Thyroid Cancer*, Singapore: World Scientific, 1999.
6. Eng C. Familial papillary thyroid cancer: many syndromes, too many genes? *J Clin Endocrinol Metab* 2000; **85**: 1755.
7. Malchoff CD, Malchoff DM. Familial nonmedullary thyroid carcinoma. *Semin Surg Oncol* 1999; **16**: 16.
8. Farndon JR et al. Familial medullary thyroid carcinoma without associated endocrinopathies: a distinct clinical entity. *Br J Surg* 1986; **73**: 278.
9. Sipple JH. The association of pheochromocytoma with carcinoma of the thyroid gland. *Am J Med* 1961; **31**: 163.
10. Hawk WA, Hazard JB. The many appearances of papillary carcinoma of the thyroid. *Cleveland Clin Q* 1976; **43**: 207–216.
11. Schroder S, Bocker W et al. The encapsulated papillary carcinoma of the thyroid. A morphologic subtype of the papillary thyroid carcinoma. *Cancer* 1984; **54**: 90-93.
12. Chen KTK, Rosai J. Follicular variant of thyroid papillary carcinoma: a clinicopathologic study of six cases. *Am J Surg Pathol* 1977; **1**: 123.
13. Lindsay S. Papillary thyroid carcinoma revisited. In: Hedinger CE (ed). *Thyroid Cancer*. Heidelberg: Springer-Verlag, 1969: 29.

14. Vickery AL, Carcangiu M *et al*. Papillary carcinoma. *Semin Diagn Pathol* 1985; **2**: 90–100.
15. Johnson TL, Lloyd RV *et al*. Prognostic implications of the tall cell variant of papillary thyroid carcinoma. *Am J Surg Pathol* 1998; **12**: 22–27.
16. Sobrinho-Simoes M, Nesland JM, Johannessen JV. Columnar cell carcinoma: another variant of poorly differentiated carcinoma of the thyroid. *Am J Clin Pathol* 1988; **89**: 264.
17. Hedinger C, Williams ED, Sobin LH. *Histological Typing of Thyroid Tumours. International Histological Classification of Tumours*. World Health Organization, Vol. 11, 2nd edn. Berlin: Springer-Verlag, 1988.
18. Fleming ID *et al*. (eds). *AJCC Cancer Staging Manual*, 5th edn. Philadelphia: Lippincott-Raven, 1997.
19. Hay ID *et al*. Ipsilateral lobectomy versus bilateral lobar resection in papillary thyroid carcinoma: a retrospective analysis of surgical outcome using a novel prognostic scoring system. *Surgery* 1987; **102**: 1088.
20. Cady B, Rossi R. An expanded view of risk-group definition in differentiated thyroid carcinoma. *Surgery* 1988; **104**: 947.
21. Hay ID *et al*. Predicting outcome in papillary thyroid carcinoma: development of a reliable prognostic scoring system in a cohort of 1779 patients surgically treated at one institution during 1940 through 1989. *Surgery* 1993; **114**: 1050.
22. Grebe SKG, Hay ID. Thyroid cancer nodal metastases: biologic significance and therapeutic considerations. *Surg Oncol Clin North Am* 1996; **5**: 43.
23. Vini L, Harmer C. Management of thyroid cancer. *CME Cancer Med* 2003; **1(3)**: 71–77.
24. Matsuzuka F, Miyauchi A, Katayama S *et al*. Clinical aspects of primary thyroid lymphoma: diagnosis and treatment based on our experience of 119 cases. *Thyroid* 1993; 3: 93–99.
25. Thieblemont C, Bastion Y, Berger F *et al*. Mucosa-associated lymphoid tissue gastrointestinal and non-gastrointestinal lymphoma behaviour: analysis of 108 patients. *J Clin Oncol* 1997; 15: 1624–1630.
26. Machens A *et al*. Early malignant progression of hereditary medullary thyroid cancer. *N Engl J Med* 2003; **349**: 1517–1525.
27. Tisel LE, Hansson G, Jansson S *et al*. Re-operation in the treatment of medullary thyroid carcinoma. *Surgery* 1986; **99**: 60–66.
28. Tennvall J *et al*. Anaplastic thyroid carcinoma: doxorubicin, hyperfractionated radiotherapy and surgery, *Acta Oncol* 1990; **29**: 1025.
29. Yeung SC *et al*. Manumycin enhances the cytotoxic effect of paclitaxel on anaplastic thyroid carcinoma cells. *Cancer Res* 2000; **60**: 650.

Sudeep K. Thomas   Gordon C. Wishart

14

Parathyroid surgery

It is now almost 80 years since Felix Mandl[1] performed the first operation for primary hyperparathyroidism (pHPT). During that time, the clinical profile has shifted from a symptomatic disorder, with classical symptoms and signs at presentation, towards a more asymptomatic condition. pHPT is now being diagnosed with increased frequency, with an annual incidence of approximately 0.1%, and diagnosis has been simplified by development of a whole-molecule parathyroid hormone (PTH) assay. The annual incidence is higher, however, among middle-aged and elderly women (188 per 100 000 population), where the disorder is often associated with medical comorbidities.[2]

The diagnosis of pHPT is made following detection of hypercalcaemia in the presence of inappropriately normal or elevated circulating PTH levels. The hypercalcaemia is usually discovered on routine screening of patients with general symptoms including fatigue, depression, weakness, or less commonly now during the investigation of osteopenia or nephrolithiasis, the two main complications of pHPT.

Key point 1

- Primary hyperparathyroidism is now being diagnosed with increased frequency.

Mr Sudeep K. Thomas MS FRCS, Clinical Research Fellow, Department of General Surgery, Addenbrooke's Hospital, Cambridge, UK

Mr Gordon C. Wishart MD FRCS(Gen), Consultant Breast and Endocrine Surgeon, Department of General Surgery, Addenbrooke's Hospital, Hills Road, Cambridge CB2 2QQ, UK (for correspondence)

ANATOMY OF PARATHYROID GLANDS

Prior to any surgical procedure for pHPT, an understanding of the embryology and surgical anatomy of both normal and ectopic parathyroid glands is essential. The following simple rules may help parathyroid surgeons find an adenoma during a difficult neck exploration.

Superior parathyroid glands arise from the fourth branchial pouch, and due to their short migration can usually be found in a constant position posterior to the upper two-thirds of the thyroid gland. The superior gland lies superior to the inferior thyroid artery and dorsal to the recurrent laryngeal nerve. If ectopic, an upper gland may be found posterior to the oesophagus.

The position of the inferior parathyroid glands, however, is much more variable. Arising from the third branchial pouch, they descend with the thymus into the lower part of the neck. Due to this longer migration, they may be found at any position in the neck and mediastinum, although the majority lie within 1 cm of the lower border of the thyroid. They are normally inferior to the artery and ventral to the nerve. Although most people have four parathyroid glands, which exhibit symmetry on both sides of the neck, a range from two to six has been described in an extensive autopsy study.[3]

PHYSIOLOGY

Calcium is one of the major cations in the body and is involved in many biological processes, including nerve conduction, muscle contraction and signal transduction. The vast majority of body calcium (>99%) is located in bone, and it is the extracellular compartment concentration that is regulated to remain within a relatively narrow normal range (2.25–2.55 mmol/l). Increased extracellular calcium, detected by cell surface calcium receptors,[4] reduces PTH secretion by parathyroid cells via a negative-feedback mechanism.

Mature PTH is 84 amino acids long and binds to specific PTH receptors in kidney, bone and intestine to increase serum calcium by three different mechanisms:

- PTH increases the excretion of phosphate from the kidney by inhibiting its tubular reabsorption. This leads to an increase in the tubular reabsorption of calcium.

- PTH stimulates osteoclastic activity in bone, leading to demineralisation of bone and an increased level of calcium and phosphate in the bloodstream.

- PTH increases production of 1,25-hydroxyvitamin D by the kidney, thus increasing intestinal calcium absorption.

Increased PTH production leads to raised serum calcium, low serum phosphate and increased excretion of phosphate in the urine (Table 1). The

Table 1 Physiology of increased PTH excretion

↑ serum calcium
↓ serum phosphate
↑ phosphate excretion in urine
↑ calcium excretion in urine
↑ alkaline phosphatase (↑ osteoclast activity)

kidney fails to reabsorb the increased amount of calcium filtered, and as a result there is an overall increase in calcium excretion.

PRIMARY HYPERPARATHYROIDISM

In 85–90% of patients, pHPT is due to a solitary parathyroid adenoma; in 10% of cases multiglandular hyperplasia is present, which may be associated with multiple endocrine neoplasia (MEN) type I (pancreatic tumours, pituitary tumours, pHPT – Table 2), sporadic or induced by long-term lithium intake. A double adenoma or carcinoma each occurs in approximately 1% of cases of pHPT.

Table 2 Multiple endocrine neoplasia (MEN) syndromes

MEN syndromes present as multiple endocrine adenomas or adenocarcinomas in the same patient.

MEN type I
- Hyperparathyroidism
- Pituitary tumour (prolactinoma, corticotrophinoma (ACTH), somatotrophinoma (GH))
- Pancreatic tumour (gastrinoma, insulinoma, glucagonoma, VIPoma)
- Adrenocortical tumour, carcinoid, lipoma, angiofibroma

MEN type IIA
- Medullary thyroid carcinoma (MTC)
- Phaeochromocytoma
- Hyperparathyroidism

MEN type IIB
- Medullary thyroid carcinoma (MTC)
- Phaeochromocytoma
- Mucosal neuromas, Marfanoid appearance, megacolon

Familial MTC
- MTC without other endocrine lesions

CLINICAL FEATURES

Patients now rarely present with bone pain or fractures as a result of increased bone resorption. Plain X-rays may reveal major bone loss, especially in areas with cortical bone (e.g. the radius). The classical description of osteitis fibrosa cystica (von Recklinghausen's disease), with decalcification of bone, bone cysts and deformity, is rarely seen today, but X-rays may reveal calcification in soft tissues, arteries and the kidney tubules (nephrocalcinosis). A number of articular or peri-articular conditions may arise in pHPT, including pseudogout, subchondral erosions and synovitis.

A number of patients may still present with renal colic, urinary tract infection or haematuria secondary to renal calculi (nephrolithiasis). Deposition of calcium in the renal tubules (nephrocalcinosis) causes a reduction in the glomerular filtration rate, which may lead to elevation of blood urea and creatinine.

A number of gastrointestinal symptoms commonly occur in pHPT, including anorexia, nausea, heartburn, dyspepsia, constipation and abdominal pain. There is an association with peptic ulcer disease, and this can occasionally be due to a gastrin-producing tumour (gastrinoma), resulting in Zollinger–Ellison syndrome. This condition, part of MEN-I syndrome, can be excluded by measurement of fasting serum gastrin.

Patients may present with a variety of non-specific symptoms, including profound lethargy and worsening of any psychiatric condition (e.g. manic depression). Other symptoms may include memory loss, personality change, thirst and polyuria.

Hypertension may be noted at the initial diagnosis and is often associated with left ventricular hypertrophy. Although serum PTH correlates strongly with left ventricular mass (LVM), the reduction in LVM following parathyroidectomy is not associated with a similar reduction in blood pressure.

THRESHOLD FOR SURGICAL INTERVENTION

During the last decade, surgery for pHPT has been limited to those patients with symptoms or complications of the disease as well as younger patients under the age of 50. This approach was adopted following a National Institute of Health (NIH) consensus conference in 1990, which concluded that many patients did not require surgery as they were asymptomatic and their disease was not relentlessly progressive.[5]

Two leading articles have now questioned this conservative approach, suggesting that surgery should be considered following the initial diagnosis.[6,7] This is supported by two quality of life studies, which have shown that even patients with mild hypercalcaemia have physical or neuropsychological disabilities that improve following parathyroidectomy.[8,9] In addition, it is now recognised that the mortality among untreated patients with pHPT is increased, mainly from cardiovascular disease.[10]

This paradigm shift in the threshold for surgical intervention has now led to a second NIH Consensus Conference that has reviewed the indications for surgery in pHPT.[11] While these new guidelines go a small way towards supporting earlier surgical intervention, they may not go far enough. At present, surgery is the only curative treatment for patients with pHPT. With the introduction of unilateral or focused parathyroidectomy, often performed as a day-case procedure, the cost of surgical intervention may be less than any single hospital admission for a complication of the disease.

Key point 2

- Surgery should now be considered early in the natural history of the disease, even in 'asymptomatic' patients.

DIAGNOSTIC PITFALLS IN pHPT

Familial hypocalciuric hypercalcaemia

Familial hypocalciuric hypercalcaemia (FHH) is a rare disorder that can also present with hypercalcaemia and mildly elevated or inappropriately normal

PTH levels, and as a result it must be carefully distinguished from pHPT. FHH is transmitted in an autosomal dominant fashion and in the majority of cases is due to a heterozygous mutation in the calcium-sensing receptor (CaSR) gene that is the main regulator of parathyroid cell response to calcium. If the genetic disorder is homozygous, with two mutated CaSR genes, severe neonatal hyperparathyroidism results, which requires emergency total parathyroidectomy.

FHH can be confirmed by measurement of urinary calcium concentration as well as the calcium/creatinine (Ca/Cr) clearance ratio in the patient and family members with hypercalcaemia. In FHH the Ca/Cr clearance ratio is usually less than 0.01. In pHPT the Ca/Cr clearance ratio is typically greater than 0.02.[11]

Subclinical hyperparathyroidism

Not all patients with pHPT have hypercalcaemia each time the serum calcium is measured. In some patients the serum calcium is at the upper end of the normal range and the PTH is inappropriately elevated. This condition, sometimes called normocalcaemic HPT,[11] often comes to light when PTH is measured during the investigation of osteoporosis or intermittent hypercalcaemia. More recently there has been some evidence that the upper limit of normal for vitamin D-*sufficient* patients should be up to 30% lower than current values.[12] This is based on the assumption that the normal range for PTH was obtained from healthy adult volunteers, many of whom would have been vitamin D-*deficient*. Vitamin D deficiency may also explain a number of patients who have persistent elevation of PTH, despite normocalcaemia, following parathyroidectomy for pHPT.[13]

In patients with normocalcaemia and elevation of PTH all potential causes of secondary hyperparathyroidism should be ruled out, including renal insufficiency, vitamin D deficiency and hypercalciuria. In cases of vitamin D deficiency a trial of calcium and vitamin D supplements has been shown to markedly reduce PTH levels[14] and may thus prevent unnecessary surgery.

Acute hypercalcaemic crisis

Acute hypercalcaemic crisis secondary to pHPT often occurs in the elderly, many of whom have long-standing hypercalcaemia. Dehydration as a result of vomiting, increased sweating or anorexia will cause a further rise in serum calcium. This is often complicated by confusion, collapse and emergency admission to hospital. If not treated urgently with rehydration, diuretics and intravenous bisphosphonates, the patient may die from renal failure or cardiac arrhythmia.

Disodium pamidronate is the bisphosphonate of choice and should be given by slow intravenous infusion at a dose of 15–60 mg. In patients who show marked symptomatic improvement, secondary to a reduction in their serum calcium, preoperative localisation should be considered to assess suitability for focused parathyroidectomy. This should be performed in those patients who are fit enough for surgery within 6 weeks before the effect of pamidronate starts to wear off and serum calcium rises once more.

The main differential diagnosis is hypercalcaemia secondary to malignancy, although other causes include thyrotoxicosis, phaeochromocytoma and FHH (Table 3).

Table 3 Common causes of hypercalcaemia

Hyperparathyroidism
- Primary, secondary, tertiary

Malignancy
- Skeletal metastasis (breast, lung, kidney, prostate, thyroid)
- Multiple myeloma

Endocrine
- Thyrotoxicosis
- Adrenergic crisis
- Phaeochromocytoma

Iatrogenic
- Thiazide diuretics
- Excess vitamin D or calcium intake
- Lithium treatment (lithium-induced parathyroid hyperplasia)

Familial
- Familial hypocalciuric hypercalcaemia (FHH)

(a)

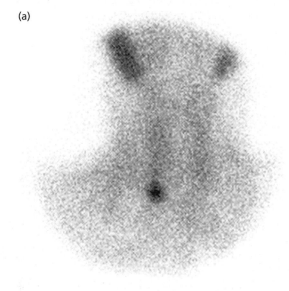

(b)

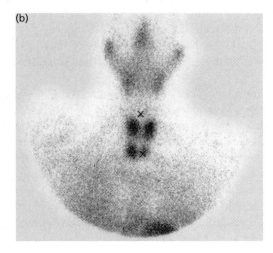

(c)

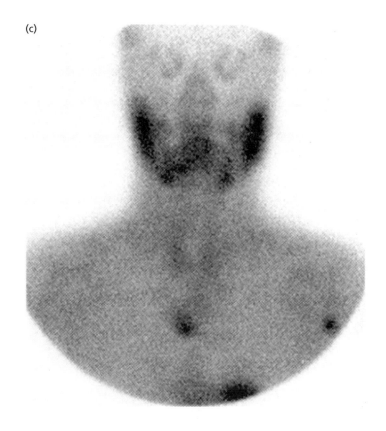

(d)

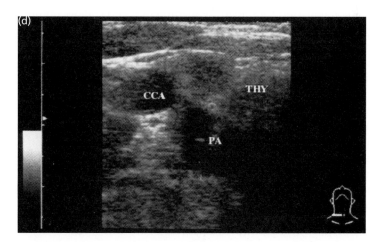

Fig. 1 (a–c) Delayed (2-hour) images taken after intravenous administration of 600 MBq
^{99m}Tc-sestamibi show delayed tracer washout: (a) at the lower pole of the right lobe of
the thyroid consistent with a parathyroid adenoma; (b) in all four glands consistent
with multigland hyperplasia; (c) in the mediastinum consistent with an ectopic
parathyroid adenoma (an incidental left axillary lymph node is also shown). (d) Neck
ultrasound showing parathyroid adenoma (PA) posterior to the thyroid gland (THY)
and adjacent to the common carotid artery (CCA).

PARATHYROIDECTOMY

For many years, parathyroid surgery has relied on experienced surgeons to distinguish an adenoma from hyperplasia of all four glands. As a result, bilateral cervical exploration has remained the preferred surgical approach, with cure rates of at least 95% in experienced hands.[15] Proponents of this technique, currently used by 97% of UK endocrine surgeons,[16] suggest that cases of hyperplasia or double adenoma are easier to recognise if bilateral neck exploration is performed.

In approximately 80–85% of cases, however, pHPT is caused by a single adenoma, and this, together with improvements in preoperative localisation techniques and the feasibility of intraoperative parathyroid hormone (iPTH) measurement, has increased the attraction of minimally invasive or unilateral surgery.

There are now several minimally invasive procedures, including focused parathyroidectomy and video-assisted and complete endoscopic techniques. Prior to the widespread introduction of any new technique, it must demonstrate equivalent outcomes, in terms of both high cure rates and low complication rates, as conventional bilateral neck exploration.

PREOPERATIVE LOCALISATION

Technetium-99m (^{99m}Tc)-sestamibi is now the agent of choice for parathyroid imaging. It can be performed either as a subtraction technique with iodine-123 (^{123}I)[17] or as a sole agent with delayed/dual-phase images.[18] The differential uptake and retention of ^{99m}Tc-sestamibi in thyroid and parathyroid tissue, which allows identification of parathyroid tissue on delayed imaging (Fig. 1), may be partly explained by the large numbers of mitochondria in parathyroid adenomas.[19] A number of techniques, including the use of collimation and single-photon emission computed tomography (SPECT), allow optimisation of the imaging technique to provide sensitivity in excess of 90%.[20] Overexpression of the multidrug-resistance protein, P-glycoprotein[21] and smaller adenoma size are both associated with false-negative scintigraphy. The combination of ^{99m}Tc-sestamibi and neck ultrasound is now recognised to be the optimum combination for pre-operative localisation, with a combined sensitivity of 94%,[22] and allows scan-directed selection of patients for either unilateral or bilateral surgery.

Other methods for parathyroid localisation have been used, including computed tomography (CT), magnetic resonance imaging (MRI) and selective venous sampling. Although they can successfully identify adenomas, the sensitivity of these techniques is extremely variable and their use is best reserved for those patients with persistent hypercalcaemia following failed neck exploration.

Key point 3

- The majority of parathyroid adenomas can be detected by preoperative localisation with ^{99m}Tc-sestamibi and/or neck ultrasound.

BILATERAL NECK EXPLORATION

Bilateral neck exploration is carried out through a collar incision 1–2 cm above the clavicle. This incision was often extended to over 10 cm in the past, but can safely be shortened to 3–6 cm without compromising access, and allows exploration of both retrothyroid spaces to detect and remove one or more enlarged glands. A number of simple rules may help in difficult cases where an adenoma cannot be found in one of the usual positions (Table 4).

If a single gland is enlarged, it is likely to be an adenoma and should be removed when the remaining glands have been visualized and are seen to be normal. In the past, frozen section was often performed on one or more glands, and although currently performed routinely by at least 73% of endocrine surgeons in the UK,[16] it is becoming less popular in Europe and North America as other peroperative techniques are increasingly used.

Bilateral neck exploration is the 'gold standard' for the surgical management of pHPT, with success rates in excess of 95% and complication rates of 1–2%.[15] It therefore provides the standard of care against which all new techniques must be compared.

UNILATERAL NECK EXPLORATION

An increasing number of surgeons are now performing unilateral surgery for pHPT based on the fact that 85–90% of patients will have single-gland disease. This change in practice has been made possible by improvements in preoperative localisation techniques using ^{99m}Tc-sestamibi scanning and/or ultrasound. A meta-analysis of ^{99m}Tc-sestamibi scanning has revealed a sensitivity and specificity of 90.7% and 98.8% respectively, suggesting that the majority of patients may be suitable for unilateral exploration.[20] A recent series of 184 patients who underwent scan-directed unilateral neck exploration reported a long-term cure rate of 98.4%.[23]

Table 4 Aid for difficult bilateral neck exploration

- The thyroid lobe should be fully mobilised, including division of a middle thyroid vein and the superior thyroid vessels, to allow full visualisation of the retrothyroid space
- The majority of glands lie within 1–2 cm of the confluence of the recurrent laryngeal nerve and the inferior thyroid artery. The artery also divides the location of superior and inferior glands
- The glands usually display symmetry, the glands on one side of the neck being located in the same position as on the other side
- An ectopic superior gland may lie posterior to the oesophagus or may only become apparent following division of the superior thyroid vessels and mobilisation of the superior thyroid pole. An ectopic inferior gland may be found in the superior horn of the thymus, the carotid sheath or high in the neck along the path of its previous descent

Unilateral exploration relies not only on the ability to localise an adenoma preoperatively but also on careful patient selection. Patients with multigland disease, MEN-related hyperplasia and renal disease are not suitable for this approach. Although a unilateral approach can be carried out through a collar incision, a number of minimally invasive techniques are now available, including focused parathyroidectomy, endoscopic parathyroidectomy and video-assisted parathyroidectomy.

Focused parathyroidectomy (FP)

Following accurate preoperative localisation of uniglandular disease, FP is carried out through a small lateral neck incision (Fig. 2a). The patient is supine, with the head in a neutral position. The surgeon develops the space between the lateral border of the strap muscles and sternomastoid to reach the retrothyroid space (Fig. 2b–d). This operation is suitable for day-case surgery and can be performed under either general or cervical block anaesthesia.

Comparison of this technique with bilateral neck exploration has shown fewer overall complications (1.2% *versus* 3.0%), a 50% reduction in operating

(a)

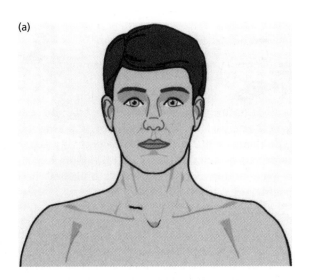

(b)

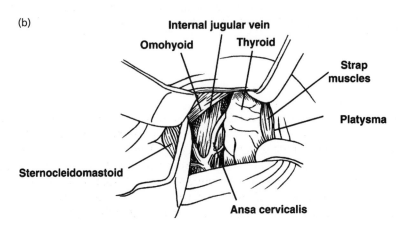

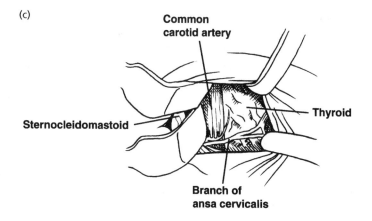

(c)

Common carotid artery

Sternocleidomastoid

Thyroid

Branch of ansa cervicalis

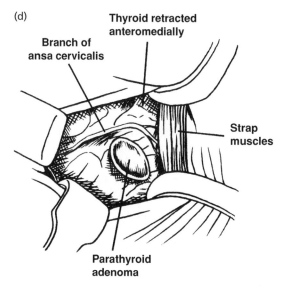

(d)

Thyroid retracted anteromedially

Branch of ansa cervicalis

Strap muscles

Parathyroid adenoma

Fig. 2 (a) Diagram showing the site of the 2.5 cm skin crease incision starting at the medial end of right sternocleidomastoid muscle. (b) Following incision of the skin, platysma and deep cervical fascia, and lateral retraction of the omohyoid, the internal jugular vein and ansa cervicalis are exposed lying lateral to the thyroid. (c) Lateral retraction of the internal jugular vein reveals the common carotid artery. A branch of the ansa cervicalis can be seen passing medially to the strap muscles. (d) Exposure of the retrothyroid space by anteromedial retraction of the thyroid and lateral retraction of the common carotid artery. The adenoma is seen inferior to a branch of the ansa cervicalis.

time and a substantial reduction in postoperative stay.[24] These data have been confirmed by a further day-case study of 50 patients undergoing focused parathyroidectomy under general anaesthesia. The procedure was suitable for all ages (mean age 63, range 33–92), was completed under general anaesthesia in a mean operating time of 30 minutes (range 16–57) and allowed early discharge within 2 hours of surgery. Furthermore, the cure rate, defined as normocalcaemia, was 100% when FP was combined with iPTH.[25]

Minimally invasive radio-guided parathyroidectomy (MIRP)

The role of sestamibi scanning has now been extended to include intraoperative adenoma localisation using a gamma-probe. Following injection of 20 mCi ^{99m}Tc-sestamibi 2 hours before surgery, a probe is used to direct the dissection according to the level of radioactivity.[26] The technique can be enhanced by addition of iPTH measurement or by measurement of the radioactivity of the removed gland.[27]

Since the use of a gamma-probe will increase radiation exposure, and may provide logistical difficulties in terms of injection timing and theatre planning, it may be utilised more appropriately in cases of persistent or recurrent HPT.

Minimally invasive endoscopic parathyroidectomy (MIEP)

Several completely endoscopic parathyroidectomy techniques have now been described.[28,29] Multiple ports are used for endoscopic dissection, the camera and gas insufflation. The gland is then retrieved via the largest incision. The technique will usually allow identification of the recurrent laryngeal nerve, and although these cases can be performed in day surgery, they do require increased operating time when compared with FP, and general anaesthesia.[30]

Minimally invasive video-assisted parathyroidectomy (MIVAP)

This technique gains access to the neck through several small incisions as for endoscopic parathyroidectomy.[31] Once identified, the gland is dissected and retrieved through the largest skin incision, following removal of the port. The procedure may be combined with iPTH measurement.

This technique requires general anaesthesia, and increased operating time when compared to FP alone, but does allow access to both sides of the neck. A recent update of 260 cases treated by this technique reported a mean operating time of 40.2 minutes (range 10–180), a conversion rate to open surgery of 7.6% (20 patients) and two cases of recurrent nerve palsy (0.8%).[32]

Endoscopic or video-assisted procedures will require general anaesthesia, and longer operating time, but may result in a cosmetic outcome that is equivalent to or better than FP. They may also allow bilateral exploration where appropriate, and the magnified view of cervical anatomy may allow better visualisation of the recurrent laryngeal nerve.

Intraoperative PTH (iPTH) measurement

The introduction of iPTH measurement by rapid PTH assay has been an important advance in the development of unilateral surgery, replacing the need for visualisation of all glands, and has been described as a 'biochemical frozen section'. Several studies have now shown that a 50% reduction in baseline, pre-excision PTH within 5–10 minutes of adenoma excision accurately predicts postoperative normocalcaemia.[33,34] There is still some uncertainty with this technique, however, since a number of cases can take up to 30 minutes to fall by 50%.[25] Experience to date does suggest that failure to achieve a 50% drop in baseline PTH does seem to predict the presence of multigland disease or a second adenoma, and can guide intraoperative decision-making about further exploration. Intraoperative PTH measurement may not be necessary for all cases of focused parathyroidectomy. When there is concordance between preoperative ^{99m}Tc-sestamibi and ultrasound scanning, the false-positive rate for adenoma localisation may be so low that iPTH measurement has little to add and is not cost-effective.

Key point 4

- Development of focused parathyroidectomy, and other minimally invasive techniques, has shown that day-case parathyroidectomy is safe and feasible.

Key point 5

- Use of intraoperative PTH measurement avoids the need for frozen section and confirms cure when combined with unilateral surgery.

PARATHYROIDECTOMY – THE FUTURE

The most important factor in the management of pHPT is that surgery should be performed by an experienced surgeon. It is unlikely that all patients will be suitable for any one technique and surgeons should ideally be able to perform a minimally invasive procedure as well as bilateral cervical exploration. The use of treatment algorithms (Fig. 3) may help select the most appropriate procedure for individual patients based on high quality preoperative imaging.

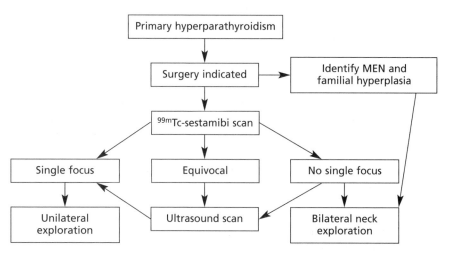

Fig. 3 Algorithm for the surgical management of primary hyperparathyroidism.

Key point 6

- Parathyroidectomy, either unilateral or bilateral, should be performed by an experienced parathyroid surgeon.

SECONDARY AND TERTIARY HYPERPARATHYROIDISM

Secondary hyperparathyroidism is the excessive production of PTH in response to low blood calcium levels caused by conditions such as renal failure and vitamin D deficiency. In chronic renal failure a decrease in glomerular filtration rate (GFR) leads to the accumulation of phosphate. This, together with a reduction in active vitamin D, stimulates PTH secretion. Symptoms include bone and joint pain, especially in the legs and feet, pruritus and an increased morbidity from cardiovascular disease. If the disease process progresses, tertiary hyperparathyroidism may develop.

In tertiary hyperparathyroidism the parathyroid glands become autonomous and function independently of calcium levels. This condition is usually associated with increased levels of PTH, calcium, alkaline phosphatase and phosphate. Symptoms often include bone pain, soft tissue calcification, tendon rupture, calciphylaxis, anaemia and pruritus.

MANAGEMENT OF SECONDARY HYPERPARATHYROIDISM

The two main strategies for management of this disease include replacement of vitamin D with oral analogues (1α-calcidol) and reduction in serum phosphate. A low phosphate diet and the use of phosphate binders such as calcium carbonate achieve phosphate reduction. Once hypercalcaemia develops, the treatment options are limited. More recently, there has been a move to consider earlier surgical intervention in these patients in an attempt to reduce their 17-fold increased cardiovascular risk.[35]

At present surgery is reserved for those patients who fail maximal medical therapy. At this stage the serum calcium and phosphate are often elevated, resulting in an increased calcium-phosphate product. The symptoms that usually improve following surgery include bone and joint pain (especially in the legs and feet), pruritus and lethargy. Current surgical options include subtotal parathyroidectomy or total parathyroidectomy with or without autotransplantation. Autotransplantation is carried out by dissection of a small portion of parathyroid tissue into 10–15 pieces that are placed into a muscle pocket in either the forearm or sternomastoid. There are increasing data, however, that show a high recurrence rate following autotransplantation in patients on long-term dialysis.[36,37] As a result, total parathyroidectomy without autotransplantation is the treatment of choice for patients unlikely to receive a renal transplant.

Key points for clinical practice

- Primary hyperparathyroidism is now being diagnosed with increased frequency.

- Surgery should now be considered early in the natural history of the disease, even in 'asymptomatic' patients.

- The majority of parathyroid adenomas can be detected by preoperative localisation with ^{99m}Tc-sestamibi and/or neck ultrasound.

- Development of focused parathyroidectomy, and other minimally invasive techniques, has shown that day-case parathyroidectomy is safe and feasible.

- Use of intraoperative PTH measurement avoids the need for frozen section and confirms cure when combined with unilateral surgery.

- Parathyroidectomy, either unilateral or bilateral, should be performed by an experienced parathyroid surgeon.

References

1. Mandl F. Therapeutischer Versuch bei Ostitis fibrosa generalisata Mittles: Exstirpation eines epithelkörperlichen Tumors. *Wien Klin Wochenshcr* 1925; **50**: 1343.
2. Heath H, Hodgson SF, Kennedy MA. Primary hyperparathyroidism: incidence, morbidity and potential impact in a community. *N Engl J Med* 1980; **302**: 189–193.
3. Gilmour JR. The embryology of the parathyroid glands, the thymus and certain associated rudiments. *J Pathol* 1937; **45**: 507.
4. Garret JE, Capuano IV, Hammerland LG *et al*. Molecular cloning and functional expression of human parathyroid calcium receptor cDNAs. *J Biol Chem* 1995; **270**: 12919–12925.
5. Potts Jr JT, Ackerman IP, Barker CF *et al*. Diagnosis and management of asymptomatic primary hyperparathyroidism: Consensus Development Conference statement. *Ann Intern Med* 1991; **114**: 593–597.
6. Utiger RD. Treatment of primary hyperparathyroidism. *N Engl J Med* 1999; **341**: 1301–1302.
7. Toft AD. Surgery for primary hyperparathyroidism – sooner rather than later. *Lancet* 2000; **355**: 1478–1479.
8. Burney RE, Jones KR, Christy B, Thompson NW. Health status improvement after surgical correction of primary hyperparathyroidism in patients with high and low preoperative calcium levels. *Surgery* 1999; **125**: 608–614.
9. Chan AK, Duh Q-Y, Katz MH, Siperstein AE, Clark OH. Clinical manifestations of primary hyperparathyroidism before and after parathyroidectomy: a case–control study. *Ann Surg* 1995; **222**: 402–414.
10. Palmer M, Adami HO, Bergstrom R, Jakobsson S, Akerstrom G, Ljunghall S. Survival and renal function in untreated hypercalcaemia. Population-based cohort study with 14 years of follow-up. *Lancet* 1987; **i**: 59–62.
11. Bilezikian JP, Potts JT, Fuleihan GE-H *et al*. Summary statement from a workshop on asymptomatic primary hyperparathyroidism: a perspective for the 21st century. *J Clin Endocrinol Metab* 2002; **87**: 5353–5361.
12. Holick MF. The parathyroid hormone D-lema. *J Clin Endocrinol Metab* 2003; **88**: 3499–3500.

13. Denizot A, Pucini M, Chagnaud C, Botti G, Henry J-FH. Normocalcaemia with elevated parathormone levels after surgical treatment of primary hyperparathyroidism. *Am J Surg* 2001; **182**: 15–19.

14. Malabanan A, Veronikis IE, Holick MF. Redefining vitamin D insufficiency. *Lancet* 1998; **351**: 805–806.

15. Chen H, Zeiger MA, Gordon TA *et al*. Parathyroidectomy in Maryland: effects of an endocrine center. *Surgery* 1996; **120**: 948–952.

16. Ozbas S, Pain S, Tang T, Wishart GC. Surgical management of primary hyperpara-thyroidism – results of a national survey. *Ann R Coll Surg Engl* 2003; **85**: 236–241.

17. O'Doherty MJ, Kettle AG, Wells PC, Collins REC, Coakley AJ. Parathyroid imaging with technetium-99m-sestamibi: preoperative localisation and tissue uptake studies. *J Nucl Med* 1992; **33**: 313–318.

18. Taillefer R, Boucher Y, Potviuc C, Lambert R. Detection and localisation of parathyroid adenomas in patients with hyperparathyroidism using a single radionuclide imaging procedure with ^{99m}Tc sestamibi (double phase study). *J Nucl Med* 1992; **33**: 1801–1807.

19. Sandrock D, Merino MJ, Norton JA, Neumann RD. Ultrastructural histology correlates of thallium-201/technetium-99m parathyroid subtraction scintigraphy. *J Nucl Med* 1993; **34**: 24–29.

20. Denham DW, Norman J. Cost-effectiveness of pre-operative sestamibi scan for primary hyperparathyroidism is dependent solely on surgeon's choice of operative procedure. *J Am Coll Surg* 1998; **186**: 293–304.

21. Kao A, Shiau YC, Tsai SC, Wang JJ, Ho ST. Technetium-99m methoxyisobutylisonitrile imaging for parathyroid adenoma: relationship to P-glycoprotein or multidrug resistance-related protein expression. *Eur J Nucl Med* 2002; **29**: 1012–1015.

22. Lumachi F, Ermani M, Basso S, Zuchetta P, Borsato N, Favia G. Localisation of parathyroid tumours in the minimally invasive era: Which technique should be chosen? Population-based analysis of 253 patients undergoing parathyroidectomy and factors affecting parathyroid gland detection. *Endocr Rel Cancer* 2001; **8**: 63–69.

23. Sidhu S, Neill AK, Russell CFJ. Long-term outcome of unilateral parathyroid exploration for primary hyperparathyroidism due to presumed solitary adenoma. *World J Surg* 2003; **27**: 339–342.

24. Udelsman R. Six hundred fifty-six consecutive explorations for primary hyperparathyroidism. *Ann Surg* 2002; **235**: 665–672.

25. Gurnell EM, Thomas SK, McFarlane I *et al*. Focused parathyroid surgery, with intraoperative parathyroid hormone (IOPTH) measurement, as an ambulatory procedure. *Br J Surg* 2004; **91**: 78–82.

26. Goldstein RE, Blevins L, Delbeke D, Martin WH. Effect of minimally invasive radioguided parathyroidectomy on efficacy, length of stay, and costs in management of primary hyperparathyroidism. *Ann Surg* 2000; **231**: 732–742.

27. Norman JG, Jaffray CE, Chheda H. The false positive parathyroid sestamibi: a real or perceived problem and a case for radioguided parathyroidectomy. *Ann Surg* 2000; **231**: 31–37.

28. Gagner M. Endoscopic subtotal parathyroidectomy in patients with primary hyperparathyroidism. *Br J Surg* 1996; **83**: 875.

29. Yeung GH. Endoscopic surgery of the neck. A new frontier. *Surg Laparosc Endosc* 1998; **8**: 227–232.

30. Lorenz K, Nguyen-Thanh H, Dralle H. Unilateral and minimally invasive procedures for primary hyperparathyroidism: a review of selective procedures. *Arch Surg* 2000; **385**: 106–117.

31. Miccoli P, Pinchera A, Ceccini G *et al*. Minimally invasive, video-assisted parathyroid surgery for primary hyperparathyroidism. *J Endocrinol Invest* 1997; **20**: 429–430.

32. Miccoli P, Bert P, Materazzi G, Picine A, Conte M, Marcocci C. Five years' experience with video-assisted parathyroidectomy. *Br J Surg* 2002; **89**: 1335.

33. Inabnet WB, Fulla Y, Richard B, Bonnichon P, Icard P, Chapuis Y. Unilateral neck exploration under local anaesthesia: the approach of choice for asymptomatic primary hyperparathyroidism. *Surgery* 1999; **126**: 1004–1010.

34. Udelsman R, Donovan PI, Sokoll LJ. One hundred minimally invasive parathyroid explorations. *Ann Surg* 2000; **232**: 331–339.

35. Ganesh SK, Stack AG, Levin NW, Hubert-Shearon T, Port FK. Association of elevated serum PO_4, $Ca \times PO_4$ product, and parathyroid hormone with cardiac mortality risk in chronic hemodialysis patients. *J Am Soc Nephrol* 2001; **12**: 2131–2138.
36. Higgins RM, Richardson AJ, Ratcliffe PJ, Woods CG, Oliver DO, Morris PJ. Total parathyroidectomy alone or with autograft for renal hyperparathyroidism. *Q J Med* 1991; **79**: 323–332.
37. Ockert S, Willeke F, Richter A *et al.* Total parathyroidectomy without autotransplantation as a standard procedure in the treatment of secondary hyperparathyroidism. *Langenbeck's Arch Surg* 2002; **387**: 204–209.

Nadey S. Hakim   Vassilios Papalois

15

Pancreas and islet transplantation

The syndrome of type I insulin-dependent diabetes mellitus (IDDM) includes not only abnormal glucose metabolism but also specific microvascular complications such as retinopathy, nephropathy and neuropathy. Diabetes mellitus is currently the leading cause of kidney failure and blindness in adults, the number one disease cause of amputations and impotence, and one of the leading chronic diseases of childhood associated with poor quality of life.

The aim of pancreas and islet transplantation is to establish the same status of glucose control that is provided by endogenous secretion of insulin from a healthy native pancreas in order to improve the quality of life and ameliorate secondary diabetic complications in patients with IDDM.

The first pancreas transplant in a human was performed by Kelly and Lillehei on 16 December 1966 at the University of Minnesota.[1]

Islet transplantation is theoretically an ideal solution for patients with IDDM since it is not a major procedure, can be performed radiologically and can be repeated several times without any major discomfort to the patient. Islet transplantation in humans has been performed systematically since 1974 and, as with pancreas transplantation, the University of Minnesota pioneered the field.[2] However, despite tedious experimental and clinical efforts over the past 25 years, long-term and consistent insulin independence has not yet been achieved.

Mr Nadey S. Hakim MD PhD FRCS FACS FICS, Consultant Surgeon and Surgical Director of the Transplant Unit, St Mary's Hospital, Praed Street, London W2 1NY

Vassilios E. Papalois MD PhD FRCS FICS, Consultant Transplant Surgeon, Transplant Unit, St Mary's Hospital, Praed Street, London W2 1NY.

INDICATIONS

Pancreas transplantation is indicated for patients with IDDM; additional selection criteria are listed in Table 1. Patient selection is aided by comprehensive multidisiplinary pretransplant evaluation with additional workup according to the specific problems of each patient. The evaluation initially confirms the diagnosis of IDDM, establishes the absence of exclusion criteria, determines the patient's ability to tolerate a major operation (based primarily on the patient's cardiovascular status) and documents end-stage organ complications for future tracking following transplantation.

In a suitable candidate, the evaluation is also needed to determine the type of pancreas transplantation, based mainly on the degree of nephropathy. The degree of renal dysfunction (creatinine clearance < 20 ml/min) is used to select patients for simultaneous pancreas–kidney transplantation (SPK) versus pancreas transplant alone (PTA) (creatinine clearance > 70 ml/min). A third option is to transplant a pancreas after a kidney (PAK) in patients with IDDM who have already had a kidney transplant and who meet the criteria for

Table 1 Selection criteria for pancreas transplantation

Inclusion criteria
- Presence of IDDM
- Well-defined secondary diabetic complications
- Ability to withstand:
    surgery
    immunosuppression
- Psychological suitability
- Good understanding of:
    therapeutic nature of pancreas transplantation
    need for long-term immunosuppression and follow-up

Exclusion criteria
- Insufficient cardiovascular reserve:
    angiography indicating non-correctable coronary artery disease
    ejection fraction below 50%
    recent myocardial infarction
- Currently significant:
    psychiatric illness
    psychological instability
    drug or alcohol abuse
    non-compliance with treatment
- Active infection
- Malignancy
- Lack of well-defined secondary diabetic complications
- Extreme obesity (> 130% of ideal body weight)

pancreas transplantation. The criteria for SPK, PTA and PAK transplants are summarised in Table 2.

Table 2 Factors determining the timing of pancreas transplantation in relation to kidney transplantation

---

Simultaneous pancreas–kidney transplant (SPK)
- Diabetic nephropathy: creatinine clearance < 20 ml/min
- Patient on dialysis or very close to starting dialysis
- Failure of previous renal allograft

Pancreas transplant alone (PTA)
- Presence of two or more diabetic complications:
  proliferative retinopathy
  early nephropathy; creatinine clearance > 70 ml/min,
    proteinuria > 150 mg/24 h but < 3 g/24 h
  presence of overt peripheral or autonomic neuropathy
  vasculopathy with accelerated atherosclerosis

- Hyperlabile diabetes with:
  severe episodes of ketoacidosis
  severe and frequent episodes of hypoglycaemia
  hypoglycaemia unawareness
  severe and frequent infections
  impairment of quality of life

Pancreas transplant after kidney transplant (PAK)
- Patients with stable function of previous renal allograft that meet the criteria for PTA

RECIPIENT OPERATION

The majority of pancreas transplants are performed in conjunction with a kidney transplant from the same donor through a midline-incision intraperitoneal approach. The same approach is used for PTA and PAK transplants. The surgical approach to pancreas transplantation is similar to that for the kidney in many aspects. The pancreas is directed with the head towards the pelvis and usually the graft vessels are anastomosed end-to-side to the recipient common or external iliac vessels using 5/0 Prolene suture for the venous and 6/0 Prolene suture for the arterial anastomosis. If possible, the vessels are anastomosed to the right iliac vessels of the recipient, which are more superficial compared with the left iliac vessels. This minimises the chances of post-transplant graft thrombosis. This type of venous anastomosis results in systemic drainage of the venous outflow of the pancreatic graft. More recently, the University of Tennessee[3] has introduced a portal drainage technique where the pancreas is placed head-up and the portal vein anastomosed to one of the mesenteric veins. This achieves a more physiological drainage into the portal circulation. This technique is possibly associated with a higher rate of technical complications while there is no clear evidence that it has better metabolic results. The only possible advantage of portal drainage is the absence of systemic hyperinsulinaemia which is characteristic of systemic drainage.

PANCREATIC DRAINAGE

Several surgical techniques have been used to manage the exocrine secretions of the pancreatic graft, including urinary drainage, enteric drainage and polymer injection. Urinary drainage is currently the most popular, but enteric drainage has recently regained popularity. Duct injection is becoming less popular, even in the European centres where it was first introduced.[4]

Urinary drainage

The duodenum is opened and anastomosed to the bladder. This is most easily achieved using a stapler. The major advantage of urinary drainage is the ability to detect pancreas rejection episodes early (before hyperglycaemia) by monitoring urinary amylase. It is, however, associated with significant morbidity, including duodenal leaks, cystitis, urethritis, reflux pancreatitis, dehydration, acidosis and electrolyte abnormalities.[5]

Enteric drainage

The duodenum is anastomosed side-to-side in two layers to a loop of proximal ileum, avoiding any tension. The enteric drainage of exocrine secretions is more physiological in view of the bowel resorption. However, urinary amylase cannot be used as a rejection maker and eventual leaks can lead to severe complications.

Duct injection

The injection of polymer into the main pancreatic duct is a very simple and fast technique, which leads eventually to the atrophy of the exocrine portion of the pancreas. Unfortunately, it can also lead to the atrophy of the endocrine tissue, resulting in graft failure.

IMMUNOSUPPRESSION

Optimal immunosuppressive strategies in pancreas transplantation aim at achieving effective control of rejection while minimising injury to the allograft as well as risk to the patient. Until recently, a standard immunosuppressive protocol consisted of cyclosporine (cyclosporin A), prednisone and azathioprine combined with an induction course of anti-T-cell monoclonal or polyclonal antibody (antilymphocyte globulin (ALG), antithymocyte globulin (ATG) or OKT3). Tacrolimus has replaced cyclosporine in 20% of centres and more recently mycophenolate mofetil (MMF) has been used instead of azathioprine.[3] These agents may be associated with higher patient and graft survival rates.

Transplantation requires a lifelong commitment to immunosuppression. However, most patients find it easier to adjust to their immunosuppressive medications than to insulin, dietary and activity restrictions.

Key point 2

- Optimal immunosuppressive strategies in pancreas transplantation aim at achieving effective control of rejection while minimising injury to the allograft as well as the risk to the patient.

RESULTS OF PANCREAS TRANSPLANTATION

From December 1966 up to date, over 16 000 pancreas transplants have been performed worldwide. The latest publication of the International Pancreas Transplant Register (IPTR) data includes 8800 pancreas transplants that had been performed from December 1966 to November 1996, including more than 6400 from the USA and more than 2300 from other countries.[6] Most of those transplants (86%) were SPK, 8% were PAK and 5% were PTA. Outside the USA most were performed in Europe (91%). The leading country was France (19%), followed by Germany (16%), Sweden (10%) and Spain (7%).

GRAFT SURVIVAL

For the 4592 bladder-drained pancreas transplants performed in the USA between October 1987 and November 1996, the patient survival rates at 1, 2, 3 and 5 years were 92%, 89%, 86% and 81% respectively. The graft survival rates at 1, 2, 3 and 5 years were 76%, 71%, 67% and 61% for all cases. When only the 4062 technically successful cases were considered, the 1-, 2-, 3- and 5-year graft survival rates were 85%, 81%, 76% and 72% respectively. Patient and graft survival according to recipient category are presented in Table 3. The patient survival rate was not significantly different ($P > 0.22$) between the three recipient categories. Graft survival was significantly different between the three categories ($P = 0.0001$). The outcome was significantly better for SPK than for PTA but there was no difference between PTA and PAK ($P = 0.83$). The technical failure rate was lower in the SPK category compared with PTA. There was no significant difference between 1-year graft survival rates for primary versus retransplants in the SPK (79% *versus* 77%; $P > 0.10$) and PTA (57% *versus* 51%; $P > 0.8$) categories. In contrast, for PAK transplants, the 1-year graft survival rate was higher in primary transplants than in retransplants (62% *versus* 47%; $P < 0.0001$).

The results of pancreas transplantation in European and other non-US centres are comparable to those in the USA. The 1-year patient survival rates for SPK in the USA, Europe and other countries were 92%, 91% and 86% respectively ($P = 0.08$). The 1-year graft survival rates for bladder-drained SPK in the USA, Europe and other countries were 79%, 73% and 70% respectively. Likewise, the 1-year graft survival rates for enterically drained SPK in the USA, Europe and other countries were 72%, 63% and 72% respectively.

Table 3 The 1-, 2-, 3- and 5-year patient and graft survival rates following pancreas transplantation according to recipient category

	Patient survival (%)			Graft survival (%)		
	SPK	PAK	PTA	SPK	PAK	PTA
1-year	92	91	90	79	58	56
2-year	89	87	88	75	45	48
3-year	86	82	86	71	38	40
5-year	81	74	81	65	27	32

SPK, simultaneous pancreas–kidney transplant (3989 cases); PAK, pancreas after kidney transplant (375 cases); PTA, pancreas transplant alone (229 cases).

EFFECT OF PANCREAS TRANSPLANTATION ON SECONDARY COMPLICATIONS OF IDDM

The results of patient and graft survival after pancreas transplantation have significantly improved in the last decade. Pancreas transplantation is not a life-saving procedure, and the assessment of its effect on the progress of the secondary diabetic complications as well as the overall quality of life of pancreas transplant recipients is of great importance.

One major problem in studying the effects of pancreas transplantation on halting or, even more, reversing the progress of secondary diabetic complications is that many pancreas transplant recipients have end-stage degenerative diabetic complications, for which there is no hope for improvement. In addition, since the majority of pancreas transplants are performed simultaneously with a kidney, it is difficult to differentiate and attribute any positive development after SPK to the effect of the normal status of glucose metabolism rather than to the corrected uraemia. Finally, most of the studies that deal with the effect of pancreas transplantation on diabetic complications are not multicentre prospective randomised trials with large numbers of patients and long-term follow-up from which reliable conclusions could be reached.

Key point 3

- Pancreas transplantation is not a life-saving procedure, and the assessment of its effect on the progress of the secondary diabetic complications as well as the overall quality of life of pancreas transplant recipients is of great importance.

Retinopathy

There is some controversy about the effect of pancreas transplantation on diabetic retinopathy. Most of these studies were performed in patients already affected by proliferative retinopathy. In one of these studies with follow-up of 4 or more years after transplantation, stabilisation of retinopathy was observed – more than that observed in patients followed for the same period of time but whose pancreas transplants had failed.[7] In another study two groups of diabetic patients were included: in the first group the patients underwent SPK and in the second a kidney transplant alone.[8] The status of diabetic retinopathy remained unchanged in 88% and 90% of these patients respectively. The results were similar in another study performed in diabetic patients who underwent PTA; the post-transplant euglycaemia did not change the course of diabetic retinopathy.[9]

Nephropathy

In one study of diabetic patients who underwent pancreas transplantation after having had a successful kidney transplant, it was demonstrated that pancreas transplantation prevents, to some extent, recurrence of diabetic nephropathy and that the diabetic glomerular lesions were less severe compared with diabetic patients who underwent a kidney transplant alone.[10] However, studies performed on patients who received a PTA showed that the diabetic glomerular lesions did not improve even after several years of achieving an insulin-independent euglycaemic state with pancreas transplantation.[11]

Key point 4

- Pancreas transplantation prevents, to some extent, recurrence of diabetic nephropathy. The diabetic glomerular lesions after combined transplantation were less severe compared with diabetic patients who underwent a kidney transplant alone.

Neuropathy

A number of studies have reported improvements in both motor and sensory nerve function as assessed by nerve conduction velocity in patients after SPK compared with recipients of kidney transplant alone and with patients with pancreatic graft failure.[12,13] These studies clearly demonstrated that although the correction of uraemia by a simultaneous kidney transplant, or a kidney transplant alone, significantly improves motor and sensory nerve conduction, the presence of a pancreatic graft has an additional and important positive effect in improving peripheral neuropathy. Studies of the effect of pancreas transplantation on autonomic neuropathy were performed in PTA and compared with non-transplanted patients or patients after pancreas graft failure.[14] These studies demonstrated that, after PTA, patients with a functioning pancreatic graft had better survival rates compared with recipients with a failed pancreatic graft and with diabetics who were not transplanted. However, other studies of autonomic function following pancreas transplantation are less clear. In some, pancreas transplantation was associated with greater improvement in autonomic symptoms, even if they were accompanied by little objective evidence.[15,16]

Key point 5

- A number of studies have reported improvements in both motor and sensory nerve function as assessed by nerve conduction velocity after combined transplantation compared both with recipients of kidney transplant alone and with patients with pancreatic graft failure.

QUALITY OF LIFE AFTER PANCREAS TRANSPLANTATION

Patient and graft survival rates, the incidence of complications and the effect of transplantation on the secondary diabetic complications are important in evaluating the results. What is perhaps of even greater significance is the effect that pancreas transplantation has on the overall quality of life of diabetic patients. The effect on the quality of life is important for the evaluation of all modern therapeutic interventions, but this is particularly so in the case of a non-life-saving organ transplant that carries a non-negligible risk and involves many social and financial aspects. It is encouraging that it is in the field of quality of life that many studies agree that pancreas transplantation has a very positive effect.

A detailed study evaluated the effect of pancreas transplantation on many different aspects of life quality of 157 diabetic patients.[17] The results indicated a much better quality of life (satisfaction with physical capacity as well as leisure time activities) in recipients of SPK compared with pretransplant predialysis diabetic patients.

In an interesting study, authors reported on the benefit of SPK compared with kidney transplant alone.[18] After SPK, 90% of recipients had full-time occupations, compared with 50% of recipients of kidney transplant alone. In addition, lost working days decreased by 44% compared to the pre-transplant situation in the SPK, whereas in recipients of kidneys only there was no change. Furthermore, SPK was associated with a better quality of life in physical well-being, sole functioning and perception of self.

In another extensive analysis 131 recipients of pancreatic transplant were studied 1–11 years after transplant.[19] Patients with functioning pancreatic grafts were compared with recipients with failed grafts who had good kidney function. The recipients with functioning grafts reported more satisfaction with the overall quality of life (68% *versus* 48%), felt healthier (89% *versus* 25%) and were able to care for themselves and their daily activities (78% *versus* 56%).

In a prospective study with 1-year follow-up using the Medical Outcome Study Health Survey 36-Item Short Form (SF-36) and comparing SPK recipients with kidney transplants alone and IDDM patients who did not receive a transplant, improvements in general health perception, social function, vitality and pain were seen in both transplanted groups. However, physical limitations improved only in SPK recipients.[20] In addition, financial situation, physical capacity, occupational status, sexual and leisure time activities improved significantly for SPK recipients.[21]

Key point 6

- Patients experience a much better quality of life (satisfaction with physical capacity as well as leisure time activities) after combined kidney–pancreas transplant, compared with pretransplant predialysis diabetic patients.

ISLET TRANSPLANTATION

ADVANTAGES AND PROBLEMS OF ISLET TRANSPLANTATION

As previously mentioned, islet transplantation is in theory an ideal solution for patients with IDDM since it is not a major procedure, can be performed radiologically and can be repeated several times without any major discomfort to the patient. Unfortunately, there are many problems related to islet transplantation, the most difficult being the availability of human organs for islet allotransplantation. Indeed, of approximately 5000 donors available each year in the USA, only a small proportion are suitable for pancreas or islet transplantation, and most of those are used for whole-organ pancreas transplantation. The technique for islet isolation has to be meticulous in order to obtain a good yield of viable islets. There is great difficulty in early detection of islet allograft rejection, even when they are transplanted simultaneously with a kidney. Finally, the islets are very sensitive to the currently used drugs in the standardised immunosuppressive regimens, such as steroids, cyclosporine and tacrolimus.

Key point 7

- The technique for islet isolation has to be meticulous in order to obtain a good yield of viable islets. There is great difficulty in early detection of islet allograft rejection, even when they are transplanted simultaneously with a kidney.

HUMAN ISLET ALLOGRAFTS

After many years of research, it was only in the late 1980s that it became possible to perform islet allotransplants with some success. Islets obtained from cadaveric donors were transplanted into the liver via the portal vein. Initial results were encouraging, but were later disappointing as it became obvious that most recipients remained hyperglycaemic. By the end of 1995, 270 patients with IDDM who received adult islet allografts were reported to the International Islet Transplant Registry (IITR).[22] Of these, only 27 (10%) became insulin-independent for less than 1 week, 14 (5%) were insulin-independent for more than 1 week, 14 (5%) were insulin-independent for more than 1 year, and 1 patient was insulin-independent for more than 4 years. Factors related to short-term insulin independence are detailed in Table 4. In addition to the classical immunosuppressive protocols, induction therapy with 15-deoxyspergualin is an important factor for achieving relatively long-term insulin independence. The reason is the ability of 15-deoxyspergualin to minimise the macrophage-mediated attack that islet allografts (as well as autografts) undergo post transplant and that causes the phenomenon of islet primary non-function.[23] Although the IITR results for long-term insulin

Table 4 Factors related to insulin independence after islet allotransplantation

- Preservation time less than 8 hours
- Transplantation of more than 6000 islet equivalents (number of islets if all had a diameter of 150 μm) per kilogram of body weight
- Transplantation into the liver via the portal vein
- Induction immunosuppression with anti-T-cell agents and 15-deoxyspergualin

independence are not good, it is important to emphasise that many of the insulin-dependent islet recipients have had persisting C-peptide secretion, a reduction of insulin dose and an improvement in the stability of glucose control, which correlated with less dangerous hypoglycaemic episodes. This means that it is possible for some of the transplanted islets to survive a long time. With improvements in islet isolation techniques, as well as improvements in detection of rejection and immunosuppression, long-term insulin independence with islet allotransplantation might become a reality.

Patients who underwent pancreatectomy and hepatectomy for extensive abdominal cancer followed by simultaneous islet and liver grafts had very good islet function post transplant.[22] Indeed, 9 out of 15 (60%) became insulin-independent. Ultimately, all patients succumbed to their malignancy, one of them having remained insulin-independent for 5 years until her death. The reasons for these better results compared with the results of islet transplants in patients with IDDM are not clear. A possible explanation is that islets only had to overcome allograft rejection and not the autoimmune response associated with IDDM. The fact that these patients had cancer could have compromised their immunity and finally the simultaneous liver transplant could have had a protective element.

THE FUTURE OF PANCREAS AND ISLET TRANSPLANTATION

Advances in immunosuppressive strategies and diagnostic technology will only enhance the already-good results achieved with pancreas transplantation. Further documentation of the long-term benefits and effects of pancreas transplantation may lead to its wider availability and acceptance. Prevention of rejection and effective control with earlier diagnosis may soon permit solitary pancreas transplantation to become an acceptable option in diabetic patients without advanced secondary complications or diabetes. During the past decade, significant advances have been achieved in islet transplantation.[24] The success of islet autografts indicates that successful engraftment and function of human islets is possible, and, with some advancements in rejection monitoring and immunosuppression, results of islet allotransplantation will also improve. Recent developments in the field of islet xenotransplantation and microencapsulation enhance the belief that islet transplantation will become an ideal option for the treatment of IDDM. Currently, however, islet transplantation cannot compete with the results obtained with whole-organ pancreas transplantation. Therefore, while continuing with the tedious but promising research work to improve the results of islet transplantation, every patient with IDDM who meets the criteria should be offered the option of pancreas transplantation.

Key point 8

- Until islet transplantation results improve, every patient with IDDM who meets the criteria for transplantation should be offered the option of pancreas transplantation.

Key points for clinical practice

- The aim of pancreas and islet transplantation is to establish the same status of glucose control that is provided by endogenous secretion of insulin from a healthy native pancreas in order to improve the quality of life and ameliorate secondary diabetic complications in patients with IDDM.

- Optimal immunosuppressive strategies in pancreas transplantation aim at achieving effective control of rejection while minimising injury to the allograft as well as the risk to the patient.

- Pancreas transplantation is not a life-saving procedure, and the assessment of its effect on the progress of the secondary diabetic complications as well as the overall quality of life of pancreas transplant recipients is of great importance.

- Pancreas transplantation prevents, to some extent, recurrence of diabetic nephropathy. The diabetic glomerular lesions after combined transplantation were less severe compared with diabetic patients who underwent a kidney transplant alone.

- A number of studies have reported improvements in both motor and sensory nerve function as assessed by nerve conduction velocity after combined transplantation compared both with recipients of kidney transplant alone and with patients with pancreatic graft failure.

- Patients experience a much better quality of life (satisfaction with physical capacity as well as leisure time activities) after combined kidney–pancreas transplant, compared with pretransplant predialysis diabetic patients.

- The technique for islet isolation has to be meticulous in order to obtain a good yield of viable islets. There is great difficulty in early detection of islet allograft rejection, even when they are transplanted simultaneously with a kidney.

- Until islet transplantation results improve, every patient with IDDM who meets the criteria for transplantation should be offered the option of pancreas transplantation.

References

1. Kelly W, Lillehi R, Merkel F. Allotransplantation of the pancreas and duodenum along with the kidney in diabetic nephropathy. *Surgery* 1967; **61**: 827–835.
2. Najarian J, Sutherland DER, Steffes M. Isolation of human islets of Langerhans for transplantation. *Transplant Proc* 1975; **7**: 611–613.
3. Stratta R. Pancreas transplantation in the 1990s. In: Hakim NS, Stratta RJ, Dubernard JM (eds). *Proceedings of the Second British Symposium on Pancreatic Transplantation (ICSS 232)*. London: Royal Society of Medicine, 1998: 103–121.
4. Dubernard JM. Improving morbidity rates of reno-pancreatic transplantation by modification of the technique. In: Hakim NS, Stratta RJ, Dubernard JM (eds). *Proceedings of the Second British Symposium on Pancreatic Transplantation (ICSS 232)*. London: Royal Society of Medicine, 1998; 21–26.

5. Hakim NS, Gruessner A, Papalois VE *et al*. Duodenal complications in bladder-drained pancreas transplants. *Surgery* 1997; **121**: 618–624.

6. Gruessner A, Sutherland DER, Goetz F *et al*. Pancreas transplantation in the United States (US) and non-US as reported to the United Network for Organ Sharing (UNOS) and the International Pancreas Transplant Registry (IPTR). In: Terasaki P, Cecka J (eds). *Clinical Transplants 1996*. Los Angeles: LA Tissue Typing Laboratory, 1996: 47–67.

7. Bandello F, Vigano C *et al*. Influence of successful pancreatorenal transplantation on diabetic retinopathy: a 20 cases report. *Diabetologia* 1991; **34 (Suppl I)**: 92–94.

8. Caldara R, Bandello F, Vigano C *et al*. Influence of successful pancreatorenal transplantation on diabetic nephropathy. *Transplant Proc* 1994; **26**: 490.

9. Ransay RC, Frederich CB, Sutherland DER *et al*. Progression of diabetic retinopathy after pancreas transplantation for insulin-dependent diabetes mellitus. *N Engl J Med* 1988; **318**: 208–214.

10. Billus RW, Mauer SM, Sutherland DER *et al*. The effect of pancreas transplantation on the glomerular structure of renal allografts in patients with insulin-dependent diabetes. *N Engl J Med* 1989; **321**: 80–85.

11. Fioretto P, Mauer SM, Bilou RW *et al*. Effects of pancreas transplantation on glomerular structure in insulin-dependent diabetic patients with their own kidneys. *Lancet* 1993; **342**: 1193–1196.

12. Comi G, Galardi G, Amadio S *et al*. Neurophysiological study of the effect of combined kidney and pancreas transplantation on diabetic neuropathy: a 2-year follow-up evaluation. *Diabetologia* 1991; **34 (Suppl I)**: 103–107.

13. Solders G, Tyden G, Persson A *et al*. Improvement of nerve conduction in diabetic nephropathy. *Diabetes* 1992; **41**: 946–951.

14. Navarro X, Kennedy WR, Goetz FGC *et al*. Influence of pancreas transplantation on cardiorespiratory reflexes, nerve conduction, and mortality in diabetes mellitus. *Diabetes* 1990; **39**: 802–806.

15. Nusser J, Scheuer R, Abendroth D *et al*. Effect of pancreatic transplantation and/or renal transplantation on diabetic autonomic neuropathy. *Diabetologia* 1991; **34 (Suppl I)**: 118–120.

16. Hathaway DK, Abell T, Cardoso S *et al*. Improvement in autonomic and gastric function following pancreas–kidney versus kidney-alone transplantation and the correlation with quality of life. *Transplantation* 1994; **57**: 816–822.

17. La Rocca E, Secchi A, Galardi G *et al*. Kidney and pancreas transplantation improves hypertension in type I diabetic patients. In: *Abstract Book, 7th Congress of the European Society for Organ Transplantation, ESOT '95, Vienna*. October 3–7 1995: 362.

18. Piehlmeier W, Bullinger M, Nusser J *et al*. Quality of life in type I (insulin dependent) diabetic patients prior to and after pancreas and kidney transplantation in relation to organ function. *Diabetologia* 1991; **34 (Suppl I)**: 150–157.

19. Zehrer CL, Gross CR. Quality of life of pancreas transplantation recipients. *Diabetologia* 1991; **34 (Suppl I)**: 145–149.

20. Zehrer CL, Gross CR. Comparison of quality of life between pancreas/kidney and kidney transplant recipients. 1 year follow-up. *Transplant Proc* 1994; **26**: 508–509.

21. Sutherland DER, Goetz FC, Najarian JS. Living-related donor segmental pancreatectomy for transplantation. *Transplant Proc* 1994; **26**: 508–509.

22. Hering BJ. Insulin independence following islet transplantation in man – a comparison of different recipient categories. *International Islet Transplantation Registry* 1996; **6**: 5–19.

23. Kaufman DB, Field MJ, Gruber SA *et al*. Extended functional survival of murine islet allograft with 15-deoxyspergualin. *Transplant Proc* 1992; **24**: 1045–1047.

24. Shapiro AMJ, Lakey JRT, Ryan EA *et al*. Islet transplantation in seven patients with type I diabetes mellitus using a glucocortocoid-free immunosuppressive regimen. *N Engl J Med* 2000; **343**: 230–238.

Robert A. Reichert Nigel P.M. Sacks

16

Strategies for breast cancer prevention

Breast cancer survival has greatly increased over the past 20 years due to earlier detection and improved multidisciplinary treatments.[1] However, a significant number of women still die from this disease: 11 500 in England and Wales in 2002.[2]

As with any malignancy, the prevention of breast cancer would be better than a search for the best cure. Are there ways that we can prevent this disease, which is the most common cancer in women, and thus make an even greater impact on improved survival, especially in those at high risk? In this chapter we aim to outline and summarise the current status of breast cancer prophylaxis with emphasis on what a surgeon needs to know to address these issues with the patients he or she sees in day-to-day practice.

Prophylaxis implies total prevention of disease. No strategy yet exists that can totally prevent breast cancer, as we do not know the cause in the vast majority of cases. It is therefore better to use the term *risk reduction*, as all the modalities that will be discussed in this chapter can reduce but not completely eliminate risk. As our understanding of the genetics, aetiology, and biology of breast cancer grows, further strategies for prevention will be developed based on that greater understanding.

In developing a risk-reduction strategy, it is important that we know what risk we wish to reduce. The primary goal may not necessarily be the reduction of the risk of the development of breast cancer, but instead the reduction of risk of death and to a lesser extent morbidity from breast cancer.[3] As we shall see, some strategies reduce the absolute incidence of breast cancer, but appear to reduce only the incidence of early, favourable cancers, which are easily curable and increase the risk of other significant comorbidities.[4]

Robert A. Reichert MD FACS, Surgical Fellow, Academic Surgery, Breast Unit, Royal Marsden Hospital

Mr Nigel P.M. Sacks MS FRCS FRACS, Consultant Surgeon, Royal Marsden Hospital, Fulham Road, London SW3 6JJ, UK

RISK ASSESSMENT

Before any risk-reduction methods are employed, the relative risk of developing breast cancer in each patient must be assessed. Current risk-reducing techniques have different morbidities, and it is therefore necessary to be able to determine if each woman's risk is great enough to warrant the side-effects of a specific risk-reduction method. The patient must be aware of the risk/benefit ratio of each risk-reduction strategy.

The marked increase in the early detection of breast cancer means that most women are aware of their risk of developing this disease. In addition, the publicity in the media of various drugs that increase risk, most recently HRT,[5,6] or decrease risk, most recently aromatase inhibitors,[7] has also increased awareness of breast cancer risk and the desire to reduce that risk.

Breast-care specialists are often asked by their patients what their own individual risk is and what steps they can take to reduce it. Most women, particularly those with a family history, greatly overestimate their risk of breast cancer.[8] Therefore it is imperative that breast-care specialists know how to evaluate risk and understand the limitations of risk assessment; so that they can reassure those not at risk and further counsel or refer those that may be at increased risk.

Key point 2

• Most women, particularly those with a family history, greatly overestimate their risk of breast cancer.

The link between breast cancer and heredity has long been known. It is now clear that all sporadic cancers, including breast cancer, have genetic alterations in just the cancer cells (somatic mutations) that cause invasive behaviour. These alterations do not occur in the remainder of the individual's cells outside the tumour. However, about 5–10% of common cancers, including those of the breast, are known to be due to inherited genetic alterations that are present in all an individual's cells (germline mutations).

Two specific high-penetrance breast cancer-associated (*BRCA*) gene mutations, *BRCA1* and *BRCA2*, have been identified, and are responsible for about half the hereditary cancers or 5% of all breast cancers. *BRCA1* has been mapped to chromosome 17q and *BRCA2* to 13q. Thus neither is X-linked and can be passed to an individual's offspring by standard Mendelian inheritance (each child has a 50% risk of carrying the mutation). A particular mutation in the *BRCA1* gene is found in high frequency in Ashkenazi Jews. There appears to be at least one other high-penetrance breast cancer-associated gene (*BRCAX*) and many other low-penetrance genes, which have not yet been identified, that contribute to breast cancer risk.[9]

Women who carry a *BRCA* gene mutation have about a 50% risk of developing breast cancer by the age of 50 and about an 85% chance by age 70.[9] Clinicians caring for carriers or suspected carriers of *BRCA* mutations should be aware that *BRCA1* and 2 are also associated with a high risk of ovarian and some other cancers.

Presently, tests to identify *BRCA1* and 2 mutations are available. Table 1 lists the probabilities of a patient carrying such a gene based on family and personal history. This table can be used to determine which women need to be referred for genetic counselling and testing. It is not within the scope of this chapter to discuss the issues surrounding gene testing and counselling. Presently available tests are accurate if positive. However, a negative result does not ensure that an individual does not carry a gene mutation, as that person may have a gene that has yet to be mapped. Therefore women who have clinical criteria that would make them possible gene carriers should be treated as such unless they have tested negative for a gene known to be present in other family members.

Table 1 Risk of *BRCA* mutation in a family[9]

Chance that a mutation is present (%)	Family history
< 10	• A single case of breast or ovarian cancer, any age
10	• Single breast cancer < 35 years old
> 10–30	• 2 breast cancers < 50 years old • 1 breast cancer < 40 years old in an Ashkenazi Jew
> 30–50	• 3 breast cancers < 50 years old • 4 or 5 breast cancers, no ovarian cancer • 1 breast and ovarian cancer in the same person
> 50	• > 1 breast cancer and ovarian cancer • ≥ 4 cases of female/male breast cancer • > 6 female breast cancers

Key point 3

- 5–10% of breast cancers are known to be due to inherited genetic alterations that are present in all an individual's cells (germline mutations), and can be passed to at least half of an individual's offspring by standard Mendelian inheritance.

Key point 4

- Two specific high-penetrance breast cancer-associated (*BRCA*) gene mutations, *BRCA1* and *BRCA2*, have been identified, and are responsible for about half the hereditary cancers or 5% of all breast cancers.

In those not at high risk of being gene carriers, many well-established factors that increase the risk of sporadic breast cancer have been identified. (Table 2). The relative contribution of each of these factors to overall risk is much harder to assess.

To this end, various risk-assessment models have been devised. The two most widely used are the Claus[10] and Gail[11] models. These models have been developed by studying factors that appear to increase risk in large populations, and assessing the relative contribution of each factor. Each of these models has significant limitations. They can only be applied to women from similar populations to those used to derive the model. For example, the Gail model was restricted to Caucasian women over the age of 35 who had annual screening mammograms. Each model only evaluates certain factors, so that the influence of factors other than those included in the specific model is not assessed.

Most importantly, all of these models assess population risk, not individual risk. They are very accurate at determining the overall risk of a population of women with a specific set of risk factors, but not the risk of an individual woman with those specific risk factors. In other words, when a woman is determined to have a risk of 1.7% of developing breast cancer in 5 years by one

Table 2 Magnitude of known lifetime breast cancer risk factors[3]

Relative risk < 2	Relative risk 2–4	Relative risk > 4
Early menarche, age < 11	One 1st-degree relative with breast cancer	Two 1st-degree relatives with breast cancer
Late menopause, age < 55	Radiation exposure	Mantle radiation for Hodgkin's disease ages 15–35
Nulliparity	Prior breast cancer	Lobular carcinoma *in situ*
Age > 35 at first birth	Mammographic dense breast	Ductal carcinoma *in situ*
Hormone replacement > 5 years (combined E+P>E)		Atypical hyperplasia
Postmenopausal obesity		
Alcohol use, > 2 units/day		
Proliferative benign breast disease		

of these models, it means that she is in a population of women with similar risk factors, 1.7% of whom will develop breast cancer. Her individual risk could be much greater or less.[3]

> ## Key point 5
>
> - Before any risk-reduction methods are employed, the relative risk of developing breast cancer in each patient must be assessed. However, all risk-assessment models assess population risk, not individual risk.

The prior diagnosis of ductal carcinoma *in situ* (DCIS), lobular carcinoma *in situ* (LCIS) and atypical ductal hyperplasia (ADH) all significantly increase risk.[12] The Gail model takes this into account, but some others do not. Models are constantly being refined, and new models are being proposed that are likely to increase the accuracy of determining an individual's risk.[13,14]

> ## Key point 6
>
> - The prior diagnosis of ductal carcinoma *in situ* (DCIS), lobular carcinoma *in situ* (LCIS) and atypical ductal hyperplasia (ADH) all significantly increase risk.

RISK-REDUCTION STRATEGIES

CHANGING EXOGENOUS FACTORS

While most of the exogenous factors that increase breast cancer risk do not have a major impact on that risk, they are the only ones within a patient's control (Table 2). Obviously, reduction of alcohol intake and avoidance of obesity are goals that have health benefits beyond and above the reduction of breast cancer risk, but attaining these goals can be difficult for many.

Issues surrounding parity are more difficult. There are many factors influencing a woman's decisions about childbirth, and usually these decisions are made long before breast cancer risk reduction becomes a concern, so regulation of parity is not a realistic risk-reduction strategy.

The relation of hormone replacement therapy (HRT) to the development of breast cancer has long been debated. It is now generally accepted that prolonged use of HRT does increase breast cancer risk. The recent publications of the Women's Health Initiative (WHI) study in the USA and the Million Women study in the UK support this conclusion. Both studies showed an increase in the risk of breast cancer with the use of combined oestrogen/progesterone HRT preparations: 24% in the WHI study and double in the Million Women study. While the Million Women study showed a smaller but significant increased risk for oestrogen alone, a significant difference has yet to emerge in the WHI study, which continues to follow this group.[5,6] Thus breast-care specialists are frequently asked to address the effect of HRT use on breast cancer risk. While it is easy to simply advise women not to use HRT, this is one case that clearly illustrates the necessity of evaluating risk/benefit ratio. A significant number of women still benefit – although not as greatly as was once believed – from HRT. Therefore, it is important that the clinician make clear the level of these competing risks to each patient so that she can make an informed decision.

SCREENING

If risk reduction is defined as reducing the risk of dying from breast cancer then screening strategies clearly are a major form of risk reduction. The pros and cons of mammographic screening in general have been extensively reviewed elsewhere. However, with respect to women under 50 years of age with high risk due to family history, mammographic screening finds as many breast cancers per 1000 women as the regular NHS breast screening programme.[15] For this reason, patients with a strong family history of breast cancer have been recommended to begin annual mammographic screening from the age of 35. Obviously, gene carriers are included, as are those at moderate risk of being a gene carrier (Table 1). However, no evidence exists that screening this group increases survival.[16] Annual mammographic screening is also recommended for those diagnosed with DCIS, LCIS and ADH.

Other forms of screening for high-risk patients are being investigated. The most promising to date is the use of magnetic resonance imaging (MRI).[17] Duct lavage and duct endoscopy may play a role in the future in screening high-risk women, but these methods are purely investigational.[18]

Key point 7

- If risk reduction is defined as reducing the risk of dying from breast cancer then screening strategies are clearly a major form of risk reduction.

CHEMOPREVENTION

Endogenous oestrogen has a pivotal role in promoting the development of most breast cancers.[19] Since the introduction of tamoxifen over 20 years ago, the possibility that an anti-oestrogen drug could be used to prevent the onset of breast cancer has been considered. This was supported by studies that showed a 30–40% relative reduction in the incidence of contralateral breast cancers in women treated with adjuvant tamoxifen.[20] In the late 1980s a feasibility study began at the Royal Marsden Hospital (RMH), which showed that tamoxifen used for risk reduction was relatively safe and well tolerated by healthy women.[21]

There have now been four trials of tamoxifen that have reported results: the RMH feasibility study, which was continued as the TAMOPLAC trial,[22] the

National Adjuvant Breast and Bowel Project (NSABP) P-1 trial,[23] the International Breast Cancer Intervention Study (IBIS)[24] and the Italian National Trial (INT).[25] The published results are somewhat contradictory. The P-1 study showed a significant reduction in oestrogen-receptor (ER)-positive tumours, whilst the Tamoplac and INT trials did not (Table 3). These results raised more questions than answers, and led to divergence of practice around the world. The initial results of the IBIS trial were released more recently and supported the P-1 findings. Of course none of these studies as yet has any data on the effect on breast cancer mortality.

A combined analysis of all four tamoxifen studies and an osteoporosis trial using raloxifene – another selective oestrogen receptor modulator (SERM) similar to tamoxifen but with a better side-effect profile – was recently published. Cancer incidence was a secondary endpoint in the raloxifene study. An overall risk reduction of 38% was shown, with no reduction in ER-negative tumours. Endometrial cancer was significantly increased with tamoxifen, but not with raloxifene. Thromboembolic events were significantly increased in all groups, but no significant difference in deaths from all causes was noted. These authors based in the UK feel that follow-up data are not sufficient to allow recommendation of either agent for chemoprevention.[26]

After the P-1 study was published, the US Food and Drug administration (FDA) licensed tamoxifen for chemoprevention. While at first their review board did not concur,[27] the most recent review of chemoprevention by the American Society of Clinical Oncology concludes, based on the evidence available, that tamoxifen does significantly reduce the risk of developing ER-positive breast cancers in high-risk women. However, they also point out that there is no evidence of survival benefit, and there are significant risks, particularly of endometrial cancer and thromboembolic events. This article is an excellent review of all the studies to date and of all the issues surrounding chemoprevention, and is available free on-line.[28]

With the exception of the P-1 trial, the remaining studies are continuing follow-up. The raloxifene osteoporosis study and recent evidence from the ATAC study of the effect of aromatase inhibitors on contralateral breast cancer incidence in the adjuvant setting have raised the possibility that these agents may also be effective for risk reduction.[7,29] Therefore additional studies looking at these drugs as chemoprevention (IBIS 2 and STAR) are underway, and may answer many of the questions raised so far.

BRCA gene carriers are a particular group of concern. They are clearly at the highest risk, yet data so far suggest that they may be relatively resistant to

Table 3 Randomised prospective trials of tamoxifen (Tam) for primary breast cancer risk reduction[28]

Study	No. of patients	Median follow-up (months)	Cancers Placebo	Cancers Tam	% reduction in new cancers	P
NSABP P-1	13 388	59	244	124	49	<0.00001
IBIS 1	7152	50	101	68	32	<0.013
Royal Marsden	2494	70	75	62	17	NS
Italian	5408	50	45	34	24	NS

chemoprevention.[28] Subset analyses of the chemoprevention studies done to date show that there is little if any benefit for *BRCA1* carriers, but significant benefit for *BRCA2* carriers.[30] This is not an unexpected result, as *BRCA1* carriers are much more likely to develop ER-negative tumours. However, other evidence has shown that oestrogen reduction (e.g. oophorectomy) in both *BRCA1* and 2 carriers reduces risk.[31] Investigation in this area continues; however, chemoprevention for gene carriers outside a study is not recommended at this time.

Key point 8

- Tamoxifen significantly reduces the risk of developing oestrogen receptor positive breast cancers in high risk women. However, there is no evidence of survival benefit, and there are significant risks.

RISK-REDUCTION MASTECTOMY

Bilateral mastectomy has always appeared to be an attractive alternative for risk reduction, particularly for women with the highest risk because of the lack of good alternatives. However, in the past there has been continued controversy as to effectiveness and selecting who is at sufficient risk to justify this quite radical approach. This is particularly true as the treatment for primary breast cancer has become much more conservative with much improved survival rates.[1,2] It seems somewhat paradoxical to advocate radical surgery to prevent a tumour that is largely curable with a less radical approach. Conversely, those at the highest risk, especially those who are gene carriers, are less likely to have favourable tumours and also, because they are younger with denser breasts, are less likely to have cancers detected at an early stage by screening. In addition, as techniques of breast reconstruction have improved, it is possible for women to have reasonable, although not perfect, cosmetic results.

Data to date show that while not fully preventing breast cancer, risk-reduction mastectomy does reduce that risk by 90–95%.[32–34] By specifically identifying true gene carriers, the risk reduction is increased even further.[35]

The two main areas of controversy are how to identify those at sufficient risk to benefit from bilateral mastectomy, and what is the best surgical intervention for that patient. There is no absolute indication for risk-reducing mastectomy. Generally those women who are identified as gene carriers, or who have a family history that would suggest that they have a high genetic risk, but cannot be specifically tested, are candidates; as are those with known proliferative breast lesions associated with a high risk of developing invasive breast cancer such as ADH and LCIS.

However, the problem remains of the threshold risk at which to advise surgery. For example, should a woman with a fivefold relative risk of developing breast cancer be counselled to consider prophylactic mastectomy while a woman with relative risk of two- or threefold that of the age-matched population be counselled against this form of surgery? The ultimate decision to undergo such surgery rests with the patient herself after careful consideration and appropriate counselling by the surgeon, geneticist, psychologist/ psychiatrist and breast-care nurse in the light of all the information available to her (Table 4).

A special group to consider comprise those women with high genetic risk who have already developed an invasive breast cancer in one breast. These women have a 35% chance of a contralateral cancer within 10 years of the first diagnosis and up to 64% lifetime risk.[36] The decision about contralateral mastectomy in this population is complicated by factors such as the prognosis of the original tumour and whether breast conservation has been used in the treatment of the original tumour. Many women who are at high risk are now choosing bilateral mastectomy at the time of their diagnosis of a first breast cancer as treatment for the affected side, and prophylaxis contralaterally.

The primary objective of risk-reducing mastectomy is to remove as much breast tissue as possible. The secondary objective is to achieve as good a cosmetic result as possible. Debulking procedures or reductions leave large amounts of at risk breast tissue behind (the cells of which still contain the same gene mutations), and do not reduce risk. They therefore have no role in risk reduction of breast cancer and should never be offered as such.

Table 4 Essential components of counselling prior to risk-reducing mastectomy[43]

- Accurate assessment of risk/genetic predisposition, including option of genetic testing (many centres have a threshold residual absolute breast cancer risk of 25%)
- Full knowledge of all available non-surgical options
- Full understanding of the extent of surgery and operative complications
- Appreciation of the limitations of breast reconstruction including
  - loss of sensitivity of breasts/nipples
  - possible dissatisfaction with cosmesis
  - expected durability of implants
- Understanding of the likely extent of risk reduction after surgery

Key point 9

- Risk-reducing mastectomy can reduce the risk of breast cancer by over 90% in high-risk individuals, particularly gene-mutation carriers. The primary objective of risk-reducing mastectomy is to remove as much breast tissue as possible. The secondary objective is to achieve as good a cosmetic result as possible.

The two surgical options are subcutaneous mastectomy and total mastectomy with immediate, delayed or (in some cases) no reconstruction. While the breast is a subcutaneous organ, the difference between the two operations is largely one of the underlying surgical aim. Subcutaneous mastectomy is an operation designed to remove the underlying breast parenchyma and minimise the subsequent risk of breast cancer development. The aim in total mastectomy, on the other hand, is to remove all the breast tissue, including the ducts within the nipple–areolar complex, with the intent of avoiding any subsequent breast cancer development. The techniques for both have been extensively reviewed elsewhere.[37–39]

Since subcutaneous mastectomy aims to preserve the nipple–areolar complex, an S-shaped subareolar incision with an extension laterally to help remove the axillary tail is generally used. A 10–12 cm inframammary incision may occasionally be adequate in small breasts. Up to one-third of patients may need reduction of the skin envelope to achieve optimal cosmetic results. This is usually best achieved using a wise-pattern skin incision similar to that for reduction mammoplasty.

With a total mastectomy, the entire breast gland is removed, together with a small ellipse of skin bearing the nipple–areolar complex, or with a circular skin incision placed 2–3 mm outside the areolar margin to allow maximal skin sparing.

In both techniques flaps should be made thin enough to ensure removal of all breast tissue, and attention to removing the entire axillary tail is important. Axillary dissection is not indicated, and would add significant morbidity. However, all risk-reduction surgery should be carried out with the same care and attention to removal of breast tissue as therapeutic mastectomy

Reconstruction is most commonly performed by placing an expandable prosthetic implant submuscularly. This avoids the complications of capsule contracture and implant extravasation associated with subcutaneous placement. Immediate reconstruction involves the fashioning of a submuscular pocket deep to the pectoralis major, serratus anterior and upper rectus abdominis muscles. This may be approached through an oblique incision in the pectoralis major muscle, or between the serratus anterior and pectoralis major muscle laterally. A large pocket is created with blunt dissection and a textured prosthesis is implanted. The use of a latissimus dorsi pedicled muscle flap may provide an alternative method of implant cover and has the advantage of achieving a greater degree of immediate ptosis, particularly when reconstructing the fuller breast. If the nipple–areolar complex is removed at the time of skin-sparing mastectomy or in total mastectomy, the skin island can be used to replace the nipple–areolar complex, and a new nipple constructed at a later date.

Implants used currently are silicone compound gel/saline expandable prostheses. These have the advantage of being adjustable by changing the saline volume using small subcutaneous filling ports. Once satisfactory size and symmetry have been achieved, the ports can be removed under local anaesthesia without having to replace the entire prosthesis. While there has been a great deal of concern about systemic side-effects of silicone implants, spurred by the media and the FDA ban on such implants, to date no scientific studies have shown evidence of any problem.[40]

As an alternative to implants, an autologous free tissue transfer (abdominal TRAM or DIEP flap or buttock SGAP flap) can be used for reconstruction. These have the advantage of avoiding an implant and a better long-term cosmetic result. However, these procedures are much more complex, with a longer recovery and a higher risk of complications.

Early and long-term complications of subcutaneous or total mastectomy may be considerable. These include flap and/or nipple loss, haematoma, implant exposure and infection, and have been noted in up to 20% of patients in some series.[41,42] Some years ago, the most frequent long-term complication was capsular contracture secondary to subcutaneous placement of the prosthesis. However, with submuscular placement of the implant, this complication is now very much less common, although displacement of the prosthesis (usually in an upward direction) may occur and may need later correction. The use of textured implants has helped to reduce the problems of migration and encapsulation of the implant.

The decision to undergo risk-reduction mastectomy is difficult for a number of reasons. Most specialists recommend a careful, multidisciplinary process, with detailed counselling on many occasions. Each woman must clearly understand her risk, but also understand that evaluating individual risk is quite hard. Even women who are known gene carriers may not develop breast cancer; unfortunately we are not yet able to determine who those women are on an individual basis. Women in a high-risk population must understand the alternatives to mastectomy, including screening and the risks and benefits of those alternatives. Finally, each woman should understand the complications of mastectomy and reconstruction and be provided with examples of both good and bad outcomes.

The final decision of course lies with the individual patient, but that decision can only be made with proper counselling. Conversely, the breast-care specialist must remember that each woman's needs and concerns are important in the final decision. A woman's own concern about breast cancer risk vs body image and sexual function greatly influence the final decision (Table 4).

Risk-reducing mastectomy is ideally carried out in units where expertise in these disciplines is concentrated. There is now a consensus amongst breast specialists that this form of surgery should be undertaken only by a breast or reconstructive surgeon experienced in these techniques, with the support of a full multidisciplinary team.[43]

Key point 10

- The ultimate decision to undergo risk-reduction mastectomy rests with the patient herself after careful consideration and appropriate counselling by the surgeon, geneticist, psychologist/psychiatrist and breast-care nurse in the light of all the information available to her.

CONCLUSIONS

All women are at risk for developing and dying from breast cancer. For most of these women, except for lifestyle changes that only slightly reduce risk, we can only offer early diagnosis by mammographic screening to reduce risk. There is a small group that can be clearly defined as at extremely high risk through predictive *BRCA* gene testing. This group can achieve significant risk reduction through bilateral preventative mastectomy; however, careful counselling is required for each individual patient.

There is a large group of women without a detectable gene defect who are at higher risk than the general population; however, defining the exact level of that risk is still difficult, as is their optimal management. Chemoprevention with anti-oestrogenic agents holds promise for risk reduction in these patients, but the results of ongoing studies are needed before definite recommendations can be made.

Key points for clinical practice

- No strategy yet exists that can totally prevent breast cancer. It is therefore better to use the term *risk reduction*. The primary goal may not necessarily be the reduction of the risk of the development of breast cancer, but instead the reduction of risk of death and to a lesser extent morbidity from breast cancer.

- Most women, particularly those with a family history, greatly overestimate their risk of breast cancer.

- 5–10% of breast cancers are known to be due to inherited genetic alterations that are present in all an individual's cells (germline mutations), and can be passed to at least half of an individual's offspring by standard Mendelian inheritance.

- Two specific high-penetrance breast cancer-associated (*BRCA*) gene mutations, *BRCA1* and *BRCA2*, have been identified, and are responsible for about half the hereditary cancers or 5% of all breast cancers.

- Before any risk-reduction methods are employed, the relative risk of developing breast cancer in each patient must be assessed. However, all risk-assessment models assess population risk, not individual risk.

- The prior diagnosis of ductal carcinoma *in situ* (DCIS), lobular carcinoma *in situ* (LCIS) and atypical ductal hyperplasia (ADH) all significantly increase risk.

- If risk reduction is defined as reducing the risk of dying from breast cancer then screening strategies are clearly a major form of risk reduction.

- Tamoxifen significantly reduces the risk of developing oestrogen receptor positive breast cancers in high risk women. However, there is no evidence of survival benefit, and there are significant risks.

- Risk-reducing mastectomy can reduce the risk of breast cancer by over 90% in high-risk individuals, particularly gene-mutation carriers. The primary objective of risk-reducing mastectomy is to remove as much breast tissue as possible. The secondary objective is to achieve as good a cosmetic result as possible.

Key points for clinical practice (continued)

- The ultimate decision to undergo risk-reduction mastectomy rests with the patient herself after careful consideration and appropriate counselling by the surgeon, geneticist, psychologist/psychiatrist and breast-care nurse in the light of all the information available to her.

References

1. Jemal A, Murray T, Samuels A, Ghafoor A, Ward E, Thun MJ. Cancer statistics, 2003. *CA Cancer J Clin* 2003; **53**: 5–26.
2. Statistics OfN. Breast cancer incidence rate rises while death rate falls. 2003. www.statistics.gov.uk
3. Tchou J, Morrow M. Available models for breast cancer risk assessment: how accurate are they? *J Am Coll Surg* 2003; **197**: 1029–1035.
4. Powles TJ. Breast cancer prevention. *Oncologist* 2002; **7**: 60–64.
5. Beral V. Breast cancer and hormone-replacement therapy in the Million Women Study. *Lancet* 2003; **362**: 419–427.
6. Chlebowski RT, Hendrix SL, Langer RD *et al*. Influence of estrogen plus progestin on breast cancer and mammography in healthy postmenopausal women: the Women's Health Initiative randomized trial. *JAMA* 2003; **289**: 3243–3253.
7. Cuzick J. Aromatase inhibitors in prevention – data from the ATAC (Arimidex, Tamoxifen Alone or in Combination) trial and the design of IBIS-II (the second International Breast Cancer Intervention Study). *Rec Results Cancer Res* 2003; **163**: 96–103; discussion 264–266.
8. Black WC, Nease RF Jr, Tosteson AN. Perceptions of breast cancer risk and screening effectiveness in women younger than 50 years of age. *J Natl Cancer Inst* 1995; **87**: 720–731.
9. Eeles RA. Screening for hereditary cancer and genetic testing, epitomized by breast cancer. *Eur J Cancer* 1999; **35**: 1954–1962.
10. Claus EB, Risch N, Thompson WD. Autosomal dominant inheritance of early-onset breast cancer. Implications for risk prediction. *Cancer* 1994; **73**: 643–651.
11. Gail MH, Brinton LA, Byar DP *et al*. Projecting individualized probabilities of developing breast cancer for white females who are being examined annually. *J Natl Cancer Inst* 1989; **81**: 1879–1886.
12. Page DL, Dupont WD. Anatomic markers of human premalignancy and risk of breast cancer. *Cancer* 1990; **66(6 Suppl)**: 1326–1335.
13. Amir E, Evans DG, Shenton A *et al*. Evaluation of breast cancer risk assessment packages in the family history evaluation and screening programme. *J Med Genet* 2003; **40**: 807–814.
14. Gail MH, Costantino JP. Validating and improving models for projecting the absolute risk of breast cancer. *J Natl Cancer Inst* 2001; **93**: 334–335.
15. Lalloo F, Boggis CR, Evans DG, Shenton A, Threlfall AG, Howell A. Screening by mammography, women with a family history of breast cancer. *Eur J Cancer* 1998; **34**: 937–940.
16. Eeles RA. Future possibilities in the prevention of breast cancer: intervention strategies in *BRCA1* and *BRCA2* mutation carriers. *Breast Cancer Res* 2000; **2**: 283–290.
17. Leach MO, Eeles RA, Turnbull LW *et al*. The UK national study of magnetic resonance imaging as a method of screening for breast cancer (MARIBS). *J Exp Clin Cancer Res* 2002; **21(3 Suppl)**: 107–114.
18. Dooley WC, Ljung BM, Veronesi U *et al*. Ductal lavage for detection of cellular atypia in women at high risk for breast cancer. *J Natl Cancer Inst* 2001; **93**: 1624–1632.
19. Miller AB, Bulbrook RD. The epidemiology and etiology of breast cancer. *N Engl J Med* 1980; **303**: 1246–1248.
20. Cuzick J, Baum M. Tamoxifen and contralateral breast cancer. *Lancet* 1985; **ii**: 282.

21. Powles TJ, Davey JB, McKinna A. A feasibility trial of tamoxifen chemoprevention of breast cancer in Great Britain. *Cancer Invest* 1988; **6**: 621–624.

22. Powles T, Eeles R, Ashley S *et al*. Interim analysis of the incidence of breast cancer in the Royal Marsden Hospital tamoxifen randomised chemoprevention trial. *Lancet* 1998; **352**: 98–101.

23. Fisher B, Costantino JP, Wickerham DL *et al*. Tamoxifen for prevention of breast cancer: report of the National Surgical Adjuvant Breast and Bowel Project P-1 study. *J Natl Cancer Inst* 1998; **90**: 1371–1388.

24. Cuzick J, Forbes J, Edwards R *et al*. First results from the International Breast Cancer Intervention Study (IBIS-I): a randomised prevention trial. *Lancet* 2002; **360**: 817–824.

25. Veronesi U, Maisonneuve P, Costa A *et al*. Prevention of breast cancer with tamoxifen: preliminary findings from the Italian randomised trial among hysterectomised women. Italian Tamoxifen Prevention Study. *Lancet* 1998; **352**: 93–97.

26. Cuzick J, Powles T, Veronesi U *et al*. Overview of the main outcomes in breast-cancer prevention trials. *Lancet* 2003; **361**: 296–300.

27. Chlebowski RT, Collyar DE, Somerfield MR, Pfister DG. American Society of Clinical Oncology technology assessment on breast cancer risk reduction strategies: tamoxifen and raloxifene. *J Clin Oncol* 1999; **17**: 1939–1955.

28. Chlebowski RT, Col N, Winer EP *et al*. American Society of Clinical Oncology technology assessment of pharmacologic interventions for breast cancer risk reduction including tamoxifen, raloxifene, and aromatase inhibition. *J Clin Oncol* 2002; **20**: 3328–3343.

29. Baum M, Buzdar A, Cuzick J *et al*. Anastrozole alone or in combination with tamoxifen versus tamoxifen alone for adjuvant treatment of postmenopausal women with early-stage breast cancer: results of the ATAC (Arimidex, Tamoxifen Alone or in Combination) trial efficacy and safety update analyses. *Cancer* 2003; **98**: 1802–1810.

30. King MC, Wieand S, Hale K *et al*. Tamoxifen and breast cancer incidence among women with inherited mutations in BRCA1 and BRCA2: National Surgical Adjuvant Breast and Bowel Project (NSABP-P1) Breast Cancer Prevention Trial. *JAMA* 2001; **286**: 2251–2256.

31. Rebbeck TR, Levin AM, Eisen A *et al*. Breast cancer risk after bilateral prophylactic oophorectomy in BRCA1 mutation carriers. *J Natl Cancer Inst* 1999; **91**: 1475–1479.

32. Hartmann LC, Schaid DJ, Woods JE *et al*. Efficacy of bilateral prophylactic mastectomy in women with a family history of breast cancer. *N Engl J Med* 1999; **340**: 77–84.

33. Hartmann LC, Sellers TA, Schaid DJ *et al*. Efficacy of bilateral prophylactic mastectomy in BRCA1 and BRCA2 gene mutation carriers. *J Natl Cancer Inst* 2001; **93**: 1633–1637.

34. Rebbeck TR, Friebel T, Lynch HT *et al*. Bilateral prophylactic mastectomy reduces breast cancer risk in BRAC1 and BRAC2 mutation carriers: the PROSE Study Group. *J Clin Oncol* 2004; **22**: 1055–1062.

35. Lynch HT, Lynch JF, Rubinstein WS. Prophylactic mastectomy: obstacles and benefits. *J Natl Cancer Inst* 2001; **93**: 1586–1587.

36. Chabner E, Nixon A, Gelman R *et al*. Family history and treatment outcome in young women after breast-conserving surgery and radiation therapy for early-stage breast cancer. *J Clin Oncol* 1998; **16**: 2045–2051.

37. Malata CM, McIntosh SA, Purushotham AD. Immediate breast reconstruction after mastectomy for cancer. *Br J Surg* 2000; **87**: 1455–1472.

38. Slavin SA, Schnitt SJ, Duda RB *et al*. Skin-sparing mastectomy and immediate reconstruction: oncologic risks and aesthetic results in patients with early-stage breast cancer. *Plast Reconstr Surg* 1998; **102**: 49–62.

39. Woods JE. Subcutaneous mastectomy: current state of the art. *Ann Plast Surg* 1983; **11**: 541–550.

40. Janowsky EC, Kupper LL, Hulka BS. Meta-analyses of the relation between silicone breast implants and the risk of connective-tissue diseases. *N Engl J Med* 2000; **342**: 781–790.

41. Slade CL. Subcutaneous mastectomy: acute complications and long-term follow-up. *Plast Reconstr Surg* 1984; **73**: 84–90.

42. Fisher J, Maxwell GP, Woods J. Surgical alternatives in subcutaneous mastectomy reconstruction. *Clin Plast Surg* 1988; **15**: 667–676.

43. Davidson TI, Sack NPM. Risk reducing mastectomy. In: Eeles R (ed). *Genetic Predisposition to Cancer*. London: Chapman and Hall, 2004.

Abhay Chopada Irving Taylor

17

Randomised controlled trials in General Surgery

Increasing enthusiasm for evidence-based surgery has resulted in an increasing number of surgical approaches undergoing evaluation by randomised controlled trials both for traditional and evolving new techniques.

BREAST SURGERY

Poggi *et al.*[1] reported a 19-year follow-up on 237 women randomised to modified radical mastectomy (*n*=116) or breast-conservation therapy (BCT) (*n* = 121) between 1979 and 1987. At a median of 18.4 years there was no detectable difference in overall survival or disease-free survival between the two groups. For BCT patients, long-term in-breast failures continued to occur throughout the duration of follow-up. There was no statistically significant difference in the incidence of contralateral breast carcinoma between the two treatment groups.

Veronesi *et al.*[2] reported data from 516 patients randomised to either sentinel-node biopsy and total axillary dissection (axillary group) (*n* = 257) or to sentinel-node biopsy followed by axillary dissection only if the sentinel node contained metastases (the sentinel-node group) (*n* = 259). A sentinel node was positive in 83 of the 257 patients in the axillary-dissection group (32.3%) and in 92 of the 259 patients in the sentinel-node group (35.5%). In the axillary-dissection group, the overall accuracy of the sentinel-node status was 96.9%, sensitivity 91.2% and specificity 100%. Among the 167 patients who did not undergo axillary dissection, there were no cases of overt axillary metastasis

Abhay Chopada MSc FRCS, Department of Surgery, Royal Free and University College London Medical School, London, UK

Prof. Irving Taylor MD ChM FRCS FMedSci FRCPS(Glas)Hon, Vice-Dean and Director of Clinical Studies, Royal Free and University College London Medical School, Charles Bell House, 67–73 Riding House Street, London W1W 7EJ, UK

during follow-up. Veronesi *et al.* therefore conclude that sentinel node biopsy appears to be a safe and acceptable method of screening for axillary disease.

Rahusen *et al.*[3] randomised patients with non-palpable breast cancer to undergo either a wire-guided ($n = 23$) or an ultrasound (US)-guided excision ($n = 26$). Mean tumour diameter, specimen weight and operating time were similar in both groups. The excision was adequate in 24 (89%) of 27 US-guided excisions and 12 (55%) of 22 wire-guide excisions ($P = 0.007$). US-guided excision therefore appears to be superior to wire localisation.

The role of octreotide in minimising lymphorrhoea following axillary dissection was evaluated by Carcoforo *et al.*[4] Patients were randomised to either a control group ($n = 136$) or a treatment group ($n = 125$) that received 0.1 mg octreotide subcutaneously three times a day for 5 days, starting on the first postoperative day. In the control group the mean quantity of lymphorrhoea was 94.6 ± 19 ml per day for an average of 16.7 ± 3.0 days. In comparison, the mean quantity of lymphorrhoea in the treatment group was 65.4 ± 21.1 ml ($P < 0.0001$) per day and the average duration was 7.1 ± 2.9 days ($P < 0.0001$).

Key point 1

- At 19 years of follow-up, there was no detectable difference in overall survival or disease-free survival in patients with early-stage breast carcinoma who were treated with mastectomy compared with those treated with BCT.

Key point 2

- Sentinel-node biopsy is a safe and accurate method of screening the axillary nodes for metastasis.

Key point 3

- US-guided excision seems to be superior to wire-guided excision with respect to margin clearance of mammographically detected and US-visible non-palpable breast cancers.

GENERAL SURGERY AND CRITICAL CARE

Nathens *et al.*[5] randomised 595 patients admitted to an intensive care unit (91% trauma victims) to receive supplementation with antioxidants in the form of α-tocopherol and ascorbic acid. Multiple organ failure was significantly less likely to occur in patients receiving antioxidants than in patients receiving standard care, with a relative risk of 0.43 (95% confidence interval 0.19–0.96). Patients randomised to antioxidant supplementation also had a shorter duration of mechanical ventilation and length of intensive care unit stay. Nathens *et al.* therefore recommended early supplementation with antioxidants in this group of surgical intensive care patients.

Sandham *et al.*[6] compared goal-directed therapy guided by a pulmonary-artery catheter ($n = 997$) with standard care without the use of a pulmonary-artery catheter ($n = 997$). The study was conducted in high-risk patients 60 years of age or older, with American Society of Anesthesiologists (ASA) class III or IV risk, who were scheduled for urgent or elective major surgery, followed by a stay in an intensive care unit. There was a higher rate of pulmonary embolism in the catheter group than in the standard-care group (8 *versus* 0; $P = 0.004$). Survival was similar in both groups. Elective use of a pulmonary artery catheter with directed therapy does not appear to benefit elderly, high-risk surgical patients requiring intensive care.

Kosmadakis *et al.*[7] evaluated the role of recombinant erythropoietin (r-HuEPO) in patients with gastrointestinal cancers and mild anaemia. Thirty-one cancer patients received subcutaneous r-HuEPO at a dose of 300 IU/kg body weight plus 100 mg iron intravenously (study group) and 32 patients received placebo medication and iron (control group) for 7 days. Patients in the study group needed significantly fewer perioperative transfusions. Postoperatively, the study group had significantly higher hematocrit, haemoglobin and reticulocyte count values compared with the control group. The use of erythropoietin was also associated with a reduced number of postoperative complications and improved 1-year survival.

Thomas *et al.*[8] randomised 74 patients with undiagnosed abdominal pain to morphine or placebo. Morphine analgesia did not affect diagnostic accuracy or clinical course.

Key point 4

- Supplementation with α-tocopherol and ascorbic acid reduces the incidence of organ failure and shortens length of intensive care stay.

Key point 5

- Use of pulmonary catheter and directed therapy is of no benefit over standard care in elderly, high-risk surgical patients requiring intensive care and may increase the risk of pulmonary embolism.

Key point 6

- Perioperative erythropoietin administration in patients with gastrointestinal tract cancer and mild anaemia reduces transfusion requirements and provides favourable outcome.

COLORECTAL SURGERY

Use of the contrast agent Gastrografin was evaluated in the setting of adhesive small bowel obstruction (SBO) by Biondi et al.[9] Eighty-three patients with suspected adhesive obstruction were randomised to receive oral Gastrografin or conservative management alone. Patients with evidence of partial obstruction with contrast in the colon at 24 hours were fed orally. Among patients treated conservatively, hospital stay was shorter in the Gastrografin group ($P < 0.001$). All patients in whom contrast medium reached the colon tolerated an early oral diet. Gastrografin does seem to benefit patients with adhesive partial SBO.

Sandler et al.[10] evaluated the role of daily aspirin in the prevention of colorectal adenomas in patients treated for previous colorectal cancer. In this study, which included 635 patients, 325 mg aspirin daily for a minimum of 1 year reduced the risk of finding further polyps on colonoscopy from 27% to 17% ($P = 0.004$). Aspirin may therefore have a long-term role in prevention of metachronous lesions.

The traditional role of mechanical bowel preparation in colonic surgery was challenged by Zmora et al.[11] Three hundred and eighty-seven patients undergoing elective colon and rectal resections with primary anastamosis were prospectively randomised into a mechanical bowel preparation group with polyethylene glycol before surgery ($n = 187$) and a group without preoperative mechanical bowel preparation ($n = 193$). Wound infection, anastamotic leak and intra-abdominal abscess rate were similar in both groups, suggesting that bowel surgery may be carried out safely without mechanical bowel preparation.

Quah et al.[12] reassessed patients from their previous laparoscopic *versus* open anterior resection trial to evaluate the effect of the surgical approach on pelvic nerve injury resulting in bladder or bowel dysfunction. Available data suggested a higher rate of male sexual dysfunction in the laparoscopic assisted anterior resection group (7 of 15) compared with the open group (1 of 22). Bladder function was similar in both groups. All the patients with sexual dysfunction had bulky or low rectal tumours. Hence caution was urged in the choice of approach in sexually active male patients with bulky or low tumours.

Machado et al.[13] randomised 100 patients with rectal cancer undergoing total mesorectal excision and colo-anal anastomosis to receive either a colonic pouch or a side-to-end anastomosis using the descending colon. On functional assessment at 6 months and 1 year, only the ability to evacuate the bowel in less than 15 minutes at 6 months reached a significant difference in favour of the pouch procedure. Hence it was concluded that colonic pouch or side-to-end anastamosis are both equally acceptable alternatives.

The role of GTN (glyceryl trinitrate) ointment in shortening the healing time and decreasing postoperative pain following haemorrhoidectomy was analysed by Hwang-do et al.[14] 110 patients were randomised to receive GTN ointment or placebo. The GTN group did show reduced need for analgesia and more rapid healing.

Davies et al.[15] analysed the role of botulinum toxin injection following haemorrhoidectomy. Fifty patients were randomised to receive either injection with 20 U Botox or normal saline to the internal sphincter following surgery. The Botox group demonstrated reduced postoperative pain and analgesic requirements.

Cheetham et al.[16] compared the immediate and long-term results of stapled haemorrhoidectomy with diathermy haemorrhoidectomy in patients with prolapsing internal haemorrhoids in an intended day-care setting. Patients were randomised to diathermy technique ($n = 16$) or stapled procedure ($n = 15$). The total pain score was significantly higher in the diathermy group: 50 (range 9.8–79.9) versus 19.6 (range 1.3–89.5) ($P = 0.03$). At long-term follow-up, three patients (all in the stapled group) developed new symptoms of faecal urgency and anal pain, and three patients required further surgery to remove symptomatic external haemorrhoids after stapled haemorrhoidectomy. Hence caution is urged, especially with regard to long-term safety of the stapled haemorrhoidectomy procedure.

Holzer et al.[17] reported results of use of a new gentamicin collagen fleece (Septocoll) after surgical treatment of a pilonidal sinus. Fifty-one patients were randomised to gentamicin fleece plus primary closure and 52 patients to open treatment alone. The median interval to wound healing was 17 days in the treatment group and 68 days in the open group ($P = 0.0001$).

Tjandra et al.[18] compared the results of a direct end-to-end repair of the anal sphincter with an overlapping repair for a localised anterior defect of external anal sphincter after obstetric trauma. Twenty-three patients were randomised. Improvement in continence scores, maximum squeeze pressure and functional anal canal length were similar in both groups. In the overlap group, one patient developed a unilaterally prolonged pudendal nerve terminal motor latency that was persistent 22 months after surgery, and two patients had impaired faecal evacuation postoperatively. Tjandra et al. concluded that while both techniques are effective, overlapping repair might be associated with more difficulties with faecal evacuation and a prolonged pudendal nerve terminal motor latency postoperatively.

Key point 8

- Oral Gastrografin helps in the management of patients with adhesive SBO and allows a shorter hospital stay.

Key point 9

- Daily aspirin reduces the risk of colorectal adenomas in patients with previous colorectal cancer.

Key point 10

- Colon and rectal surgery can be safely performed without preoperative mechanical bowel preparation.

Key point 11

- Colonic J-pouch or side-to-end colo-colic anastomosis in low-anterior resection with total mesorectal excision has similar functional and surgical results at 1 year.

Key point 12

- Laparoscopically assisted rectal resection may be associated with a higher rate of male sexual dysfunction, but not bladder dysfunction, compared with the open approach.

Key point 13

- Haemorrhoids:
  - GTN accelerates healing after haemorrhoidectomy
  - Botox reduces pain after haemorrhoidectomy
  - Stapled haemorrhoidectomy may result in new symptoms such as faecal urgency and anal pain at long-term follow-up.

Key point 14

- *Pilonidal disease*: combination of gentamicin collagen fleece (Septocoll) with primary closure of pilonidal sinus excision wound results in a shorter period to healing than the open technique.

Key point 15

- *Anal surgery*: direct end-to-end repair may be better than overlapping repair, as overlapping repair might be associated with more difficulties with faecal evacuation and a prolonged pudendal nerve terminal motor latency postoperatively.

UPPER GI AND HEPATICOPANCREATOBILIARY SURGERY

Parilla *et al.*[19] published long-term efficacy data comparing medical management with surgical treatment of Barrett's oesophagus. One hundred and one patients were randomised. At 5 years satisfactory clinical results (excellent to good) were achieved in 39 of the 43 patients (91%) undergoing medical treatment and in 53 of the 58 patients (91%) following antireflux surgery. The persistence of added inflammatory lesions was significantly higher in the medical treatment group. The metaplastic segment did not disappear in any patient. High-grade dysplasia appeared in 2 of the 43 patients (5%) in the medical treatment group and in 2 of the 58 patients (3%) in the surgical treatment group. In the latter, both patients presented with clinical and pH-metric recurrence. There was no case of malignancy after successful antireflux surgery.

Yoo et al.[20] assessed the need for routine nasogastric decompression after extensive resection in patients with gastric cancer. One hundred and thirty-six patients with gastric cancer who underwent radical gastrectomy with D2 or more lymph node dissection were included. Time to passage of first flatus, time to taking liquid diet, length of operation and postoperative hospital stay were all significantly shorter in the no-decompression group. Two patients in each group required subsequent nasogastric decompression. There were no significant differences between the two groups with regard to the presence of postoperative fever, nausea, vomiting, anastamotic leaks or pulmonary or wound complications. Hence routine nasogastric decompression may not be necessary in operations for gastric cancer.

Partial fundoplication is believed to be associated with a lower incidence of postoperative dysphagia, and consequently is more suitable for patients with gastro-oesophageal reflux disease (GERD) and impaired oesophageal body motility. Chryos et al.[21] randomised 33 consecutive patients with proven GERD and less than 30 mmHg amplitude of peristalsis at 5 cm proximal to lower oesophageal sphincter (LES) to undergo either laparoscopic Toupet fundoplication (TF) ($n = 19$) or laparoscopic Nissen fundoplication (NF) ($n = 14$). Both TF and NF efficiently controlled reflux in patients with GERD and low amplitude of oesophageal peristalsis. Early in the postoperative period, TF is associated with fewer functional symptoms, although 1 year after surgery similar symptoms are reported after either procedure.

Figueras et al.[22] carried out a randomised study of hilar dissection and the 'glissonean' approach with stapling of the pedicle for major hepatectomies to contrast their feasibility, safety, amount of haemorrhage, postoperative complications, operative times and costs. Eighty patients were randomised to the study. Both techniques were equally effective for treating hilar structures. En bloc stapling transection was faster, but hilar dissection was associated with a shorter pedicular clamping time and less necrosis and was less costly.

Jang et al.[23] evaluated the trophic effect of serum gastrin on the pancreatic parenchyma by inducing artificial hypergastrinemia following pancreatic resection. Fifty-six patients who underwent pylorus-preserving pancreato-duodenectomy for periampullary neoplasms were randomised to receive oral lansoprazole for 12 weeks or control group. Serum gastrin level was elevated in the lansoprazole group and the mean volume of the distal pancreas was reduced by only 10% after pylorus-preserving pancreatoduodenectomy, whereas severe pancreatic atrophy occurred in the control group. Postoperative insulin and stool elastase levels were higher in the lansoprazole group than in the control group. Induced hypergastrinaemia may have a role to play in the treatment or prevention of pancreatic insufficiency following resection or injury.

Sarr[24] reported on behalf of the Pancreatic Surgery Group the role of the somatostatin analogue vapreotide after elective pancreatectomy. Two hundred and seventy-five procedures were included. Vapreotide did not affect the rate of pancreatic complications (30.4% *versus* 26.4% with placebo) or overall complications (40% *versus* 42% respectively).

Key point 16

- At 5 years medical and surgical treatment of Barrett's oesophagus yield similar clinical and functional results.

Key point 17

- Nasogastric decompression is not necessary in operations for gastric cancer.

Key point 18

- Toupet fundoplication is associated with fewer functional symptoms in the early postoperative period, but the results of total and partial fundoplication are similar at 1 year in GERD patients with impaired oesophageal peristalsis.

Key point 19

- Hilar dissection is as effective as the 'glissonean' approach and stapling of the pedicle for major hepatectomies.

Key point 20

- Induced hypergastrinaemia with oral proton pump inhibitors may prevent pancreatic atrophy after pancreatoduodenectomy.

Key point 21

- Vapreotide does not decrease pancreas-specific complications after elective pancreatectomy.

VASCULAR SURGERY

Klinkert *et al.*[25] reported 5 years of follow-up in 151 patients operated for above-knee femoropopliteal bypass. Patients were randomised to receive either a PTFE graft ($n = 76$) or autologous saphenous vein bypass ($n = 75$). Saphenous vein bypass had better patency rates at all intervals and needed fewer reoperations. The saphenous vein should be the graft material of choice for above-knee femoropopliteal bypasses and should not be reserved for reinterventions. Polytetrafluoroethylene (PTFE) is an acceptable alternative if the saphenous vein is not available.

Ridker[26] randomised 508 patients to low-intensity warfarin (INR 1.5–2) given after standard 6-month anticoagulation for venous thromboembolic disease. The risk of recurrent thrombosis was reduced by 64% (hazard ratio 0.36; 95% confidence interval 0.19–0.67; $P < 0.001$).

Key point 22

- Above-knee femoropopliteal bypass using the saphenous vein has better patency rates and needs fewer re-operations compared with PTFE grafts.

Key point 23

- Long-term, low-intensity warfarin therapy significantly reduces the risk of recurrent venous thromboembolism.

THYROID SURGERY

Bellantone et al.[27] randomised 75 patients undergoing a total thyroidectomy to receive standard treatment, supplementation with oral calcium or supplementation with oral calcium and vitamin D for 7 days. The groups receiving supplemental calcium and/or vitamin D demonstrated a significantly reduced risk of symptomatic hypocalcemia. Hence the authors conclude that supplementation with calcium and vitamin D may allow a safe and early discharge from the hospital.

Miccolli et al.[28] selected a total of 33 patients with a thyroid nodule proven to be a papillary thyroid carcinoma who underwent a near-total thyroidectomy. They were randomly assigned to minimally invasive video-assisted thyroidectomy (MIVAT) ($n = 16$) or conventional open surgery ($n = 17$). Iodine-131 (^{131}I) thyroid bed uptake and serum thyroglobulin were measured 1 month after operation. Mean ^{131}I uptake was $5.1\% \pm 4.9\%$ in the MIVAT group and $4.6 \pm 6.7\%$ in the open group. Mean thyroglobulin serum levels were also similar in both groups. Hence Miccoli et al. concluded that MIVAT was as effective as open surgery in achieving completeness of resection in papillary carcinoma of thyroid.

Key point 24

- Routine supplementation therapy with oral calcium or vitamin D effectively prevents symptomatic hypocalcaemia after total thyroidectomy.

Key point 25

- Minimally invasive video-assisted thyroidectomy is as effective as open surgery in achieving completeness of resection in papillary carcinoma thyroid.

Key points for clinical practice

- At 19 years of follow-up, there was no detectable difference in overall survival or disease-free survival in patients with early-stage breast carcinoma who were treated with mastectomy compared with those treated with BCT.

- Sentinel-node biopsy is a safe and accurate method of screening the axillary nodes for metastasis.

- US-guided excision seems to be superior to wire-guided excision with respect to margin clearance of mammographically detected and US-visible non-palpable breast cancers.

- Supplementation with α-tocopherol and ascorbic acid reduces the incidence of organ failure and shortens length of intensive care stay.

- Use of pulmonary catheter and directed therapy is of no benefit over standard care in elderly, high-risk surgical patients requiring intensive care and may increase the risk of pulmonary embolism.

- Perioperative erythropoietin administration in patients with gastrointestinal tract cancer and mild anaemia reduces transfusion requirements and provides favourable outcome.

- Morphine analgesia did not affect diagnostic accuracy or clinical course of abdominal pain in acute admission.

- Oral Gastrografin helps in the management of patients with adhesive SBO and allows a shorter hospital stay.

- Daily aspirin reduces the risk of colorectal adenomas in patients with previous colorectal cancer.

- Colon and rectal surgery can be safely performed without preoperative mechanical bowel preparation.

- Colonic J-pouch or side-to-end colo-colic anastomosis in low-anterior resection with total mesorectal excision has similar functional and surgical results at 1 year.

- Laparoscopically assisted rectal resection may be associated with a higher rate of male sexual dysfunction, but not bladder dysfunction, compared with the open approach.

Key points for clinical practice (continued)

- Haemorrhoids:
  - GTN accelerates healing after haemorrhoidectomy
  - Botox reduces pain after haemorrhoidectomy
  - Stapled haemorrhoidectomy may result in new symptoms such as faecal urgency and anal pain at long-term follow-up.

- *Pilonidal disease*: combination of gentamicin collagen fleece (Septocoll) with primary closure of pilonidal sinus excision wound results in a shorter period to healing than the open technique.

- *Anal surgery*: direct end-to-end repair may be better than overlapping repair, as overlapping repair might be associated with more difficulties with faecal evacuation and a prolonged pudendal nerve terminal motor latency postoperatively.

- At 5 years medical and surgical treatment of Barrett's oesophagus yield similar clinical and functional results.

- Nasogastric decompression is not necessary in operations for gastric cancer.

- Toupet fundoplication is associated with fewer functional symptoms in the early postoperative period, but the results of total and partial fundoplication are similar at 1 year in GERD patients with impaired oesophageal peristalsis.

- Hilar dissection is as effective as the 'glissonean' approach and stapling of the pedicle for major hepatectomies.

- Induced hypergastrinaemia with oral proton pump inhibitors may prevent pancreatic atrophy after pancreatoduodenectomy.

- Vapreotide does not decrease pancreas-specific complications after elective pancreatectomy.

- Above-knee femoropopliteal bypass using the saphenous vein has better patency rates and needs fewer re-operations compared with PTFE grafts.

- Long-term, low-intensity warfarin therapy significantly reduces the risk of recurrent venous thromboembolism.

- Routine supplementation therapy with oral calcium or vitamin D effectively prevents symptomatic hypocalcaemia after total thyroidectomy.

- Minimally invasive video-assisted thyroidectomy is as effective as open surgery in achieving completeness of resection in papillary carcinoma thyroid.

References

1. Poggi MM *et al*. Eighteen-year results in the treatment of early breast carcinoma with mastectomy versus breast conservation therapy: the National Cancer Institute Randomised Trial. *Cancer* 2003; **98**: 697–702.

2. Veronesi U *et al.* A randomised comparison of sentinel-node biopsy with routine axillary dissection in breast cancer. *N Engl J Med* 2003; **349**: 546–553.

3. Rahusen FD *et al.* Ultrasound-guided lumpectomy of nonpalpable breast cancer versus wire-guided resection: a randomised clinical trial. *Ann Surg Oncol* 2002; **9**: 994–998.

4. Carcoforo P *et al.* Octreotide in the treatment of lymphorrhea after axillary node dissection: a prospective randomised controlled trial. *J Am Coll Surg* 2003; **196**: 365–369.

5. Nathens AB *et al.* Randomised, prospective trial of antioxidant supplementation in critically ill surgical patients. *Ann Surg* 2002; **236**: 814–822.

6. Sandham JD *et al.* A randomised, controlled trial of the use of pulmonaryartery catheters in high-risk surgical patients. *N Engl J Med* 2003; **348**: 5–14.

7. Kosmadakis N *et al.* Perioperative erythropoietin administration in patients with gastrointestinal tract cancer: prospective randomised double-blind study. *Ann Surg* 2003; **237**: 417–421.

8. Thomas SH *et al.* Effects of morphine analgesia on diagnostic accuracy in emergency department patients with abdominal pain: a prospective, randomised trial. *J Am Coll Surg* 2003; **196**: 18–31.

9. Biondi S *et al.* Randomised clinical study of Gastrografin administration in patients with adhesive small bowel obstruction. *Br J Surg* 2003; **90**: 542–546.

10. Sandler R *et al.* A randomised trial of aspirin to prevent colorectal adenomas in patients with previous colorectal cancer. *N Engl J Med* 2003; **348**: 883–890.

11. Zmora O *et al.* Colon and rectal surgery without mechanical bowel preparation: a randomised prospective trial. *Ann Surg* 2003; **237**: 363–367.

12. Quah HM, Jayne DG, Eu KW, Seow-Choen F. Bladder and sexual dysfunction following laparoscopically assisted and conventional open mesorectal resection for cancer. *Br J Surg* 2002; **89**: 1551–1556.

13. Machado M, Nygren J, Goldman S, Ljungqvist O. Similar outcome after colonic pouch and side-to-end anastomosis in low anterior resection for rectal cancer: a prospective randomised trial. *Ann Surg* 2003; **238**: 214–220.

14. Hwang-do Y, Yoon SG, Kim HS, Lee JK, Kim KY. Effect of 0.2 percent glyceryl trinitrate ointment on wound healing after a hemorrhoidectomy: results of a randomised, prospective, double-blind, placebo-controlled trial. *Dis Colon Rectum* 2003; **46**: 950–954.

15. Davies J *et al.* Botulinum toxin (Botox) reduces pain after hemorrhoidectomy: results of a double-blind, randomised study. *Dis Colon Rectum* 2003; **46**: 1097–1102.

16. Cheetham MJ, Cohen CR, Kamm MA, Phillips RK. A randomised, controlled trial of diathermy hemorrhoidectomy vs. stapled hemorrhoidectomy in an intended day-care setting with longer-term follow-up. *Dis Colon Rectum* 2003; **46**: 491–497.

17. Holzer B *et al.* Efficacy and tolerance of a new gentamicin collagen fleece (Septocoll) after surgical treatment of a pilonidal sinus. *Colorectal Dis* 2003; **5**: 222–227.

18. Tjandra JJ, Han WR, Goh J, Carey M, Dwyer P. Direct repair vs. overlapping sphincter repair: a randomised, controlled trial. *Dis Colon Rectum* 2003; **46**: 937–942.

19. Parrilla P *et al.* Long-term results of a randomised prospective study comparing medical and surgical treatment of Barrett's esophagus. *Ann Surg* 2003; **237**: 291–298.

20. Yoo CH, Son BH, Han WK, Pae WK. Nasogastric decompression is not necessary in operations for gastric cancer: prospective randomised trial. *Eur J Surg* 2002; **168**: 379–383.

21. Chrysos E *et al.* Laparoscopic surgery for gastroesophageal reflux disease patients with impaired esophageal peristalsis: total or partial fundoplication? *J Am Coll Surg* 2003; **197**: 8–15.

22. Figueras J *et al.* Hilar dissection versus the 'glissonean' approach and stapling of the pedicle for major hepatectomies: a prospective, randomised trial. *Ann Surg* 2003; **238**: 111–119.

23. Jang JY *et al.* Randomised prospective trial of the effect of induced hypergastrinemia on the prevention of pancreatic atrophy after pancreatoduodenectomy in humans. *Ann Surg* 2003; **237**: 522–529.

24. Sarr MG, on behalf of the Pancreatic Surgery Group. The potent somatostatin analogue vapreotide does not decrease pancreas-specific complications after elective pancreatectomy: a prospective, multicenter, double-blinded, randomised, placebo-controlled trial. *J Am Coll Surg* 2003; **196**: 556–564.

25. Klinkert P, Schepers A, Burger DH, van Bockel JH, Breslau PJ. Vein versus polytetrafluoroethylene in above-knee femoropopliteal bypass grafting: five year results of a randomised controlled trial. *J Vasc Surg* 2003; **37**: 149–155.

26. Ridker PM. Long-term, low-intensity warfarin therapy for the prevention of recurrent venous thromboembolism. *N Engl J Med* 2003; **348**: 1425–1434.

27. Bellantone R *et al*. Is routine supplementation therapy (calcium and vitamin D) useful after total thyroidectomy? *Surgery* 2002; **132**: 1109–1112.

28. Miccoli P *et al*. Minimally invasive video-assisted thyroidectomy for papillary carcinoma: a prospective study of its completeness. *Surgery* 2002; **132**: 1070–1073.

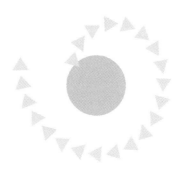

Index

Page numbers in **bold** indicate tables; those in *italics*, illustrations